Mediterranean Diet Cookbook For Beginners

600 Easy & Healthy Recipes - 21-Day Diet Meal Plan - 8 Grocery Shopping Tips

By Emily Wagner

Table of Contents

Introduction

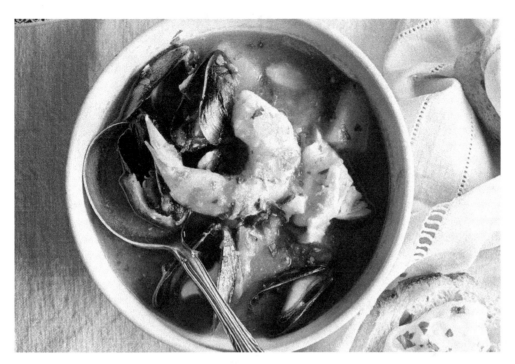

We all know that there are many factors affecting our physical and mental health, the most important of which is diet. Therefore, regardless of whether our body is currently healthy or not, we should choose a healthy diet to keep our body healthy for a long time, so that we have more energy to do what we want to do. Don't wait for the illness to come and lie in the hospital bed in pain.

The diet we recommend today is one of the best diets recognized in the world-the Mediterranean diet.

The Mediterranean Diet is based on the eating foods that people from countries such as Greece and Italy way before processed foods became popular. Many studies have revealed that the Mediterranean Diet is exceptionally healthy compared to the Standard American Diet (SAD) and it can benefit those who are at high risk of developing cardiovascular diseases, stroke, diabetes, and other metabolic diseases. Unlike other types of diets, the Mediterranean Diet incorporates healthy eating habit and a splash of deliciousness as they still allow the consumption of olive oil as well as a glass of wine. It is also not too limiting compared to other diets such as Atkins or Keto; thus, people who try this diet can enjoy eating their food more because their food choices are not limited.

In this recipe book, we provide a large number of recipes, which are categorized by main ingredients. Considering the particularity of the Mediterranean diet, most of the recipes are pasta, beans, vegetables, fruits, etc. There are only a few meat recipes. When you are using this book, you must be clear that making a certain recipe does not mean that this meal can only eat this recipe. You can also choose other vegetable and fruit recipes according to the characteristics of the Mediterranean. In this book, we will give you a sample recipe for 3 weeks for your reference.

There may be some flaws in some of the recipes in this book, but the introduction of the Mediterranean diet is accurate, because it does not have strict restrictions on food, so you only need to follow the rules of the Mediterranean diet, you will definitely get a very healthy body. We will also continuously upgrade the quality of recipes and create new recipes so that you can buy the best delicious recipes.

Chapter 1 Understanding the Mediterranean Diet

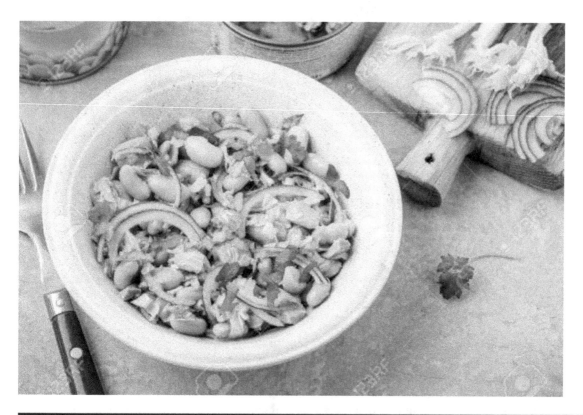

What is the Mediterranean Diet?

The Mediterranean diet is one of the best diets in the world. The Mediterranean generally refers to southern European countries such as Greece, Spain, France, and southern Italy on the Mediterranean coast. Studies have shown that the residents of this region are far more likely to suffer from cardiovascular diseases, diabetes and other rich diseases Lower than other European and American countries.

UNESCO has designated this diet as a World Cultural Heritage and considers it a great contribution to the world. The symbol of this diet is rich in plant-based foods, fresh fruits and desserts daily after meals. Olive oil is the main source of fat, mainly dairy products such as cheese and yogurt, small amounts of fish and poultry. Eat one to four eggs per week, a small amount of red meat, and a small amount of wine.

The main characteristics of this diet are that more than 50% of calories come from high-quality carbohydrates, 30% to 35% of calories come from fat (mainly provided by olive oil), and the remaining 12% of calories come from protein, dairy products and white meat.

Edible olive oil is a feature of the Mediterranean diet. Olive oil contains a lot of monounsaturated fatty acids, most notably oleic acid. Epidemiological studies have confirmed that it is closely related to the reduction of the risk of coronary heart disease. There is evidence that the antioxidant effect of olive oil can improve cholesterol metabolism, reduce blood density of low-density lipoprotein, lower blood pressure in patients with hypertension, and also have anti-inflammatory effects, which is obviously beneficial for patients with rheumatoid arthritis.

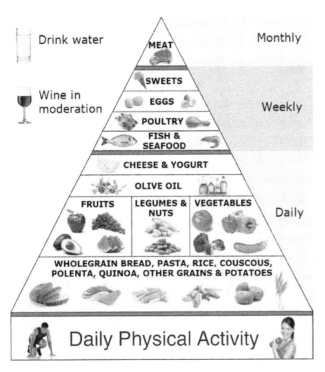

Drink water

Wine in moderation

MEAT — Monthly

SWEETS

EGGS — Weekly

POULTRY

FISH & SEAFOOD

CHEESE & YOGURT

OLIVE OIL

FRUITS | LEGUMES & NUTS | VEGETABLES — Daily

WHOLEGRAIN BREAD, PASTA, RICE, COUSCOUS, POLENTA, QUINOA, OTHER GRAINS & POTATOES

Daily Physical Activity

The Mediterranean Diet Pyramid

Why is the Mediterranean diet so healthy and popular? Then we have to start with its diet. The Mediterranean diet was not invented by one person, but a dietary habit of the locals. The proportion of what they eat every day is like a pyramid, so we call this the "Mediterranean diet pyramid"

This diet pyramid is based on the habits of healthy, long-living adults in the Mediterranean region. On the right of Pyramid, it shows the recommended amounts of food that you need to eat to stay healthy. At the bottom of the pyramid is physical activity and although not related to food, the Mediterranean Diet encourages its dieters to always engage in physical activities. In fact, people from the Mediterranean region age healthily because they are always doing some physical activities. Physical activities, such as doing exercises, should be done daily.

Eat Fruits and Vegetable Daily

One of the most important things that people should remember while following this diet is to eat vegetables and fruits at every meal. The premise here is that eating fruits and vegetables that are darker in color contain more antioxidants. These include green leafy vegetables, legumes, beans, citrus, berries, and a wide variety of products to choose from. It is also crucial to eat whole grains and nuts in your diet. Olive oil is also included here as the principal source of fat.

Eat Fish and Seafood Twice A Week

Fish is a good source of protein, and it is allowed in this particular diet regimen. However, it is crucial for dieters only to consume fish at least twice a week. This is also true for other types of shellfish such as crabs, shrimps, clams, squid, and many others. Now the size of the seafood does not really matter as long as you only eat it twice a week.

Eat Moderate Portions Daily to Weekly

Those who love dairy and egg will not feel restricted with this diet regimen as it still allows its consumption but in moderate portions. These include poultry and dairy products. On the other hand, wine lovers will definitely rejoice with the Mediterranean Diet as it allows people to drink red wine, typically with meals. However, the amount varies such that women are required to drink one (1) glass daily while men can take two (2) glasses. Red wine is the only alcoholic beverage that is allowed for this diet and not anything else.

Eat Less of These

The Mediterranean Diet is unlike any other diet regimens that you will ever encounter as it is not too restrictive. You can still enjoy eating red meat but, sweets, and saturated fat once in a while but only in limited amounts. For instance, you can eat all kinds of red meat (not the processed ones) as long as they are matchbox size. When eating these foods, you may consider it as your "cheat" day.

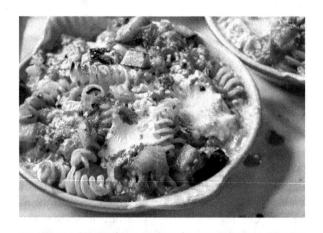

Characteristics of The Mediterranean Diet

In the first paragraph, I have said that the main characteristics of this diet are that more than 50% of calories come from high-quality carbohydrates, 30% to 35% of calories come from fat (mainly provided by olive oil). Now I want to tell you some characteristics of this diet.

Olive oil: When referring to the Mediterranean diet, we cannot fail to mention olive oil, because this is the most obvious feature that distinguishes this diet from other diet. Its advantages are low intake of saturated fatty acids and high levels of unsaturated fatty acids, which can reduce the risk of cardiovascular disease and prevent multiple malignant cancers. EFSA, the European Food Safety Association, also published a document in 2011 confirming the cardiovascular benefits of olive oil, and recommended a daily intake of 5 mg of hydroxytyrosol from olive oil. If you are going to shopping, the extra virgin olive oil is the best choice for you.

Eat plenty of fruits and vegetables : Vegetables and fruits are rich in vitamin C and vitamin E, which have the function of anti-oxidation and protection of cardiovascular and cerebrovascular, and improve human immunity. People in the Mediterranean region need to eat more than 500g of fruits and vegetables every day.

Red Wine: Red wine contains a substance that is good for the human body-salicylic acid. The content of salicylic acid in red wine is almost double that of white wine. Drinking red wine in moderation for a long time has the function of preventing thrombosis and preventing myocardial infarction.

No-strict food: Unlike other diets, this one can't eat, that one can't eat too. The Mediterranean diet allows you to eat many different foods, but you need to control the proportion of some meat foods to reduce the intake of saturated fatty acids.

The Benefits of The Mediterranean Diet

The Mediterranean Diet is dubbed as one of the healthiest diet regimens as it has so many benefits for our body health. Studies showed that this particular diet regimen could help lower the levels of low-density lipoprotein (LDL) cholesterol, which is also known as the "bad" cholesterol. The build-up of bad cholesterol often leads to the build-up of fat deposits on the arteries.

Secondly , more than help improving heart health, this particular diet regimen also can low cancer incidence and prevent Parkinson's disease. Both cancer and Parkinson's diseases are inflammation-related diseases. If you have other inflammation-related diseases, you also can try this diet.

Moreover, this particular diet regimen can also increase longevity and reduce overall mortality, This is the reason why these places are dubbed as the "blue zone" – places with the highest longevity.

Because it has so many defense functions, it is not only suitable for the elderly, but also for most young people. When you maintain this Mediterranean diet for a long time, you will always maintain a very healthy body.

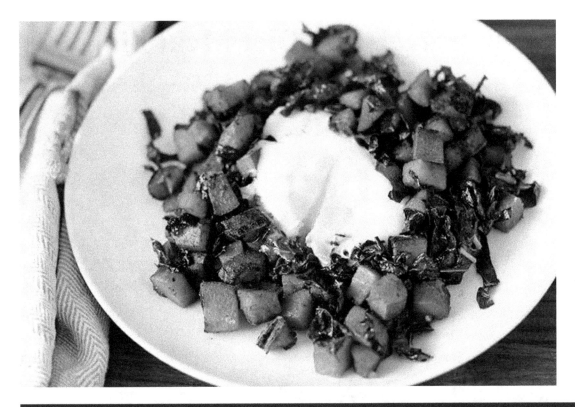

Grocery Shopping Tips

Grocery shopping is easy if you are planning to adopt the Mediterranean Diet. The best thing about shopping to fill your pantry with Mediterranean Diet-approved ingredients is that it is very easy as you can find whole food ingredients just about anywhere. But, it is still important to know which foods you need to stock on.

- **Vegetables:** All kinds of vegetables, such as green leafy kinds, tubers, root crops, and many others are allowed in your pantry. However, make sure that they are organic.
- **Fruits:** Fruits of all colors are encouraged for this diet as long as it is organic and pesticide-free.
- **Grains:** Whole grain foods such as whole-grain pasta, brown rice, and others should occupy your pantry.
- **Frozen Vegetables:** Frozen vegetables are good because they are good alternatives to fresh produce, especially if you cannot find them near you.
- **Legumes:** Legumes such as beans, pulses, and lentils are good sources of protein, and they have long shelf-life
- **Nuts and seeds:** Nuts and seeds are good sources of fats and energy. Snack on them instead of your usual favorite sweet treats.
- **Condiments:** Always opt for natural condiments like sea salt, cinnamon, and other herbs and spices.
- **Meats:** When opting for meats, go for fish that are wild caught. If you choose for chicken or poultry, make sure that they are pasture-raised.

Chapter 2 21 Day Diet Meal Plan

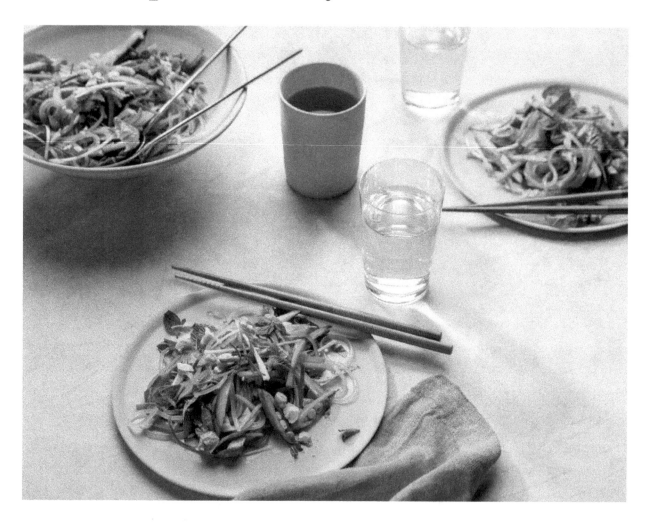

Meal Plan	Breakfast	Lunch	Dinner	Snacks
Day-1	Breakfast Egg on Avocado	Amazingly Good Parsley Tabbouleh	Avocado Peach Salsa on Grilled Swordfish	Amazing Avocado Smoothie
Day-2	Brussels Sprouts Chips	Baked Parmesan and Eggplant Pasta	Coconut Salsa on Chipotle Fish Tacos	Apple and Walnut Salad
Day-3	Brekky Egg-Potato Hash	Creamy Alfredo Fettuccine	Baked Cod Crusted with Herbs	Banana Kale Smoothie
Day-4	Zucchini Tomato Frittata	Bell Peppers on Chicken Breasts	Asian Steamed Broccoli	Banana-Peanut Butter Oatmeal Smoothie
Day-5	Curried Veggies and Poached Eggs	Fresh Herbs and Clams Linguine	Dill Relish on White Sea Bass	Beetroot Apple Smoothie

Day-6	Dill and Tomato Frittata	Instant Pot Quinoa Pilaf	Easy Fish Curry	Blueberry Frozen Yogurt
Day-7	Dill, Havarti & Asparagus Frittata	Ancestral Roasted Chicken	Fresh and No-Cook Oysters	Greek Yogurt Muesli Parfaits
Day-8	Egg and Ham Breakfast Cup	Garlicky Peas and Clams on Veggie Spiral	Healthy Poached Trout	Five Berry Mint Orange Infusion
Day-9	Scrambled Eggs with Feta 'n Mushrooms	Balsamic Chicken with Roasted Tomatoes	Orange Herbed Sauced White Bass	Delectable Mango Smoothie
Day-10	Spiced Breakfast Casserole	Cucumber Salad with Rice and Asparagus	Pecan Crusted Trout	Delectable Strawberry Popsicle
Day-11	Brussels Sprouts Chips	Escarole and Cannellini Beans on Pasta	Pesto and Lemon Halibut	Easy Fruit Compote
Day-12	Zucchini Tomato Frittata	Artichokes, Olives & Tuna Pasta	Roasted Halibut with Banana Relish	Melon Cucumber Smoothie
Day-13	Banana-Coconut Breakfast	Brussels Sprouts and Paprika Chicken Thighs	Seafood Stew Cioppino	Dragon Fruit, Pear, and Spinach Salad
Day-14	Blue Cheese, Fig and Arugula Salad	Bulgur and Chicken Skillet	Mustard Chops with Apricot-Basil Relish	Mediterranean Style Fruit Medley
Day-15	Butternut Squash Stir Fry	Mushroom Chickpea Marsala	Peas and Ham Thick Soup	Peanut Banana Yogurt Bowl
Day-16	Comforting Vegetable Potpie	Chicken and Hazelnut Mash	Baked Cod Crusted with Herbs	Pomegranate and Lychee Sorbet
Day-17	Delicious Stuffed Squash	Chicken Breasts with Stuffing	Yummy Salmon Panzanella	Pomegranate Granita with Lychee
Day-18	Garlicky Rosemary Potatoes	Garlicky Peas and Clams on Veggie Spiral	Ratatouille Pasta Style	Soothing Red Smoothie
Day-19	Veggie Jamaican Stew	Cranberry and Roasted Squash Delight	Tasty Tuna Scaloppine	Strawberry and Avocado Medley
Day-20	Tomato Basil Cauliflower Rice	Escarole and Cannellini Beans on Pasta	Simple Cod Piccata	Smoothie Bowl with Dragon Frui
Day-21	Tasty Avocado Sauce over Zoodles	Yummy Turkey Meatballs	Seafood Stew Cioppino	Summertime Fruit Salad

Chapter 3 Eggs Recipes

Breakfast Egg on Avocado

Serves: 6 , Cooking Time: 15 minutes

Ingredients:

- 1 tsp garlic powder
- 1/2 tsp sea salt
- 1/4 cup Parmesan cheese (grated or shredded)
- 1/4 tsp black pepper
- 3 medium avocados (cut in half, pitted, skin on)
- 6 medium eggs

Directions for Cooking:

1) Prepare muffin tins and preheat the oven to 350 degrees F.
2) To ensure that the egg would fit inside the cavity of the avocado, lightly scrape off 1/3 of the meat.
3) Place avocado on muffin tin to ensure that it faces with the top up.
4) Evenly season each avocado with pepper, salt, and garlic powder.
5) Add one egg on each avocado cavity and garnish tops with cheese.
6) Pop in the oven and bake until the egg white is set, about 15 minutes.
7) Serve and enjoy.

Nutrition Information:

Calories per serving: 252; Protein: 14.0g; Carbs: 4.0g; Fat: 20.0g

Breakfast Egg-Artichoke Casserole

Serves: 8 , Cooking Time: 35 minutes

Ingredients:

- 16 large eggs
- 14 ounce can artichoke hearts, drained
- 10-ounce box frozen chopped spinach, thawed and drained well
- 1 cup shredded white cheddar
- 1 garlic clove, minced
- 1 teaspoon salt
- 1/2 cup parmesan cheese
- 1/2 cup ricotta cheese
- 1/2 teaspoon dried thyme
- 1/2 teaspoon crushed red pepper
- 1/4 cup milk
- 1/4 cup shaved onion

Directions for Cooking:

1) Lightly grease a 9x13-inch baking dish with cooking spray and preheat the oven to 350 degrees F.
2) In a large mixing bowl, add eggs and milk. Mix thoroughly.
3) With a paper towel, squeeze out the excess moisture from the spinach leaves and add to the bowl of eggs.
4) Into small pieces, break the artichoke hearts and separate the leaves. Add to the bowl of eggs.
5) Except for the ricotta cheese, add remaining ingredients in the bowl of eggs and mix thoroughly.
6) Pour egg mixture into the prepared dish.
7) Evenly add dollops of ricotta cheese on top of the eggs and then pop in the oven.
8) Bake until eggs are set and doesn't jiggle when shook, about 35 minutes.
9) Remove from the oven and evenly divide into suggested servings. Enjoy.

Nutrition Information:

Calories per serving: 302; Protein: 22.6g; Carbs: 10.8g; Fat: 18.7g

Brekky Egg-Potato Hash

Serves: 2, Cooking Time: 25 minutes

Ingredients:

- 1 zucchini, diced
- 1/2 cup chicken broth
- ½ pound cooked chicken
- 1 tablespoon olive oil
- 4 ounces shrimp
- salt and ground black pepper to taste
- 1 large sweet potato, diced
- 2 eggs
- 1/4 teaspoon cayenne pepper
- 2 teaspoons garlic powder
- 1 cup fresh spinach (optional)

Directions for Cooking:

1) In a skillet, add the olive oil.
2) Fry the shrimp, cooked chicken and sweet potato for 2 minutes.
3) Add the cayenne pepper, garlic powder and salt and toss for 4 minutes.
4) Add the zucchini and toss for another 3 minutes.
5) Whisk the eggs in a bowl and add to the skillet.
6) Season using salt and pepper. Cover with the lid.
7) Cook for 1 minute and add the chicken broth.
8) Cover and cook for another 8 minutes on high heat.
9) Add the spinach and toss for 2 more minutes.
10) Serve immediately.

Nutrition Information:

Calories per serving: 190; Protein: 11.7g; Carbs: 2.9g; Fat: 12.3g

Cooked Beef Mushroom Egg

Serves: 2, Cooking Time: 15 minutes

Ingredients:

- ¼ cup cooked beef, diced
- 6 eggs
- 4 mushrooms, diced
- Salt and pepper to taste
- 12 ounces spinach
- 2 onions, chopped
- A dash of onion powder
- ¼ green bell pepper, chopped
- A dash of garlic powder

Directions for Cooking:

1) In a skillet, toss the beef for 3 minutes or until crispy.
2) Take off the heat and add to a plate.
3) Add the onion, bell pepper, and mushroom in the skillet.
4) Add the rest of the ingredients.
5) Toss for about 4 minutes.
6) Return the beef to the skillet and toss for another minute.
7) Serve hot.

Nutrition Information:

Calories per serving: 213; Protein: 14.5g; Carbs: 3.4g; Fat: 15.7g

Curried Veggies and Poached Eggs

Serves: 4, Cooking Time: 45 minutes

Ingredients:

- 4 large eggs
- ½ tsp white vinegar
- 1/8 tsp crushed red pepper – optional
- 1 cup water
- 1 14-oz can chickpeas, drained
- 2 medium zucchinis, diced
- ½ lb sliced button mushrooms
- 1 tbsp yellow curry powder
- 2 cloves garlic, minced
- 1 large onion, chopped
- 2 tsps extra virgin olive oil

Directions for Cooking:

1) On medium-high fire, place a large saucepan and heat oil.
2) Sauté onions until tender around four to five minutes.
3) Add garlic and continue sautéing for another half minute.

4) Add curry powder, stir and cook until fragrant around one to two minutes.
5) Add mushrooms, mix, cover and cook for 5 to 8 minutes or until mushrooms are tender and have released their liquid.
6) Add red pepper if using, water, chickpeas and zucchini. Mix well to combine and bring to a boil.
7) Once boiling, reduce fire to a simmer, cover and cook until zucchini is tender around 15 to 20 minutes of simmering.
8) Meanwhile, in a small pot filled with 3-inches deep of water, bring to a boil on high fire.
9) Once boiling, reduce fire to a simmer and add vinegar.
10) Slowly add one egg, slipping it gently into the water. Allow to simmer until egg is cooked, around 3 to 5 minutes.
11) Remove egg with a slotted spoon and transfer to a plate, one plate one egg.
12) Repeat the process with remaining eggs.
13) Once the veggies are done cooking, divide evenly into 4 servings and place one serving per plate of egg.
14) Serve and enjoy.

Nutrition Information:
Calories per serving: 215; Protein: 13.8g; Carbs: 20.6g; Fat: 9.4g

Dill and Tomato Frittata

Serves: 6, Cooking Time: 35 minutes

Ingredients:
- pepper and salt to taste
- 1 tsp red pepper flakes
- 2 garlic cloves, minced
- ½ cup crumbled goat cheese – optional
- 2 tbsp fresh chives, chopped
- 2 tbsp fresh dill, chopped
- 4 tomatoes, diced
- 8 eggs, whisked
- 1 tsp olive oil

Directions for Cooking:
1) Grease a 9-inch round baking pan and preheat oven to 325 degrees F.
2) In a large bowl, mix well all ingredients and pour into prepped pan.
3) Pop into the oven and bake until middle is cooked through around 30-35 minutes.
4) Remove from oven and garnish with more chives and dill.

Nutrition Information:
Calories per serving: 163; Protein: 12.0g; Carbs: 4g; Fat: 11g

Dill, Havarti & Asparagus Frittata

Serves: 4, Cooking Time: 20 minutes

Ingredients:
- 1 tsp dried dill weed or 2 tsp minced fresh dill
- 4-oz Havarti cheese cut into small cubes
- 6 eggs, beaten well
- Pepper and salt to taste
- 1 stalk green onions sliced for garnish
- 3 tsp. olive oil
- 2/3 cup diced cherry tomatoes
- 6-8 oz fresh asparagus, ends trimmed and cut into 1 ½-inch lengths

Directions for Cooking:
1) On medium-high fire, place a large cast-iron pan and add oil. Once oil is hot, stir-fry asparagus for 4 minutes.
2) Add dill weed and tomatoes. Cook for two minutes.
3) Meanwhile, season eggs with pepper and salt. Beat well.
4) Pour eggs over the tomatoes.
5) Evenly spread cheese on top.
6) Preheat broiler.
7) Lower the fire to low, cover pan, and let it cook for 10 minutes until the cheese on top has melted.
8) Turn off the fire and transfer pan in the oven and broil for 2 minutes or until tops are browned.
9) Remove from the oven, sprinkle sliced green onions, serve, and enjoy.

Nutrition Information:
Calories per serving: 244; Protein: 16.0g; Carbs: 3.7g; Fat: 18.3g

Egg and Ham Breakfast Cup

Serves: 12, Cooking Time: 12 minutes
Ingredients:
- 2 green onion bunch, chopped
- 12 eggs
- 6 thick pieces nitrate free ham

Directions for Cooking:
1) Grease a 12-muffin tin and preheat oven to 400 degrees F.
2) Add 2 hams per muffin compartment, press down to form a cup and add egg in middle. Repeat process to remaining muffin compartments.
3) Pop in the oven and bake until eggs are cooked to desired doneness, around 10 to 12 minutes.
4) To serve, garnish with chopped green onions.

Nutrition Information:
Calories per serving: 92; Protein: 7.3g; Carbs: 0.8g; Fat: 6.4g

Egg Muffin Sandwich

Serves: 2, Cooking Time: 10 minutes
Muffin Ingredients:
- 1 large egg, free-range or organic
- 1/4 cup almond flour
- 1/4 cup flax meal
- 1/4 cup grated cheddar cheese
- 1/4 tsp baking soda
- 2 tbsp heavy whipping cream or coconut milk
- 2 tbsp water
- pinch salt

Filing Ingredients:
- 2 tbsp cream cheese for spreading
- 1 tbsp olive oil
- 1 tsp Dijon mustard
- 2 large eggs, free-range or organic
- 2 slices cheddar cheese or other hard type cheese
- Optional: 1 cup greens (lettuce, kale, chard, spinach, watercress, etc.)
- salt and pepper to taste

Directions for Cooking:
1) Make the Muffin: In a small mixing bowl, mix well almond flour, flax meal, baking soda, and salt. Stir in water, cream, and eggs. Mix thoroughly.
2) Fold in cheese and evenly divide in two single-serve ramekins.
3) Pop in the microwave and cook for 75 seconds.
4) Make the filing: on medium fire, place a small nonstick pan, heat olive oil and cook the eggs to the desired doneness. Season with pepper and salt.
5) To make the muffin sandwiches, slice the muffins in half. Spread cream cheese on one side and mustard on the other side.
6) Add egg and greens. Top with the other half of sliced muffin.
7) Serve and enjoy.

Nutrition Information:
Calories per serving: 639; Protein: 26.5g; Carbs: 10.4g; Fat: 54.6g

Eggs over Kale Hash

Serves: 4, Cooking Time: 20 minutes
Ingredients:
- 4 large eggs
- 1 bunch chopped kale
- Dash of ground nutmeg
- 2 sweet potatoes, cubed
- 1 14.5-ounce can of chicken broth

Directions for Cooking:
1) In a large non-stick skillet, bring the chicken broth to a simmer. Add the sweet potatoes and season slightly with salt and pepper. Add a dash of nutmeg to improve the flavor.
2) Cook until the sweet potatoes become soft, around 10 minutes. Add kale and season with

salt and pepper. Continue cooking for four minutes or until kale has wilted. Set aside.
3) Using the same skillet, heat 1 tablespoon of olive oil over medium-high heat.
4) Cook the eggs sunny side up until the whites become opaque and the yolks have set. Top

the kale hash with the eggs. Serve immediately.

Nutrition Information:
Calories per serving: 158; Protein: 9.8g; Carbs 18.5g; Fat: 5.6g

Eggs with Dill, Pepper, and Salmon

Serves: 6, Cooking Time: 15 minutes
Ingredients:
- pepper and salt to taste
- 1 tsp red pepper flakes
- 2 garlic cloves, minced
- ½ cup crumbled goat cheese
- 2 tbsp fresh chives, chopped
- 2 tbsp fresh dill, chopped
- 4 tomatoes, diced
- 8 eggs, whisked
- 1 tsp olive oil

Directions for Cooking:

1) In a big bowl whisk the eggs. Mix in pepper, salt, red pepper flakes, garlic, dill and salmon.
2) On low fire, place a nonstick fry pan and lightly grease with oil.
3) Pour egg mixture and whisk around until cooked through to make scrambled eggs.
4) Serve and enjoy topped with goat cheese.

Nutrition Information:
Calories per serving: 141; Protein: 10.3g; Carbs: 6.7g; Fat: 8.5g

Fig and Walnut Skillet Frittata

Serves: 4, Cooking Time: 15 minutes
Ingredients:
- 1 cup figs, halved
- 4 eggs, beaten
- 1 teaspoon cinnamon
- A pinch of salt
- 2 tablespoons almond flour
- 2 tablespoons coconut flour
- 1 cup walnut, chopped
- 2 tablespoons olive oil
- 1 teaspoon cardamom
- 6 tablespoons raw honey

Directions for Cooking:
1) In a mixing bowl, beat the eggs.

2) Add the coconut flour, almond flour, cardamom, honey, salt and cinnamon.
3) Mix well. Heat the olive oil in a skillet over medium heat.
4) Add the egg mixture gently.
5) Add the walnuts and figs on top.
6) Cover and cook on medium low heat for about 10 minutes.
7) Serve hot with more honey on top.

Nutrition Information:
Calories per serving: 221; Protein: 12.7g; Carbs: 5.9g; Fat: 16.3g

Frittata with Dill and Tomatoes

Serves: 4, Cooking Time: 35 minutes
Ingredients:
- pepper and salt to taste
- 1 tsp red pepper flakes
- 2 garlic cloves, minced
- ½ cup crumbled goat cheese – optional
- 2 tbsp fresh chives, chopped
- 2 tbsp fresh dill, chopped
- 4 tomatoes, diced
- 8 eggs, whisked
- 1 tsp olive oil

Directions for Cooking:
1) Grease a 9-inch round baking pan and preheat oven to 325 degrees F.

2) In a large bowl, mix well all ingredients and pour into prepped pan.
3) Pop into the oven and bake until middle is cooked through around 30-35 minutes.

4) Remove from oven and garnish with more chives and dill.

Nutrition Information:
Calories per serving: 309; Protein: 19.8g; Carbs: 8.0g; Fat: 22.0g

Italian Scrambled Eggs

Serves: 1, Cooking Time: 7 minutes
Ingredients:
- 1 teaspoon balsamic vinegar
- 2 large eggs
- ¼ teaspoon rosemary, minced
- ½ cup cherry tomatoes
- 1 ½ cup kale, chopped
- ½ teaspoon olive oil

Directions for Cooking:
1) Melt the olive oil in a skillet over medium-high heat.
2) Sauté the kale and add rosemary and salt to taste. Add three tablespoons of water to prevent the kale from burning at the bottom of the pan. Cook for three to four minutes.
3) Add the tomatoes and stir.
4) Push the vegetables on one side of the skillet and add the eggs. Season with salt and pepper to taste.
5) Scramble the eggs then fold in the tomatoes and kales.

Nutrition Information:
Calories per serving: 230; Protein: 16.4g; Carbs: 15.0g; Fat: 12.4g

Kale and Red Pepper Frittata

Serves: 4, Cooking Time: 23 minutes
Ingredients:
- Salt and pepper to taste
- ½ cup almond milk
- 8 large eggs
- 2 cups kale, rinsed and chopped
- 3 slices of crispy bacon, chopped
- 1/3 cup onion, chopped
- ½ cup red pepper, chopped
- 1 tablespoon olive oil

Directions for Cooking:
1) Preheat the oven to 350 degrees F.
2) In a medium bowl, combine the eggs and almond milk. Season with salt and pepper. Set aside.
3) In a skillet, heat the olive oil over medium flame and sauté the onions and red pepper for three minutes or until the onion is translucent. Add in the kale and cook for 5 minutes more.
4) Add the eggs into the mixture along with the bacon and cook for four minutes or until the edges start to set.
5) Continue cooking the frittata in the oven for 15 minutes.

Nutrition Information:
Calories per serving: 242; Protein: 16.5g; Carbs: 7.0g; Fat: 16.45g

Lettuce Stuffed with Eggs 'n Crab Meat

Serves: 8, Cooking Time: 10 minutes
Ingredients:
- 24 butter lettuce leaves
- 1 tsp dry mustard
- ¼ cup finely chopped celery
- 1 cup lump crabmeat, around 5 ounces
- 3 tbsp plain Greek yogurt
- 2 tbsp extra virgin olive oil
- ¼ tsp ground pepper
- 8 large eggs
- ½ tsp salt, divided
- 1 tbsp fresh lemon juice, divided
- 2 cups thinly sliced radishes

Directions for Cooking:

1) In a medium bowl, mix ¼ tsp salt, 2 tsps. juice and radishes. Cover and chill for half an hour.
2) On medium saucepan, place eggs and cover with water over an inch above the eggs. Bring the pan of water to a boil. Once boiling, reduce fire to a simmer and cook for ten minutes.
3) Turn off fire, discard hot water and place eggs in an ice water bath to cool completely.
4) Peel eggshells and slice eggs in half lengthwise and remove the yolks.
5) With a sieve on top of a bowl, place yolks and press through a sieve. Set aside a tablespoon of yolk.
6) On remaining bowl of yolks add pepper, ¼ tsp salt and 1 tsp juice. Mix well and as you are stirring, slowly add oil until well incorporated. Add yogurt, stir well to mix.
7) Add mustard, celery and crabmeat. Gently mix to combine. If needed, taste and adjust seasoning of the filling.
8) On a serving platter, arrange 3 lettuce in a fan for two egg slices. To make the egg whites sit flat, you can slice a bit of the bottom to make it flat. Evenly divide crab filling into egg white holes.
9) Then evenly divide into eight servings the radish salad and add on the side of the eggs, on top of the lettuce leaves. Serve and enjoy.

Nutrition Information:
Calories per serving: 121; Protein: 10.0g; Carbs: 1.6g; Fat: 8.3g

Mixed Greens and Ricotta Frittata

Serves: 8, Cooking Time: 35 minutes

Ingredients:
- 1 tbsp pine nuts
- 1 clove garlic, chopped
- ¼ cup fresh mint leaves
- ¾ cup fresh parsley leaves
- 1 cup fresh basil leaves
- 8-oz part-skim ricotta
- 1 tbsp red-wine vinegar
- ½ + 1/8 tsp freshly ground black pepper, divided
- ½ tsp salt, divided
- 10 large eggs
- 1 lb chopped mixed greens
- Pinch of red pepper flakes
- 1 medium red onion, finely diced
- 1/3 cup + 2 tbsp olive oil, divided

Directions for Cooking:
1) Preheat oven to 350 degrees F.
2) On medium-high fire, place a nonstick skillet and heat 1 tbsp oil. Sauté onions until soft and translucent, around 4 minutes. Add half of greens and pepper flakes and sauté until tender and crisp, around 5 minutes. Remove cooked greens and place in colander. Add remaining uncooked greens in skillet and sauté until tender and crisp, when done add to colander. Allow cooked veggies to cool enough to handle, then squeeze dry and place in a bowl.
3) Whisk well ¼ tsp pepper, ¼ tsp salt, Parmesan and eggs in a large bowl.
4) In bowl of cooked vegetables, add 1/8 tsp pepper, ricotta and vinegar. Mix thoroughly. Then pour into bowl of eggs and mix well.
5) On medium fire, place same skillet used previously and heat 1 tbsp oil. Pour egg mixture and cook for 8 minutes or until sides are set. Turn off fire, place skillet inside oven and bake for 15 minutes or until middle of frittata is set.
6) Meanwhile, make the pesto by processing pine nuts, garlic, mint, parsley and basil in a food processor until coarsely chopped. Add 1/3 cup oil and continue processing. Season with remaining pepper and salt. Process once again until thoroughly mixed.
7) To serve, slice the frittata in 8 equal wedges and serve with a dollop of pesto.

Nutrition Information:
Calories per serving: 280; Protein: 14g; Carbs: 8g; Fat: 21.3g

Mushroom Tomato Frittata

Serves: 8, Cooking Time: 8 minutes

Ingredients:

- ¼ cup mushroom, sliced
- 10 eggs
- 1 cup cherry tomatoes
- Salt
- Pepper
- 1 teaspoon olive oil

Directions for Cooking:

1) Whisk the eggs in a bowl.
2) Add the eggs in a skillet.
3) Add the mushroom, cherry tomatoes and season using salt and pepper.
4) Cover with lid and cook for about 5 to 8 minutes on low heat.

Nutrition Information:

Calories per serving: 190; Protein: 11.7g; Carbs: 2.9g; Fat: 12.3g

Mushroom, Spinach and Turmeric Frittata

Serves: 6, Cooking Time: 35 minutes

Ingredients:

- ½ tsp pepper
- ½ tsp salt
- 1 tsp turmeric
- 5-oz firm tofu
- 4 large eggs
- 6 large egg whites
- ¼ cup water
- 1 lb fresh spinach
- 6 cloves freshly chopped garlic
- 1 large onion, chopped
- 1 lb button mushrooms, sliced

Directions for Cooking:

1) Grease a 10-inch nonstick and oven proof skillet and preheat oven to 350 degrees F.
2) Place skillet on medium-high fire and add mushrooms. Cook until golden brown.
3) Add onions, cook for 3 minutes or until onions are tender.
4) Add garlic, sauté for 30 seconds.
5) Add water and spinach, cook while covered until spinach is wilted, around 2 minutes.
6) Remove lid and continue cooking until water is fully evaporated.
7) In a blender, puree pepper, salt, turmeric, tofu, eggs and egg whites until smooth. Pour into skillet once liquid is fully evaporated.
8) Pop skillet into oven and bake until the center is set around 25-30 minutes.
9) Remove skillet from oven and let it stand for ten minutes before inverting and transferring to a serving plate.
10) Cut into 6 equal wedges, serve and enjoy.

Nutrition Information:

Calories per serving: 166; Protein: 15.9g; Carbs: 12.2g; Fat: 6.0g

Paleo Almond Banana Pancakes

Serves: 3, Cooking Time: 10 minutes

Ingredients:

- ¼ cup almond flour
- ½ teaspoon ground cinnamon
- 3 eggs
- 1 banana, mashed
- 1 tablespoon almond butter
- 1 teaspoon vanilla extract
- 1 teaspoon olive oil
- Sliced banana to serve

Directions for Cooking:

1) Whisk the eggs in a mixing bowl until they become fluffy.
2) In another bowl mash the banana using a fork and add to the egg mixture.
3) Add the vanilla, almond butter, cinnamon and almond flour.
4) Mix into a smooth batter.
5) Heat the olive oil in a skillet.
6) Add one spoonful of the batter and fry them from both sides.

7) Keep doing these steps until you are done with all the batter.
8) Add some sliced banana on top before serving.

Nutrition Information:
Calories per serving: 306; Protein: 14.4g; Carbs: 3.6g; Fat: 26.0g

Scrambled Eggs with Feta 'n Mushrooms

Serves: 1 , Cooking Time: 6 minutes
Ingredients:
- Pepper to taste
- 2 tbsp feta cheese
- 1 whole egg
- 2 egg whites
- 1 cup fresh spinach, chopped
- ½ cup fresh mushrooms, sliced
- Cooking spray

Directions for Cooking:
1) On medium-high fire, place a nonstick fry pan and grease with cooking spray.
2) Once hot, add spinach and mushrooms.
3) Sauté until spinach is wilted, around 2-3 minutes.
4) Meanwhile, in a bowl whisk well egg, egg whites, and cheese. Season with pepper.
5) Pour egg mixture into pan and scramble until eggs are cooked through, around 3-4 minutes.
6) Serve and enjoy with a piece of toast or brown rice.

Nutrition Information:
Calories per serving: 211; Protein: 18.6g; Carbs: 7.4g; Fat: 11.9g

Scrambled eggs with Smoked Salmon

Serves: 1, Cooking Time: 8 minutes
Ingredients:
- 1 tbsp olive oil
- Pepper and salt to taste
- 1/8 tsp red pepper flakes
- 1/8 tsp garlic powder
- 1 tbsp fresh dill, chopped finely
- 4 oz smoked salmon, torn apart
- 2 whole eggs + 1 egg yolk, whisked

Directions for Cooking:
1) In a big bowl whisk the eggs. Mix in pepper, salt, red pepper flakes, garlic, dill and salmon.
2) On low fire, place a nonstick fry pan and lightly grease with oil.
3) Pour egg mixture and whisk around until cooked through to make scrambled eggs, around 8 minutes on medium fire.
4) Serve and enjoy.

Nutrition Information:
Calories per serving: 366; Protein: 32.0; Carbs: 1.0g; Fat: 26.0g

Spiced Breakfast Casserole

Serves: 6, Cooking Time: 35 minutes
Ingredients:
- 1 tablespoon nutritional yeast
- ¼ cup water
- 6 large eggs
- 1 teaspoon coriander
- 1 teaspoon cumin
- 8 kale leaves, stems removed and torn into small pieces
- 2 sausages, cooked and chopped
- 1 large sweet potato, peeled and chopped

Directions for Cooking:
1) Preheat the oven to 375 degrees F.
2) Grease an 8" x 8" baking pan with olive oil and set aside.
3) Place sweet potatoes in a microwavable bowl and add ¼ cup water. Cook the chopped sweet potatoes in the microwave for three to five minutes. Drain the excess water then set aside.
4) Fry in a skillet heated over medium flame the sausage and cook until brown. Mix in the kale and cook until wilted.

5) Add the coriander, cumin and cooked sweet potatoes.
6) In another bowl, mix together the eggs, water and nutritional yeast. Add the vegetable and meat mixture into the bowl and mix completely.
7) Place the mixture in the baking dish and make sure that the mixture is evenly distributed within the pan.
8) Bake for 20 minutes or until the eggs are done.
9) Slice into squares.

Nutrition Information:
Calories per serving: 137; Protein: 10.1g; Carbs: 10.0g; Fat: 6.6g

Spinach, Mushroom and Sausage Frittata

Serves: 4, Cooking Time: 30 minutes
Ingredients:
- Salt and pepper to taste
- 10 eggs
- ½ small onion, chopped
- 1 cup mushroom, sliced
- 1 cup fresh spinach, chopped
- ½ pound sausage, ground
- 2 tablespoon olive oil

Directions for Cooking:
1) Preheat the oven to 350 degrees F.
2) Heat a skillet over medium-high flame and add the olive oil.
3) Sauté the onions until softened. Add in the sausage and cook for two minutes
4) Add in the spinach and mushroom. Stir constantly until the spinach has wilted.
5) Turn off the stove and distribute the vegetable mixture evenly.
6) Pour in the beaten eggs and transfer to the oven.
7) Cook for twenty minutes or until the eggs are completely cooked through.

Nutrition Information:
Calories per serving: 383; Protein: 24.9g; Carbs: 8.6g; Fat: 27.6g

Zucchini Tomato Frittata

Serves: 8, Cooking Time: 30 minutes
Ingredients:
- 3 lbs tomatoes, thinly sliced crosswise
- ¾ cup cheddar cheese, shredded
- ¼ cup milk
- 8 large eggs
- 1 tbsp fresh thyme leaves
- 3 zucchinis, cut into ¼-inch thick rounds
- 1 onion, finely chopped
- 1 tbsp olive oil
- Salt and pepper to taste

Directions for Cooking:
1) Preheat the oven to 425 degrees Fahrenheit.
2) Prepare a non-stick skillet and heat it over medium heat.
3) Sauté the zucchini, onion and thyme. Cook and stir often for 8 to 10 minutes. Let the liquid in the pan evaporate and season with salt and pepper to taste. Remove the skillet from heat.
4) In a bowl, whisk the milk, cheese, eggs, salt and pepper together. Pour the egg mixture over the zucchini in the skillet. Lift the zucchini to allow the eggs to coat the pan. Arrange the tomato slices on top.
5) Return to the skillet and heat to medium low fire and cook until the sides are set or golden brown, around 7 minutes.
6) Place the skillet inside the oven and cook for 10 to 15 minutes or until the center of the frittata is cooked through. To check if the egg is cooked through, insert a wooden skewer in the middle and it should come out clean.
7) Remove from the oven and loosen the frittata from the skillet. Serve warm.

Nutrition Information:
Calories per serving: 175; Protein: 12.0g; Carbs: 13.6g; Fat: 8.1g

Chapter 4 Vegetable Recipes

Asian Steamed Broccoli

Serves: 6, Cooking Time: 10 minutes
Ingredients:

- 3 tablespoons olive oil
- 3 cloves of garlic, minced
- 2 tablespoons ginger, sliced
- 2 heads of broccoli, cut into florets
- 3 tablespoons sesame oil
- 2 tablespoons coconut aminos

Directions for Cooking:

1) Heat olive oil in a pot.
2) Sauté the garlic and ginger until fragrant, around 3 minutes.
3) Add the rest of the ingredients.
4) Stir fry until tender, around 7 minutes.

Nutrition Information:
Calories per serving: 128; Carbs: 1.4g; Protein: 0.6g; Fat: 13.6g

Asparagus with Raspberry Vinaigrette

Serves: 4, Cooking Time: 15 minutes
Ingredients:

- A dash of ground pepper
- 1 tbsp flat-leaf parsley, chopped
- 1 tbsp olive oil
- 1/3 cup grapeseed oil
- 2 small shallots, chopped
- ½ cup raspberry vinegar
- Salt to taste
- 2 bunches of asparagus, woody portion trimmed

Directions for Cooking:

1) In a large skillet, bring water to a boil. Add a pinch of salt and cook the asparagus spears for two minutes. Submerge in cold water and drain. Set aside.
2) In a saucepan, mix the shallots and vinegar. Bring to a simmer and remove. Let it cool and set aside.
3) Add the grapeseed oil to the vinegar mixture and whisk. Add the parsley and season the vinaigrette with salt and pepper to taste.
4) Arrange the cooked asparagus spears on a plate and pour the vinaigrette.

Nutrition Information:
Calories per Serving: 93; Carbs: 2.2g; Protein: 0.4g; Fat: 8.9g

Banana-Coconut Breakfast

Serves: 4, Cooking Time: 3 minutes
Ingredients:

- 1 ripe banana
- 1 cup desiccated coconut
- 1 cup coconut milk
- 3 tablespoons raisins, chopped
- 2 tablespoon ground flax seed
- 1 teaspoon vanilla
- A dash of cinnamon
- A dash of nutmeg
- Salt to taste

Directions for Cooking:

1) Place all ingredients in a deep pan.
2) Allow to simmer for 3 minutes on low heat.
3) Place in individual containers.
4) Put a label and store in the fridge.
5) Allow to thaw at room temperature before heating in the microwave oven.

Nutrition Information:
Calories per serving:279; Carbs: 25.46g; Protein: 6.4g; Fat: g; Fiber: 5.9g

Basil and Tomato Soup

Serves: 2, Cooking Time: 25 minutes

Ingredients:

- Salt and pepper to taste
- 2 bay leaves
- 1 ½ cups almond milk, unsweetened
- ½ tsp raw apple cider vinegar
- 1/3 cup basil leaves
- ¼ cup tomato paste
- 3 cups tomatoes, chopped
- 1 medium celery stalk, chopped
- 1 medium carrot, chopped
- 1 medium garlic clove, minced
- ½ cup white onion
- 2 tbsp chicken broth

Directions for Cooking:

1) Heat the vegetable broth in a large saucepan over medium heat.
2) Add the onions and cook for 3 minutes. Add the garlic and cook for another minute.
3) Add the celery and carrots and cook for 1 minute.
4) Mix in the tomatoes and bring to a boil. Simmer for 15 minutes.
5) Add the almond milk, basil and bay leaves. Season with salt and pepper to taste.

Nutrition Information:
Calories per Serving: 213; Carbs: 42.0g; Protein: 6.9g; Fat: 3.9g

Blue Cheese, Fig and Arugula Salad

Serves: 4, Cooking Time: 0 minutes

Ingredients:

- ¼ cup crumbled blue cheese
- 1 tsp Dijon mustard
- 1-pint fresh figs, quartered
- 2 bags arugula
- 3 tbsp Balsamic Vinegar
- 3 tbsp olive oil
- Pepper and salt to taste

Directions for Cooking:

1) Whisk thoroughly together pepper, salt, olive oil, Dijon mustard, and balsamic vinegar to make the dressing. Set aside in the ref for at least 30 minutes to marinate and allow the spices to combine.
2) On four serving plates, evenly arrange arugula and top with blue cheese and figs.
3) Drizzle each plate of salad with 1 ½ tbsp of prepared dressing.
4) Serve and enjoy.

Nutrition Information:
Calories per serving: 202; Protein: 2.5g; Carbs: 25.5g; Fat: 10g

Braised Cauliflower with Ginger

Serves: 2, Cooking Time: minutes

Ingredients:

- Pepper to taste
- 2 minced scallions
- 2 tbsp rice vinegar
- 2 tbsp soy sauce
- ¼ cup water
- 1 ½ tbsp olive oil
- 1 tsp toasted sesame oil
- 2 cloves of garlic, minced
- 2 tbsp grated ginger
- 1 head cauliflower, cored and cut into florets

Directions for Cooking:

1) In a mixing bowl, combine garlic, ginger and sesame oil. Set aside.
2) In a skillet, heat vegetable oil over medium-high heat.
3) Add the cauliflowers and cook while stirring occasionally.
4) Make a clearing at the center of the skillet and add the ginger mixture.
5) Stir in the cauliflowers.
6) Reduce the heat to low and add water, soy sauce, and vinegar.
7) Cook until tender.

Nutrition Information:
Calories per Serving: 183; Carbs: 12.8g; Protein: 4.9g; Fat: 13.6g

Braised Kale and Carrots

Serves: 2, Cooking Time: 6 minutes
Ingredients:
- 1 tablespoon olive oil
- 1 onion, sliced thinly
- 5 cloves of garlic, minced
- 3 medium carrots, sliced thinly
- 10 ounces of kale, chopped
- ½ cup water
- Salt and pepper to taste
- A dash of red pepper flakes

Directions for Cooking:
1) Heat oil in a skillet over medium flame and sauté the onion and garlic until fragrant.
2) Toss in the carrots and stir for 1 minute. Add the kale and water. Season with salt and pepper to taste.
3) Close the lid and allow to simmer for 5 minutes.
4) Sprinkle with red pepper flakes.
5) Place in individual containers.
6) Put a label and store in the fridge.
7) Allow to warm at room temperature before heating in the microwave oven.

Nutrition Information:
Calories per serving: 161; Carbs: 19.9g; Protein: 7.5g; Fat: 8.2g; Fiber: 5.9g

Broccoli and Leek Soup

Serves: 2, Cooking Time: 5 minutes
Ingredients:
- 1 tbsp lemon juice
- 1 tbsp tamari
- 1 avocado, peeled and pitted
- 1 medium-sized leek, chopped
- 2 cups water
- 1 head broccoli, chopped

Directions for Cooking:
1) Bring a pot of water to a boil. Add broccoli and cook for 5 minutes. Drain and cool.
2) Place all ingredients in a blender and pulse until smooth.
3) Place in a bowl and top with broccoli and leek stalks.

Nutrition Information:
Calories per Serving: 221; Carbs: 20.9g; Protein: 5.8g; Fat: 15.2g

Brussels Sprouts Chips

Serves: 3, Cooking Time: 20 minutes
Ingredients:
- ½ pounds Brussels sprouts, sliced thinly
- 4 tablespoons olive oil
- 2 tablespoons mozzarella cheese, grated
- 1 teaspoon garlic powder
- Salt and pepper to taste

Directions for Cooking:
1) Preheat the oven to 400 degrees F.
2) In a bowl, combine all ingredients.
3) Toss to coat the ingredients
4) Place in a baking sheet and bake for 20 minutes or until golden brown.
5) Place in individual containers.
6) Put a label and store in the fridge.
7) Allow to warm at room temperature before heating in the microwave oven.

Nutrition Information:
Calories per serving:227; Carbs: 5.1g; Protein:15.2 g; Fat: 20.5g; Fiber:3.1 g

Butternut Squash Hummus

Serves: 8, Cooking Time: 15 minutes

Ingredients:

- 2 pounds butternut squash, seeded and peeled
- 1 tablespoon olive oil
- ¼ cup tahini
- 2 tablespoons lemon juice
- 2 cloves of garlic, minced
- Salt and pepper to taste

Directions for Cooking:

1) Heat the oven to 3000F.
2) Coat the butternut squash with olive oil.
3) Place in a baking dish and bake for 15 minutes in the oven.
4) Once the squash is cooked, place in a food processor together with the rest of the ingredients.
5) Pulse until smooth.
6) Place in individual containers.
7) Put a label and store in the fridge.
8) Allow to warm at room temperature before heating in the microwave oven.
9) Serve with carrots or celery sticks.

Nutrition Information:

Calories per serving: 115; Carbs: 15.8g; Protein: 2.5g; Fat:5.8g; Fiber: 6.7g

Butternut Squash Risotto

Serves: 4, Cooking Time: 25 minutes

Ingredients:

- ¾ cup bone broth
- 1 teaspoon apple cider vinegar
- Salt and pepper to taste
- ¼ cup sage, minced
- 3 garlic cloves, minced
- 1 cup mushrooms, chopped
- ½ yellow onion, chopped
- 1 tablespoon cooking fat
- 1 ½ pounds butternut squash, peeled and cubed

Directions for Cooking:

1) Place the butternut squash in a food processor and pulse for 20 seconds or until it has a coarse consistency. Set aside.
2) Heat a skillet over medium heat and add the cooking fat. Once it is melted, sauté the mushrooms and onions for five minutes. Add the sage and garlic and season with salt. Cook for another two minutes.
3) Mix in the apple cider vinegar and add the processed squash. Mix in the bone broth and cook for 15 minutes.
4) Serve warm.

Nutrition Information:

Calories per Serving: 383; Carbs: 94.9g; Protein: 11.0g; Fat: 2.0g

Butternut Squash Stir Fry

Serves: 4, Cooking Time: 10 minutes

Ingredients:

- 1 tablespoon olive oil
- 3 cloves of garlic, minced
- 1 butternut squash, seeded and sliced
- 1 tablespoon coconut aminos
- 1 tablespoon lemon juice
- 1 tablespoon water
- Salt and pepper to taste

Directions for Cooking:

1) Heat oil over medium flame and sauté the garlic until fragrant.
2) Stir in the squash for another 3 minutes before adding the rest of the ingredients.
3) Close the lid and allow to simmer for 5 more minutes or until the squash is soft.
4) Place in individual containers.
5) Put a label and store in the fridge.
6) Allow to thaw at room temperature before heating in the microwave oven.

Nutrition Information:

Calories per serving:152; Carbs: 31.4g; Protein:2.9g; Fat: 3.7g; Fiber: 4.3g

Cajun Jambalaya Soup

Serves: 6, Cooking Time: 6 hours
Ingredients:

- ¼ cup Frank's red hot sauce
- 3 tbsp Cajun seasoning
- 2 cups okra
- ½ head of cauliflower
- 1 pkg spicy Andouille sausage
- 4 oz chicken, diced
- 1 lb. large shrimps, raw and deveined
- 2 bay leaves
- 2 cloves garlic, diced
- 1 large can organic diced tomatoes
- 1 large onion, chopped
- 4 pepper
- 5 cups chicken stock

Directions for Cooking:

1) In slow cooker, place the bay leaves, red hot, Cajun seasoning, chicken, garlic, onions, and peppers.
2) Set slow cooker on low and cook for 5 ½ hours.
3) Then add sausages cook for 10 minutes.
4) Meanwhile, pulse cauliflower in food processor to make cauliflower rice.
5) Add cauliflower rice into slow cooker. Cook for 20 minutes.
6) Serve and enjoy.

Nutrition Information:
Calories per Serving: 155; Carbs: 13.9g; Protein: 17.4g; Fat: 3.8g

Cardamom and Carrot soup

Serves: 4, Cooking Time: 45 minutes
Ingredients:

- Freshly ground black pepper
- ½ cup full-fat coconut milk
- 4 cups chicken stock or Bone Broth
- ½ teaspoon ground cardamom
- 1 teaspoon minced fresh ginger
- ¼ cup diced Cortland apple, Empire, McIntosh, or Braeburn
- 1 ½ pounds peeled large carrots, cut into ½ inch coins
- Kosher Salt
- 2 large green onions, green and white ends only, trimmed and cleaned, and thinly sliced
- 1 tablespoon olive oil

Directions for Cooking:

1) On medium fire, place large saucepan and olive oil.
2) Sauté salt and leeks for 5 minutes or until translucent.
3) Add cardamom, ginger, apple, and carrot. Sauté for 3 minutes.
4) Add broth and boil on high fire.
5) When boiling, lower heat to a simmer, cover, and cook for 30 minutes or until carrots and apples are soft.
6) Add coconut milk, turn off fire, and mix.
7) With an immersion blender, puree soup.
8) Season to taste with pepper and salt.
9) Serve while warm.

Nutrition Information:
Calories per Serving: 185; Carbs: 20.6g; Protein: 3.1g; Fat: 11.6g

Cauliflower Hash Brown

Serves: 12, Cooking Time: 6 minutes
Ingredients:

- 12 eggs, beaten
- ½ cup coconut milk
- ½ teaspoon dry mustard
- Salt and pepper to taste
- 1 head cauliflower, shredded
- 2 cups shredded cheese

Directions for Cooking:

1) Place all ingredients in a mixing bowl until well combined.
2) Put enough oil for frying in a skillet and heat over medium flame.

3) Add a large dollop of cauliflower mixture in the skillet and flatten with the back of a fork.
4) Fry until golden brown.
5) Place in a plate lined with a kitchen towel to absorb excess oil.
6) Place in individual containers.
7) Put a label and store in the fridge.
8) Allow to thaw at room temperature before heating in the microwave oven.

Nutrition Information:
Calories per serving:340; Carbs: 5.22g; Protein: 22.81g; Fat: 25.07g; Fiber: 1.9g

Cauliflower Mash

Serves: 2, Cooking Time: 0 minutes
Ingredients:
- Crushed red pepper to taste
- 1 tsp fresh thyme
- 2 tsp chopped chives
- 2 tbsp nutritional yeast
- 2 tbsp filtered water
- 1 garlic clove, peeled
- 1 lemon, juice extracted
- ¼ cup pine nuts
- 3 cups cauliflower, chopped

Directions for Cooking:
1) Mix all ingredients in a blender or food processor. Pulse until smooth.
2) Scoop into a bowl and add crushed red peppers.

Nutrition Information:
Calories per Serving: 224; Carbs: 19.8g; Protein: 10.5g; Fat: 13.6g

Cheese and Broccoli Balls

Serves: 4, Cooking Time: 5 minutes
Ingredients:
- ¾ cup almond flour
- 2 large eggs
- 2 teaspoons baking powder
- 4 ounces fresh broccoli
- 4 ounces mozzarella cheese
- 7 tablespoons flaxseed meal
- Salt and Pepper to taste

Sauce Ingredients:
- ¼ cup fresh chopped dill
- ¼ cup mayonnaise
- ½ tablespoon lemon juice
- Salt and pepper to taste

Directions for Cooking:
1) To make the cheese and broccoli balls: Place broccoli in food processor and pulse into small pieces. Transfer to a bowl.
2) Add baking powder, ¼ cup flaxseed meal, almond flour, and cheese. Season with pepper and salt if the desired. Mix well. Place remaining flaxseed meal in a small bowl.
3) Add eggs and combine thoroughly. Roll the batter into 1-inch balls. And then roll in flaxseed meal to coat the balls.
4) Cook balls in a 375 degrees F deep fryer until golden brown, about 5 minutes. Transfer cooked balls on to a paper towel lined plate.
5) Meanwhile, make the sauce by combining all ingredients in a medium bowl.
6) Serve cheese and broccoli balls with the dipping sauce on the side.

Nutrition Information:
Calories per serving: 312; Protein: 18.4g; Carbs: 9.6g; Fat: 23.2g

Chinese Soy Eggplant

Serves: 2, Cooking Time: 10 minutes
Ingredients:
- 4 tablespoons olive oil
- 2 eggplants, sliced into 3-inch in length
- 4 cloves of garlic, minced
- 1 onion, chopped
- 1 teaspoon ginger, grated
- ¼ cup coconut aminos
- 1 teaspoon lemon juice, freshly squeezed

Directions for Cooking:

1) Heat oil in a pot.
2) Pan-fry the eggplants for 2 minutes on all sides.
3) Add the garlic and onions until fragrant, around 3 minutes.
4) Stir in the ginger, coconut aminos, and lemon juice.
5) Add a ½ cup of water and bring to a simmer. Cook until eggplant is tender.

Nutrition Information:
Calories per serving: 409; Carbs: 40.8g; Protein: 6.6g; Fat: 28.3g

Coconut Curry with Vegetables

Serves: 2, Cooking Time: 20 minutes
Ingredients:
- ¼ medium onion
- ½ cup coconut cream (or coconut milk)
- 1 cup broccoli florets
- 1 large handful of spinach
- 1 tablespoon red curry paste
- 1 teaspoon minced garlic
- 1 teaspoon minced ginger
- 2 teaspoons Fish sauce
- 2 teaspoons soy sauce
- 4 tablespoons olive oil

Directions for Cooking:
1) On medium-high fire, place a medium pot and heat 2 tablespoons of olive oil.
2) Once hot, sauté onions until nearly translucent, about 4 minutes. Add garlic and cook for a minute.
3) Lower the fire to medium-low, stir in broccoli, and cook for 2 minutes.
4) Move veggies to the side and on the empty side of pot, sauté a tablespoon of red curry paste for a minute or two.
5) Then mix pot. Add spinach and mix well.
6) Pour in coconut cream and mix again.
7) Stir in ginger, soy sauce, fish sauce, and remaining olive oil. Mix well.
8) Cover and let it simmer for 10 minutes.
9) Serve and enjoy.

Nutrition Information:
Calories per serving: 398; Protein: 3.9g; Carbs: 9.9g; Fat: 7.9g

Cold Cucumber Soup

Serves: 4, Cooking Time: minutes
Ingredients:
- Chopped fresh dill
- Pepper and salt to taste
- 1 cup fat-free plain yogurt
- 1 ½ cups fat-free half and half
- 1 ½ cups low-sodium chicken broth
- Juice of 1 lemon
- ½ cup chopped fresh parsley
- 6 medium cucumbers, peeled, halved lengthwise, seeds scraped out and chopped

Directions for Cooking:
1) In a blender, puree lemon juice, parsley and cucumbers.
2) Pour half of puree in a bowl and put aside.
3) In blender, add yogurt plus half and half on remaining pureed cucumber. Mix with a spoon before pureeing to mix well.
4) Pour back into blender the cucumber puree in a bowl, puree again to mix.
5) Season with pepper and salt.
6) Puree to mix.
7) Refrigerate for at least two hours before serving cold.

Nutrition Information:
Calories per Serving: 140; Carbs: 21.3g; Protein: 8.0g; Fat: 3.0g

Cold Veggie Udon

Serves: 2, Cooking Time: 10 minutes
Ingredients:
- 2 cups Jicama, spiral
- 1/3 cup Mentsuyu, diluted 2-3 times depending on preference

Topping Ingredients:
- wasabi
- ¼ tsp roasted white sesame seeds
- 4 grape tomatoes, halved
- 1 soft hardboiled egg
- ½ cup tenkasu/agedama - optional
- 2 –inch daikon radish, peeled, grated and excess water squeezed
- 1 Japanese cucumber, peeled, sliced thinly and diagonally, then julienned
- 1 green onion, sliced thinly
- 2 tsp wakame seaweed
- ½ package of medium firm tofu, cut into ½ inch cubes

Directions for Cooking:
1) Bring a pot of water to boil.
2) Meanwhile, in a small bowl, soak for 15 minutes the wakame seaweed in water. Once done, squeeze out water and put aside.
3) Then boil Jicama noodles and tofu for a minute or two, strain and discard hot water. Place in an ice bath until totally cold before straining again.
4) Then in a separate bowl, dilute Mentsuyu with 1/3 to 2/3s cup of water to taste. Add 3-4 ice cubes to keep Mentsuyu cold.
5) To serve, arrange noodles and tofu into two bowls. Garnish with 4 slices tomatoes, half of cucumber, half of seaweed, half of egg, half of green onion, half of sesame seeds, half of radish and half of tenkasu if using per bowl.
6) Serve with Mentsuyu on the side.

Nutrition Information:
Calories per serving: 324; Carbs: 38.9g; Protein: 24.8g; Fat: 10.1g

Cold Watermelon Gazpacho

Serves: 2, Cooking Time: 0 minutes
Ingredients:
- 2 basil leaves
- ¼ cup coconut sugar
- 1 tsp kosher salt
- ¼ cup vinegar
- 1 Thai Chili
- ¼ cup green bell pepper, chopped
- ¼ cup red onion, chopped
- ¼ cup cucumber, chopped
- 2 cups ripe tomatoes, chopped
- 2 cups watermelon, chopped

Directions for Cooking:
1) Combine the tomato, watermelon, onion, cucumber, bell pepper, vinegar, chili, salt and pepper to taste. Blend to a coarse texture.
2) Chill for an hour. Serve cold.

Nutrition Information:
Calories per Serving: 133; Carbs: 32.2g; Protein: 1.6g; Fat: 0.3g

Collard Green Wrap Greek Style

Serves: 4, Cooking Time: 0 minutes
Wrap Ingredients:
- ½ block feta, cut into 4 (1-inch thick) strips (4-oz)
- ½ cup purple onion, diced
- ½ medium red bell pepper, julienned
- 1 medium cucumber, julienned
- 4 large cherry tomatoes, halved
- 4 large collard green leaves, washed
- 8 whole kalamata olives, halved

Tzatziki Sauce Ingredients:
- 1 cup full-fat plain Greek yogurt
- 1 tablespoon white vinegar
- 1 teaspoon garlic powder
- 2 tablespoons minced fresh dill
- 2 tablespoons olive oil
- 2.5-ounces cucumber, seeded and grated (¼-whole)

- Salt and pepper to taste

Directions for Cooking:

1) Make the Tzatziki sauce first: make sure to squeeze out all the excess liquid from the cucumber after grating. In a small bowl, mix all sauce ingredients thoroughly and refrigerate.
2) Prepare and slice all wrap ingredients.
3) On a flat surface, spread one collard green leaf. Spread 2 tablespoons of Tzatziki sauce on middle of the leaf.
4) Layer ¼ of each of the tomatoes, feta, olives, onion, pepper, and cucumber. Place them on the center of the leaf, like piling them high instead of spreading them.
5) Fold the leaf like you would a burrito. Repeat process for remaining ingredients.
6) Serve and enjoy.

Nutrition Information:

Calories per serving: 165.3; Protein: 7.0g; Carbs: 9.9g; Fat: 11.2g

Creamy Carrot Chowder

Serves: 8, Cooking Time: 40 minutes

Ingredients:

- 8 fresh mint sprigs
- ½ cup 2% Greek Style Plain yogurt
- 1 tsp fresh ginger, peeled and grated
- 2 cups chicken broth
- 1 lb. baby carrots, peeled and cut into 2-inch lengths
- 1/3 cup sliced shallots
- 2 tsp sesame oil

Directions for Cooking:

1) On medium fire, place a medium heavy bottom pot and heat oil.
2) Sauté shallots until tender around 2 minutes.
3) Add carrots and sauté for another 4 minutes.
4) Pour broth, cover and bring to a boil. Once soup is boiling, slow fire to a simmer and cook carrots until tender around 22 minutes.
5) Add ginger and continue cooking while covered for another eight minutes.
6) Turn off fire and let it cool for 10 minutes.
7) Pour mixture into blender and puree. If needed, puree carrots in batches then return to pot.
8) Heat pureed carrots until heated through around 2 minutes.
9) Turn off fire and evenly pour into 8 serving bowls.
10) Serve and enjoy. Or you can store in the freezer in 8 different lidded containers for a quick soup in the middle of the week.

Nutrition Information:

Calories per Serving: 47; Carbs: 6.5g; Protein: 2.2g; Fat: 1.6g

Creamy Kale and Mushrooms

Serves: 3, Cooking Time: 15 minutes

Ingredients:

- 3 tablespoons olive oil
- 3 cloves of garlic, minced
- 1 onion, chopped
- 1 bunch kale, stems removed and leaves chopped
- 5 white button mushrooms, chopped
- 1 cup coconut milk
- Salt and pepper to taste

Directions for Cooking:

1) Heat oil in a pot.
2) Sauté the garlic and onion until fragrant for 2 minutes.
3) Stir in mushrooms. Season with pepper and salt. Cook for 8 minutes.
4) Stir in kale and coconut milk. Simmer for 5 minutes.
5) Adjust seasoning to taste.

Nutrition Information:

Calories per serving: 365; Carbs: 17.9g; Protein: 6g; Fat: 33.5g

Crunchy Kale Chips

Serves: 8, Cooking Time: 2 hours
Ingredients:
- 2 tbsp filtered water
- ½ tsp sea salt
- 1 tbsp raw honey
- 2 tbsp nutritional yeast
- 1 lemon, juiced
- 1 cup sweet potato, grated
- 1 cup fresh cashews, soaked 2 hours
- 2 bunches green curly kale, washed, ribs and stems removed, leaves torn into bite sized pieces

Directions for Cooking:
1) Prepare a baking sheet by covering with an unbleached parchment paper. Preheat oven to 150oF.
2) In a large mixing bowl, place kale.
3) In a food processor, process remaining ingredients until smooth. Pour over kale.
4) With your hands, coat kale with marinade.
5) Evenly spread kale onto parchment paper and pop in the oven. Dehydrate for 2 hours and turn leaves after the first hour of baking.
6) Remove from oven; let it cool completely before serving.

Nutrition Information:
Calories per Serving: 209; Carbs: 13.0g; Protein: 7.0g; Fat: 15.9g

Delicious and Healthy Roasted Eggplant

Serves: 6, Cooking Time: 30 minutes
Ingredients:
- Pinch of sugar
- ¼ tsp salt
- ¼ tsp cayenne pepper or to taste
- 1 tbsp parsley, flat leaf and chopped finely
- 2 tbsp fresh basil, chopped
- 1 small chili pepper, seeded and minced, optional
- ½ cup red onion, finely chopped
- ½ cup Greek feta cheese, crumbled
- ¼ cup extra virgin olive oil
- 2 tbsp lemon juice
- 1 medium eggplant, around 1 lb.

Directions for Cooking:
1) Preheat broiler and position rack 6 inches away from heat source.
2) Pierce the eggplant with a knife or fork. Then with a foil, line a baking pan and place the eggplant and broil. Make sure to turn eggplant every five minutes or until the skin is charred and eggplant is soft which takes around 14 to 18 minutes of broiling. Once done, remove from heat and let cool.
3) In a medium bowl, add lemon. Then cut eggplant in half, lengthwise, and scrape the flesh and place in the bowl with lemon. Add oil and mix until well combined. Then add salt, cayenne, parsley, basil, chili pepper, bell pepper, onion and feta. Toss until well combined and add sugar to taste if wanted.

Nutrition Information:
Calories per Serving: 97; Carbs: 7.4g; Protein: 2.9g; Fat: 6.7g

Delicious Stuffed Squash

Serves: 4 servings, Cooking Time: 30minutes
Ingredients:
- ¼ cup sour cream
- ½ cup shredded cheddar
- 3 tbsp taco sauce
- 1 small tomato, chopped
- ½ small green bell pepper, seeded and chopped
- ½ medium onion, chopped
- 1 tsp cumin
- 1 tsp onion powder

- ¼ tsp cayenne
- 1 ½ tsp chili powder
- 1 can 15-oz black beans, drained and rinsed
- 1 clove garlic, minced
- 1 tbsp olive oil
- 2 medium zucchinis
- 2 medium yellow squash
- Salt and pepper

Directions for Cooking:
1) Boil until tender in a large pot of water zucchini and yellow squash, then drain. Lengthwise, slice the squash and trim the ends. Take out the center flesh and chop.
2) On medium-high fire, place skillet with oil and sauté garlic until fragrant. Add onion and tomato and sauté for 8 minutes. Add chopped squash, bell pepper, cumin, onion powder, cayenne, chilli powder and black beans and continue cooking until veggies are tender.
3) Season with pepper and salt to taste. Remove from fire.
4) Spread 1 tsp of taco sauce on each squash shell, fill with half of the cooked filling, top with cheese and garnish with sour cream. Repeat procedure on other half of squash shell. Serve and enjoy.

Nutrition Information:
Calories per Serving: 318; Carbs: 28.0g; Protein: 21.0g; Fat: 16.0g

Eggplant Bolognese With Zucchini Noodles

Serves: 4, Cooking Time: 20 minutes
Ingredients:
- 6 leaves of fresh basil, chopped
- 1 28-ounce can plum tomatoes
- ½ cup red wine
- 1 tablespoon tomato paste
- 4 sprigs of thyme, chopped
- 2 bay leaves
- 3 cloves garlic, minced
- 1 large yellow onion, chopped
- Salt and pepper to taste
- 2 tablespoon extra-virgin olive oil
- ½ pound ground beef
- 1 ½ pounds eggplant, diced
- 2 cups zucchini noodles

Directions for Cooking:
1) Heat the skillet over medium-high heat and add oil. Sauté the onion and beef and sprinkle with salt and pepper. Sauté for 10 minutes until the meat is brown. Add in the eggplants, bay leaves, garlic and thyme. Cook for another 15 minutes.
2) Once the eggplant is tender, add the tomato paste and wine. Add the tomatoes and crush using a spoon. Bring to a boil and reduce the heat to low. Simmer for 10 minutes.
3) In a skillet, add oil and sauté the zucchini noodles for five minutes. Turn off the heat.
4) Pour the tomato sauce over the zucchini noodles and garnish with fresh basil.

Nutrition Information:
Calories per Serving: 320; Carbs: 24.8g; Protein: 19.2g; Fat: 17.0g

Feta and Roasted Eggplant Dip

Serves: 12, Cooking Time: 20 minutes
Ingredients:
- ¼ tsp salt
- ¼ tsp cayenne pepper
- 1 tbsp finely chopped flat leaf parsley
- 2 tbsp chopped fresh basil
- 1 small Chile pepper
- 1 small red bell pepper, finely chopped
- ½ cup finely chopped red onion
- ½ cup crumbled Greek nonfat feta cheese
- ¼ cup extra-virgin olive oil
- 2 tbsp lemon juice
- 1 medium eggplant, around 1 lb.

Directions for Cooking:
1) Preheat broiler, position rack on topmost part of oven, and line a baking pan with foil.
2) With a fork or knife, poke eggplant, place on prepared baking pan, and broil for 5 minutes per side until skin is charred all around.

3) Once eggplant skin is charred, remove from broiler and allow to cool to handle.
4) Once eggplant is cool enough to handle, slice in half lengthwise, scoop out flesh, and place in a medium bowl.
5) Pour in lemon juice and toss eggplant to coat with lemon juice and prevent it from discoloring.
6) Add oil; continue mixing until oil is absorbed by eggplant.
7) Stir in salt, cayenne pepper, parsley, basil, Chile pepper, bell pepper, onion, and feta.
8) Toss to mix well and serve.

Nutrition Information:
Calories per Serving: 58; Carbs: 3.7g; Protein: 1.2g; Fat: 4.6g

Garlic 'n Sour Cream Zucchini Bake

Serves: 3, Cooking Time: 20 minutes
Ingredients:
- 1/4 cup grated Parmesan cheese
- paprika to taste
- 1 tablespoon minced garlic
- 1 large zucchini, cut lengthwise then in half
- 1 cup sour cream
- 1 (8 ounce) package cream cheese, softened

Directions for Cooking:
1) Lightly grease a casserole dish with cooking spray.
2) Place zucchini slices in a single layer in dish.
3) In a bowl whisk well, remaining Ingredients: except for paprika. Spread on top of zucchini slices. Sprinkle paprika.
4) Cover dish with foil.
5) For 10 minutes, cook in preheated 390oF oven.
6) Remove foil and cook for 10 minutes.
7) Serve and enjoy.

Nutrition Information:
Calories per serving: 385; Carbs: 13.5g; Protein: 11.9g; Fat: 32.4g

Garlicky Rosemary Potatoes

Serves: 4, Cooking Time: 2 minutes.
Ingredients:
- 1-pound potatoes, peeled and sliced thinly
- 2 garlic cloves
- ½ teaspoon salt
- 1 tablespoon olive oil
- 2 sprigs of rosemary

Directions for Cooking:
1) Place a trivet or steamer basket in the Instant Pot and pour in a cup of water.
2) In a baking dish that can fit inside the Instant Pot, combine all ingredients and toss to coat everything.
3) Cover the baking dish with aluminum foil and place on the steamer basket.
4) Close the lid and press the Steam button.
5) Adjust the cooking time to 30 minutes
6) Do quick pressure release.
7) Once cooled, evenly divide into serving size, keep in your preferred container, and refrigerate until ready to eat.

Nutrition Information:
Calories per serving: 119; Carbs: 20.31g; Protein: 2.39g; Fat: 3.48g

Ginger and Spice Carrot Soup

Serves: 6, Cooking Time: 40 minutes
Ingredients:
- ¼ cup Greek yogurt
- 2 tsp fresh lime juice
- 5 cups low-salt chicken broth
- 1 ½ tsp finely grated lime peel
- 4 cups of carrots, peeled, thinly sliced into rounds
- 2 cups chopped onions
- 1 tbsp minced and peeled fresh ginger
- ½ tsp curry powder
- 3 tbsp expeller-pressed sunflower oil
- ½ tsp yellow mustard seeds
- 1 tsp coriander seeds

Directions for Cooking:
1) In a food processor, grind mustard seeds and coriander into a powder.
2) On medium-high fire, place a large pot and heat oil.
3) Add curry powder and powdered seeds and sauté for a minute.
4) Add ginger, cook for a minute.
5) Add lime peel, carrots and onions. Sauté for 3 minutes or until onions are softened.
6) Season with pepper and salt.
7) Add broth and bring to a boil. Reduce fire to a simmer and simmer uncovered for 30 minutes or until carrots are tender.
8) Cool broth slightly, and puree in batches. Return pureed carrots into pot.
9) Add lime juice, add more pepper and salt to taste.
10) Transfer to a serving bowl, drizzle with yogurt and serve.

Nutrition Information:
Calories per Serving: 129; Carbs: 13.6g; Protein: 2.8g; Fat: 7.7g

Ginger-Egg Drop Soup with Zoodle

Serves: 4, Cooking Time: 15 minutes
Ingredients:
- ½ teaspoons red pepper flakes
- 2 cups thinly sliced scallions, divided
- 2 cups, plus 1 tablespoon water, divided
- 2 tablespoons extra virgin olive oil
- 2 tablespoons minced ginger
- 3 tablespoons corn starch
- 4 large eggs, beaten
- 4 medium to large zucchini, spiralized into noodles
- 5 cups shiitake mushrooms, sliced
- 5 tablespoons low-sodium tamari sauce or soy sauce
- 8 cups vegetable broth, divided
- Salt & pepper to taste

Directions for Cooking:
1) On medium-high fire, place a large pot and add oil.
2) Once oil is hot, stir in ginger and sauté for two minutes.
3) Stir in a tablespoon of water and shiitake mushrooms. Cook for 5 minutes or until mushrooms start to give off liquid.
4) Stir in 1 ½ cups scallions, tamari sauce, red pepper flakes, remaining water, and 7 cups of the vegetable broth. Mix well and bring to a boil.
5) Meanwhile, in a small bowl whisk well cornstarch and remaining cup of vegetable broth and set aside.
6) Once pot is boiling, slowly pour in eggs while stirring pot continuously. Mix well.
7) Add the cornstarch slurry in pot and mix well. Continue mixing every now and then until thickened, about 5 minutes.
8) Taste and adjust seasoning with pepper and salt.
9) Stir in zoodles and cook until heated through, about 2 minutes.
10) Serve with a sprinkle of remaining scallions and enjoy.

Nutrition Information:
Calories per serving: 238; Protein: 10.6g; Carbs: 34.3g; Sugar: 12.8g; Fat: 8.6g

Ginger Vegetable Stir Fry

Serves: 4, Cooking Time: 5 minutes
Ingredients:
- 1 tablespoon oil
- 3 cloves of garlic, minced
- 1 onion, chopped
- 1 thumb-size ginger, sliced
- 1 tablespoon water
- 1 large carrots, peeled and julienned
- 1 large green bell pepper, seeded and julienned
- 1 large yellow bell pepper, seeded and julienned

- 1 large red bell pepper, seeded and julienned
- 1 zucchini, julienned
- Salt and pepper to taste

Directions for Cooking:
1) Heat oil in a skillet over medium flame and sauté the garlic, onion, and ginger until fragrant.
2) Stir in the rest of the ingredients and adjust the flame to high.
3) Keep on stirring for at least 5 minutes until vegetables are half-cooked.
4) Place in individual containers.
5) Put a label and store in the fridge.
6) Allow to thaw at room temperature before heating in the microwave oven.

Nutrition Information:
Calories per serving: 102; Carbs: 13.6g; Protein:0 g; Fat: 2g; Fiber: 7.6g

Gobi Masala Soup

Serves: 4, Cooking Time: 35 minutes
Ingredients:
- 1 tsp salt
- 1 tsp ground turmeric
- 1 tsp ground coriander
- 2 tsp cumin seeds
- 3 tsp dark mustard seeds
- 1 cup water
- 3 cups beef broth
- 1 head cauliflower, chopped
- 3 carrots, chopped
- 1 large onion, chopped
- 2 tbsp olive oil
- Chopped cilantro for topping
- Crushed red pepper to taste
- Black pepper to taste
- 1 tbsp lemon juice

Directions for Cooking:
1) On medium-high fire, place a large heavy bottomed pot and heat olive oil.
2) Once hot, sauté garlic cloves for a minute. Add carrots and continue sautéing for 4 minutes more.
3) Add turmeric, coriander, cumin, mustard seeds, and cauliflower. Sauté for 5 minutes.
4) Add water and beef broth and simmer for 10 to 15 minutes.
5) Turn off fire and transfer to blender. Puree until smoot and creamy.
6) Return to pot, continue simmering for another ten minutes.
7) Season with crushed red pepper, lemon juice, pepper, and salt.
8) To serve, garnish with cilantro, and enjoy.

Nutrition Information:
Calories per Serving: 148; Carbs: 16.1g; Protein: 3.7g; Fat: 8.8g

Greek Spring Soup

Serves: 4, Cooking Time: 25 minutes
Ingredients:
- 6 cups chicken broth homemade or canned
- 1 1/2 cups diced or shredded cooked chicken
- 2 Tablespoons olive oil
- 1 small onion diced about 3/4 cup
- 1 bay leaf
- 1/3 cup arborio rice
- 1 large eggs
- Juice of half of a lemon
- 1 cup chopped asparagus
- 1 cup diced carrots
- 1/2 cup of fresh chopped dill divided
- Kosher salt and fresh pepper to taste
- Fresh minced chives for garnish

Directions for Cooking:
1) Place a large pot on medium-high fire and heat for 2 minutes. Add oil and heat for another 2 minutes.
2) Stir in onions and sauté for 4 minutes.
3) Mix in bay leaf, chicken broth, and ¼ cup dill. Mix well, cover and bring to a boil.
4) Once boiling, add rice and mix well. Once boiling again, lower fire to a simmer and cook for another 10 minutes while covered.
5) Stir in asparagus and carrots. Cover and cook for another 10 minutes.

6) In the meantime, in a small bowl whisk well 2 tbsp water, lemon juice, and egg. Slowly whisk into soup. Mixing constantly until soup thickens.
7) Turn off heat and remove bay leaf.

8) Stir in remaining dill and adjust seasoning if needed.
9) Serve and enjoy.

Nutrition Information:
Calories per Serving: 263; Carbs: 21.3g; Protein: 19.6g; Fats: 10.9g

Greek Styled Veggie-Rice

Serves: 6, Cooking Time: 20 minutes

Ingredients:
- pepper and salt to taste
- ¼ cup extra virgin olive oil
- 3 tbsp chopped fresh mint
- ½ cup grape tomatoes, halved
- ½ red bell pepper, diced small
- 1 head cauliflower, cut into large florets
- ¼ cup fresh lemon juice
- ½ yellow onion, minced

Directions for Cooking:
1) In a bowl mix lemon juice and onion and leave for 30 minutes. Then drain onion and reserve the juice and onion bits.
2) In a blender, shred cauliflower until the size of a grain of rice.
3) On medium fire, place a medium nonstick skillet and for 8-10 minutes cook cauliflower while covered.

4) Add grape tomatoes and bell pepper and cook for 3 minutes while stirring occasionally.
5) Add mint and onion bits. Cook for another three minutes.
6) Meanwhile, in a small bowl whisk pepper, salt, 3 tbsp reserved lemon juice and olive oil until well blended.
7) Remove cooked cauliflower, transfer to a serving bowl, pour lemon juice mixture and toss to mix.
8) Before serving, if needed season with pepper and salt to taste.

Nutrition Information:
Calories per Serving: 120; Carbs: 8.0g; Protein: 2.3g; Fat: 9.5g

Green Vegan Soup

Serves: 6, Cooking Time: 20 minutes

Ingredients:
- 1 medium head cauliflower, cut into bite-sized florets
- 1 medium white onion, peeled and diced
- 2 cloves garlic, peeled and diced
- 1 bay leaf crumbled
- 5 oz watercress
- Fresh spinach or frozen spinach
- 4 cups vegetable stock or bone broth
- 1 cup cream or coconut milk + 6 tbsp for garnish
- 1/4 cup olive oil
- 1 tsp salt or to taste
- freshly ground black pepper
- Optional: fresh herbs such as parsley or chives for garnish

Directions for Cooking:

1) On medium-high fire, place a Dutch oven greased with olive oil. Once hot, sauté garlic for a minute. Add onions and sauté until soft and translucent, about 5 minutes.
2) Add cauliflower florets and crumbled bay leaf. Mix well and cook for 5 minutes.
3) Stir in watercress and spinach. Sauté for 3 minutes.
4) Add vegetable stock and bring to a boil.
5) When cauliflower is crisp-tender, stir in coconut milk.
6) Season with pepper and salt.
7) With a hand blender, puree soup until smooth and creamy.
8) Serve and enjoy.

Nutrition Information:
Calories per serving: 392; Protein: 4.9g; Carbs: 9.7g; Sugar: 6.8g; Fat: 37.6g

Grilled Eggplant Caprese

Serves: 4, Cooking Time: 10 minutes

Ingredients:

- 1 eggplant aubergine, small/medium
- 1 tomato large
- 2 basil leaves or a little more as needed
- 4-oz mozzarella
- good quality olive oil
- Pepper and salt to taste

Directions for Cooking:

1) Cut the ends of the eggplant and then cut it lengthwise into ¼-inch thick slices. Discard the smaller pieces that's mostly skin and short.
2) Slice the tomatoes and mozzarella into thin slices just like the eggplant.
3) On medium-high fire, place a griddle and let it heat up.
4) Brush eggplant slices with olive oil and place on grill. Grill for 3 minutes. Turnover and grill for a minute. Add a slice of cheese on one side and tomato on the other side. Continue cooking for another 2 minutes.
5) Sprinkle with basil leaves. Season with pepper and salt.
6) Fold eggplant in half and skewer with a cocktail stick.
7) Serve and enjoy.

Nutrition Information:
Calories per serving: 59; Protein: 3.0g; Carbs: 4.0g; Sugar: 2.0g; Fat: 3.0g

Grilled Zucchini Bread and Cheese Sandwich

Serves: 2, Cooking Time: 40 minutes

Ingredients:

- 1 large egg
- 1/2 cup freshly grated Parmesan
- 1/4 cup almond flour
- 2 cup grated zucchini
- 2 cup shredded Cheddar
- 2 green onions thinly sliced
- Freshly ground black pepper
- kosher salt
- Vegetable oil, for cooking

Directions for Cooking:

1) With a paper towel, squeeze dry the zucchinis and place in a bowl. Add almond flour, green onions, Parmesan, and egg. Season with pepper and salt. Whisk well to combine.
2) Place a large nonstick pan on medium fire and add oil to cover pan. Once hot, add ¼ cup of zucchini mixture and shape into a square like a bread. Add another batch as many as you can put in the pan. If needed, cook in batches. Cook for four minutes per side and place on a paper towel lined plate.
3) Once done cooking zucchinis, wipe off oil from the pan. Place one zucchini piece on the pan, spread ½ of shredded cheese, and then top with another piece of zucchini. Grill for two minutes per side. Repeat process to make 2 sandwiches.
4) Serve and enjoy.

Nutrition Information:
Calories per serving: 667; Protein: 41.5g; Carbs: 14.4g; Fat: 49.9g

Hoemade Egg Drop Soup

Serves: 4, Cooking Time: 15 minutes

Ingredients:

- 1 tbsp cornstarch
- 1 tbsp dried minced onion
- 1 tsp dried parsley
- 2 eggs
- 4 cubes chicken bouillon
- 4 cups water
- 1 cup chopped carrots
- ½ cup thinly shredded cabbage

Directions for Cooking:

1) Combine water, bouillon, parsley, cabbage, carrots, and onion flakes in a saucepan, and then bring to a boil.
2) Beat the eggs lightly and stir into the soup.

3) Dissolve cornstarch with a little water. Stir until smooth and stir into the soup. Let it boil until the soup thickens.

Nutrition Information:
Calories per serving: 98; Carbs: 6.9g; Protein: 5.1g; Fat: 5.3g

Hot and Sour Soup

Serves: 4, Cooking Time: 25 minutes

Ingredients:

- ½ tsp sesame oil
- 1 cup fresh bean sprouts
- 1 egg, lightly beaten
- 1 tsp black pepper
- 1 tsp ground ginger
- 3 tbsp white vinegar
- 3 tbsp soy sauce
- ¼ lb. sliced mushrooms
- ½ lb. tofu, cubed
- 2 tbsp corn starch
- 3 ½ cups chicken broth

Directions for Cooking:

1) Mix corn starch and ¼ cup chicken broth and put aside.

2) Over high heat place a pot then combine and boil: pepper, ginger, vinegar, soy sauce, mushrooms, tofu and chicken broth.
3) Once boiling, add the corn starch mixture. Stir constantly and reduce fire. Once concoction is thickened, drop the slightly beaten egg while stirring vigorously.
4) Add bean sprouts and for one to two minutes allow simmering.
5) Remove from fire and transfer to serving bowls and enjoy while hot.

Nutrition Information:
Calories per serving: 141; Carbs: 12.9g; Protein: 10.0g; Fat: 6.6g

Indian Bell Peppers and Potato Stir Fry

Serves: 2, Cooking Time: 15 minutes

Ingredients:

- 1 tablespoon oil
- ½ teaspoon cumin seeds
- 4 cloves of garlic, minced
- 4 potatoes, scrubbed and halved
- Salt and pepper to taste
- 5 tablespoons water
- 2 bell peppers, seeded and julienned
- Chopped cilantro for garnish

Directions for Cooking:

1) Heat oil in a skillet over medium flame and toast the cumin seeds until fragrant.
2) Add the garlic until fragrant.

3) Stir in the potatoes, salt, pepper, water, and bell peppers.
4) Close the lid and allow to simmer for at least 10 minutes.
5) Garnish with cilantro before cooking time ends.
6) Place in individual containers.
7) Put a label and store in the fridge.
8) Allow to thaw at room temperature before heating in the microwave oven.

Nutrition Information:
Calories per serving: 83; Carbs: 7.3g; Protein: 2.8g; Fat: 6.4g; Fiber:1.7 g

Indian Style Okra

Serves: 4, Cooking Time: 12 minutes

Ingredients:

- 1 lb. small to medium okra pods, trimmed
- ¼ tsp curry powder
- ½ tsp kosher salt

- 1 tsp finely chopped serrano chile
- 1 tsp ground coriander
- 1 tbsp canola oil

- ¾ tsp brown mustard seeds

Directions for Cooking:
1) On medium-high fire, place a large and heavy skillet and cook mustard seeds until fragrant, around 30 seconds.
2) Add canola oil. Add okra, curry powder, salt, chile, and coriander. Sauté for a minute while stirring every once in a while.
3) Cover and cook low fire for at least 8 minutes. Stir occasionally.
4) Uncover, increase fire to medium-high and cook until okra is lightly browned, around 2 minutes more.
5) Serve and enjoy.

Nutrition Information:
Calories per Serving: 78; Carbs: 6.4g; Protein: 2.1g; Fat: 5.7g

Instant Pot Artichoke Hearts

Serves: 6, Cooking Time: 30 minutes
Ingredients:
- 4 artichokes, rinsed and trimmed
- Juice from 2 small lemons, freshly squeezed
- 2 cups bone broth
- 1 tablespoon tarragon leaves
- 1 stalk, celery
- ½ cup extra virgin olive oil
- Salt and pepper to taste

Directions for Cooking:
1) Place all ingredients in a pressure cooker.
2) Give a good stir.
3) Close the lid and seal the valve.
4) Pressure cook for 4 minutes.
5) Allow pressure cooker to release steam naturally.
6) Then serve and enjoy.

Nutrition Information:
Calories per serving: 133; Carbs: 14.3g; Protein: 4.4g; Fat: 11.7g

Instant Pot Fried Veggies

Serves: 3, Cooking Time: 6 minutes
Ingredients:
- 1 tablespoon olive oil
- 1 onion, chopped
- 4 cloves of garlic, minced
- 2 carrots, peeled and julienned
- 1 zucchini, julienned
- 1 large potato, peeled and julienned
- ½ cup chopped tomatoes
- 1 teaspoon rosemary sprig
- Salt and pepper to taste

Instructions
1) Press the Sauté button and heat the oil.
2) Sauté the onion and garlic until fragrant.
3) Stir in the rest of the ingredients.
4) Close the lid and make sure that the vents are sealed.
5) Press the Manual button and adjust the cooking time to 1 minute.
6) Do quick pressure release.
7) Once the lid is open, press the Sauté button and continue stirring until the liquid has reduced.
8) Once cooled, evenly divide into serving size, keep in your preferred container, and refrigerate until ready to eat.

Nutrition Information:
Calories per serving: 97; Carbs: 10.4g; Protein: 0.5g; Fat: 4.2g

Instant Pot Sautéed Kale

Serves: 6, Cooking Time: minutes
Ingredients:
- 3 tablespoons olive oil
- 2 cloves of garlic, minced
- 1 onion, chopped
- 2 teaspoons crushed red pepper flakes
- 4cups kale, chopped
- ¼ cup water
- Salt and pepper to taste

Directions for Cooking:

1) Press the "Sauté" button on the Instant Pot.
2) Heat the oil and sauté the garlic and onions until fragrant.
3) Stir in the rest of the ingredients.
4) Close the lid and make sure that the steam release valve is set to "Sealing."
5) Press the "Manual" button and adjust the cooking time to 4 minutes.
6) Do quick pressure release.

Nutrition Information:
Calories per serving: 82; Carbs: 5.1g; Protein: 1.1g; Fat: 7.9g

Interestingly Good Eggplant Curry

Serves: 4 , Cooking Time: 40 minutes
Ingredients:
- ¼ bunch cilantro, chopped finely
- 1 tsp salt
- 1 fresh jalapeno Chile pepper, finely chopped
- ½ cup plain yogurt
- 1 tomato diced
- 1 tbsp curry powder
- 1 tbsp ginger garlic paste
- 1 medium onion, thinly sliced
- 1 tsp cumin seeds
- 6 tbsp olive oil
- 1 large eggplant, ribbon cut
- 1 10.5-oz package firm tofu, cut into ½-inch cubes

Directions for Cooking:
1) On medium fire, place a nonstick medium saucepan and heat 2 tbsp oil. Add ribbon eggplant, cover, stir occasionally and cook for 8-10 minutes or until slightly soft. Remove from fire, transfer to a plate and set aside.
2) On same saucepan, add 2 tbsp oil and sauté tofu on medium-high fire, around a total of 10-12 minutes or until all sides are browned. Transfer to a serving bowl and set aside
3) On the same pan, add remaining oil and sauté tomato, curry powder and ginger garlic paste for at least two minutes. Add salt, jalapeno pepper and yogurt and cook for a minute.
4) Add eggplant, mix well, cover and cook for another 10 minutes.
5) Remove from fire, pour over tofu and garnish with cilantro before serving.

Nutrition Information:
Calories per Serving: 307; Carbs: 14.4g; Protein: 9.4g; Fat: 25.5g

Lemon Basil Spaghetti Squash

Serves: 2, Cooking Time: 15 minutes
Ingredients:
- Salt and pepper to taste
- 1/8 teaspoon cayenne pepper
- ¼ cup olive oil
- 1/3 cup lemon juice
- 1 tablespoon lemon zest
- 1 cup fresh basil leaves
- 6 garlic cloves, minced
- 1 avocado, mashed
- 3 cups spaghetti squash
- 2 teaspoon olive oil
- ¼cup cherry tomatoes, halved
- 1 cup kale, chopped

Directions for Cooking:
1) In a food processor, mix together the cayenne pepper, ¼ cup olive oil, lemon juice, lemon zest, basil leaves and garlic. Blend until smooth.
2) Heat a skillet over medium-high heat and add 2 teaspoon olive oil. Sauté the tomatoes for two minutes. Add the spaghetti squash and kale and mix thoroughly.

Nutrition Information:
Calories per Serving: 527; Carbs: 28.9g; Protein: 4.7g; Fat: 47.4g

Lemon Zucchini 'n Basil Soup

Serves: 4, Cooking Time: 20 minutes

Ingredients:
- 1 medium onion, chopped
- 1/2 cup loosely packed basil
- 3 cups chicken broth
- 3-4 cloves garlic, chopped
- 4 medium zucchini, peeled and chopped into cubes
- Additional Seasonings, Optional and to Taste
- Basil leaves, chopped
- Lemon wedges
- 4 tbsp Parmesan cheese, grated
- Salt and pepper to taste
- Sour cream, dollop
- Yogurt, dollop
- Zest of 1 lemon

Directions for Cooking:

1) Place a pot on medium fire and heat oil for 2 minutes. Stir in onions and sauté for 4 minutes.
2) Add garlic and sauté for a minute.
3) Stir in zucchini and sauté for 4 minutes.
4) Mix in lemon zest and chicken broth and simmer for 10 minutes.
5) Stir in basil and puree with an immersion blender.
6) Season with pepper and salt to taste.
7) Ladle into 4 bowls and evenly topped with lemon wedges, Parmesan cheese, sour cream, and yogurt.
8) Enjoy.

Nutrition Information:
Calories per Serving: 115; Carbs: 8.6g; Protein: 5.5g; Fats: 7.0g

Lentil and Kale Soup

Serves: 4, Cooking Time: 35 minutes

Ingredients:
- 1 ½ cups celery, chopped
- ½ tsp cumin
- 1 ½ tsp dried thyme
- 1 ½ tsp black pepper
- 1 cup chopped leeks
- 1 cup red lentils
- 1 ½ tsp minced garlic
- 2 cups chopped onions
- 3 cups kale, ribs removed
- 1 ½ tbsp hot sauce
- 4 tbsp balsamic vinegar
- 1/8 cup tomato paste
- 6 cups low sodium vegetable stock
- 3 cups chopped tomatoes
- 2 cups diced sweet potatoes
- 1 ½ cup chopped carrots

Directions for Cooking:
1) Sauté onions in a pan under low heat. Add the garlic until fragrant.
2) Place onions, garlic and the rest of the ingredients in a pot.
3) Stir and cook for 30 minutes on medium fire.
4) You can also cook it in a slow cooker for 8 hours.

Nutrition Information:
Calories per Serving: 376; Carbs: 81.7g; Protein: 12.8g; Fat: 2.5g

Marinara Sauce Over Cheesy Eggplant Bake

Serves: 4, Cooking Time: 45 minutes

Ingredients:
- salt and freshly ground black pepper to taste
- 2 tablespoons shredded pepper jack cheese
- 1-1/2 teaspoons olive oil
- 1-1/2 cups prepared marinara sauce
- 1/4 teaspoon red pepper flakes
- 1/4 cup water, plus more as needed
- 1/4 cup grated Parmesan cheese
- 1/4 cup grated Parmesan cheese
- 1/4 cup and 2 tablespoons ricotta cheese
- 1/4 cup and 2 tablespoons dry breadcrumbs
- 1/2 pinch salt, or as needed
- 1 tablespoon olive oil

- 1 tablespoon olive oil
- 1 large eggplant
- 1 clove garlic, sliced

Directions for Cooking:

1) Cut eggplant crosswise in 5 pieces. Peel and chop two pieces into ½-inch cubes.
2) Lightly grease a pot 1 tbsp olive oil. For 5 minutes, heat oil over medium-high fire.
3) Add half of eggplant strips and cook for 2 minutes per side. Transfer to a casserole dish.
4) Add 1 ½ tsp olive oil and garlic. Cook for a minute. Add chopped eggplants. Season with pepper flakes and salt. Cook for 4 minutes. Lower heat to medium low and continue cooking eggplants until soft, around 8 minutes more.

5) Stir in water and marinara sauce. Cook for 8 minutes until heated through. Stirring every now and then. Transfer to a bowl.
6) In a bowl, whisk well pepper, salt, pepper jack cheese, Parmesan cheese, and ricotta. Evenly spread cheeses over eggplant strips and then fold in half.
7) Pour marinara sauce on top of eggplants in casserole dish.
8) In a small bowl whisk well olive oil, and breadcrumbs. Sprinkle all over sauce.
9) Cook for 15 minutes at a preheated 390oF oven until tops are lightly browned.
10) Serve and enjoy.

Nutrition Information:
Calories per serving: 269; Carbs: 23.4g; Protein: 9.9g; Fat: 15.8g

Marsala Roasted Carrots

Serves: 8 servings, Cooking Time: 40 minutes

Ingredients:

- Chopped fresh parsley – optional
- Pepper and salt to taste
- 2 tbsp balsamic vinegar
- 2 tbsp extra virgin olive oil
- ½ cup marsala
- 2 lbs. julienned carrots

Directions for Cooking:

1) Peel and julienne carrots.
2) Place carrots on baking sheet.

3) Add vinegar, olive oil and marsala. Toss to coat.
4) Roast carrots in oven for 30-40 minutes at 425 degrees F, while occasionally stirring.
5) Carrots are cooked once tender and lightly browned. Remove from oven and season with pepper, salt and fresh parsley.

Nutrition Information:
Calories per Serving: 100; Carbs: 12.0g; Protein: 1.0g; Fat: 4.0g

Mashed Cauliflower

Serves: 3, Cooking Time: 7 minutes

Ingredients:

- 1 cauliflower head, chopped into florets
- 2 tablespoons olive oil
- Juice from ½ lemon, freshly squeezed
- Salt and pepper to taste

Directions for Cooking:

1) Place a steam rack or trivet in your steamer and pour a cup of water.
2) Place the cauliflower florets on the steam rack.

3) Close the lid and steam cauliflower for 7 minutes.
4) Place the cauliflower in a food processor and pulse.
5) Add the rest of the ingredients.
6) Pulse until smooth.

Nutrition Information:
Calories per serving: 41; Carbs: 2.4g; Protein: 0.7g; Fat: 4.9g

Mashed Sweet Orange Potatoes and Apples

Serves: 2, Cooking Time: 35 minutes
Ingredients:
- 2 tbsp unsweetened almond milk
- 1 red apple peeled, cored and sliced
- ½ teaspoon ground allspice
- 1 teaspoon ground cinnamon
- 2 tbsp Earth Balance soy free buttery spread
- 2 large sweet orange potatoes, peeled and diced

Directions for Cooking:
1) Place sweet potatoes in medium saucepan and fill with water until potatoes are covered.
2) Bring pan to a boil and reduce fire to a simmer once boiling. Cover and simmer until potatoes are tender, around 20 minutes.
3) In a small saucepan on medium low fire melt butter. Add allspice, cinnamon and sugar. Mix in apples and cook until apples are tender, around 5 minutes. Make sure to stir frequently. Turn off fire and allow to cool for at least 10 minutes.
4) Once sweet potatoes are cooked, drain and let it cool.
5) Transfer warm sweet potatoes and apples in a blender.
6) Add milk and puree until smooth.
7) Transfer to a serving plate, serve and enjoy.

Nutrition Information:
Calories per Serving: 169; Carbs: 40.1g; Protein: 3.5g; Fat: 0.7g

Mediterranean Diet Approved Falafel Recipe

Serves: 12, Cooking Time: 15 minutes
Ingredients:
- 1 tablespoon canola oil
- 1/2 teaspoon lime juice
- 1/8 teaspoon garlic powder
- 17 oz canned chickpeas, drained
- 2 tablespoons besan/chickpea flour
- 3 large green collard leaves
- 3/4 teaspoon salt

Directions for Cooking:
1) De-stem the collard greens and wash. Put in a food processor and chop until fine.
2) Add chickpeas and process into fine pieces but not mush.
3) Pour mixture into a bowl. Season with lime juice, garlic powder, and salt. Mix well.
4) Stir in chickpea flour and form into 12 equal patties.
5) Place a pan on medium fire and heat oil for 2 minutes.
6) Pan fry falafel in batches for 5 minutes per side or until lightly browned.

Nutrition Information:
Calories per Serving: 50; Carbs: 6.0g; Protein 2.0g; Fat: 2.0g

Over-The-Top Fried Cauliflower Rice

Serves: 1, Cooking Time: 20 minutes
Ingredients:
- garlic powder, salt, and pepper
- 2 eggs
- extra virgin olive oil
- 4oz mushrooms, sliced
- 1 small handful baby spinach
- 1 green onion chopped
- 1/2 avocado
- 1/2 lemon
- 1-1/2 cups cauliflower rice

Directions for Cooking:
1) In small bowl, mash and mix pepper, salt, garlic powder, lemon juice, and avocado.
2) In another small bowl, whisk eggs. Season with pepper and salt and then whisk well.
3) On medium fire, place a medium nonstick pan and heat a drizzle of oil. Add mushrooms and sauté until liquid has evaporated. Season with pepper, salt, and garlic powder. Continue

cooking until golden brown. Transfer to a bowl.
4) In same pan, increase the fire to medium-high and add another drizzle of oil. Add cauliflower in pan and continue cooking until cauliflower is golden brown, about 5 minutes. Season with pepper, salt, and garlic powder. Mix well and transfer to a bowl.

5) In same pan, lower the fire to medium and return mushrooms. Add baby spinach and green onions and sauté for a minute.
6) Pour in eggs and scramble. Once cooked to the desired doneness, place on top of cauliflower.
7) Top with avocado salsa and enjoy.

Nutrition Information:
Calories per serving: 490; Protein: 26.3g; Carbs: 41.0g; Fat: 29.7g

Mediterranean Diet Styled Stuffed Peppers

Serves: 4, Cooking Time: 30 minutes
Ingredients:
- A handful of parsley, chopped roughly
- 0.40 lb. of feta cheese, crumbled finely
- 1 lb. of ready to eat quinoa
- 1 courgette, thinly sliced and quartered lengthwise
- 4 red peppers

Directions for Cooking:
1) Preheat oven to 400 degrees F.
2) Cut the peppers one by one lengthways and place on baking pan with the hollow side up. Remove and discard the seeds, season and drizzle with a tbsp. of olive oil. For fifteen minutes, roast the pepper.
3) In a fry pan, heat a tsp of olive oil and sauté the courgette. Before adding the parsley, feta and quinoa, remove fry pan from fire, season with pepper and mix well.
4) Then equally put the quinoa mixture into the hollow of the pepper and bake again in the oven for five more minutes.
5) Serve and enjoy while hot.

Nutrition Information:
Calories per Serving: 294; Carbs: 34.2g; Protein: 13.4g; Fat: 12.2g

Mushroom-Cauliflower Risotto

Serves: 6, Cooking Time: 30 minutes
Ingredients:
- 1 cup heavy cream
- 1 large shallot, minced
- 1 small onion, diced
- 1/2 cup grated Parmesan cheese
- 2 cup chicken stock, divided
- 2 tablespoons chopped fresh flat-leaf parsley
- 2 tablespoons olive oil
- 4 cups riced cauliflower
- 6 cloves garlic, minced
- 8 ounces cremini mushrooms, thinly sliced
- Sea salt and black pepper, to taste

Directions for Cooking:
1) On medium fire, place a large nonstick pan and heat olive oil.

2) Sauté garlic for a minute. Add onions and sauté for 5 minutes.
3) Stir in mushrooms and sauté until soft, about 8 minutes.
4) Add chicken stock and bring to a boil.
5) Stir in cauliflower and cook for ten minutes or until tender but not mushy.
6) Stir in heavy cream and lower the fire to low. Mix well.
7) Season with pepper, salt, parsley and Parmesan cheese.
8) Cook until heated through, about 5 minutes.
9) Serve and enjoy.

Nutrition Information:
Calories per serving: 297; Protein: 7.0g; Carbs: 9.7g; Fat: 26.0g

Paprika 'n Cajun Seasoned Onion Rings

Serves: 6, Cooking Time: 24 minutes

Ingredients:

- ¼ cup coconut milk
- ½ teaspoon Cajun seasoning
- ¾ cup almond flour
- 1 ½ teaspoon paprika
- 1 large white onion
- 1 teaspoon garlic powder
- 2 large eggs, beaten
- Salt and pepper to taste

Directions for Cooking:

1) Preheat a pot with oil for 8 minutes.
2) Peel the onion, cut off the top and slice into circles.
3) In a mixing bowl, combine the coconut milk and the eggs.
4) Soak the onion in the egg mixture.
5) In another bowl, combine the almond flour, paprika garlic powder, Cajun seasoning, salt and pepper.
6) Dredge the onion in the almond flour mixture.
7) Place in the pot and cook in batches until golden brown, around 8 minutes per batch.

Nutrition Information:

Calories per serving: 62; Carbs: 3.9g; Protein: 2.8g; Fat: 4.1g

Pomegranate, Squash in Quinoa Stew

Serves: 4, Cooking Time: 65 minutes

Ingredients:

- 1 tbsp finely chopped ginger
- 1 garlic clove, chopped
- 1 large onion, thinly sliced
- 2 tbsp olive oil
- 1 small butternut squash, deseeded and cubed
- Small handful of mint leaves
- Seeds from 1 pomegranate
- 600 ml vegetable stock
- Juice of 1 lemon
- 5 prunes, chopped roughly
- 200g quinoa
- 1 tsp ras-el-hanout or Middle Eastern spice mix

Directions for Cooking:

1) Preheat oven to 350 degrees F. In baking tray, place squash, drizzle with 1 tbsp oil, season with pepper and salt and bake until soft, around 30 to 35 minutes.
2) While waiting for squash, place a large fry pan on medium-high fire and heat oil. Once oil is hot, sauté ginger and garlic until garlic is lightly browned around 2 to 3 minutes. Add onions and sauté for another 4 minutes until soft and translucent.
3) Add quinoa and spices. Cook for 3 minutes. Season with pepper and salt.
4) Add soup stock, lemon juice, and prunes. Cover and bring to a boil. Once boiling, lower fire to a simmer and for 25 minutes cook quinoa.
5) If quinoa mixture is already soft and squash is not yet done, turn off fire.
6) Once squash is soft, transfer into pan of quinoa and turn on fire to medium and cook until heated through.
7) To serve, equally transfer stew into serving bowls, garnish with pomegranate seeds and enjoy.

Nutrition Information:

Calories per Serving: 318; Carbs: 50.0g; Protein: 11.0g; Fat: 8.2g

Portobello Caps Paleo Taco

Serves: 4, Cooking Time: 25 minutes

Ingredients:

- Salt to taste
- 2 tsp paleo taco seasoning
- ½ tbsp olive oil
- 1 clove garlic
- 1 red chili pepper, diced
- 1 lb. ground beef
- ¼ large onion, chopped
- 4 Portobello mushrooms

Topping Ingredients:
- ½ cup guacamole
- ½ cup Kalamata olives, sliced
- ½ cup cherry tomatoes, sliced
- 2 green onions cut finely
- Fresh cilantro to taste

Directions for Cooking:
1) On medium fire, place a medium pot and melt olive oil. Once oil is hot, add onions and sauté until soft and translucent.
2) Remove mushroom stems and spoon out insides of mushroom cap. Chop steps and spooned insides and into pot of onions.
3) Meanwhile, place caps in a foil line baking sheet and bake for ten minutes per side in a preheated 400 degrees F oven.
4) Add chili peppers and ground beef into pot and continue sautéing until browned.
5) Season with salt and taco when browned. And turn off fire.
6) When mushroom caps are done baking, add around 2 tbsp of meat in middle of cap, top with green onions, olives, tomatoes, and cilantro.
7) Add a dollop of guacamole, serve and enjoy.

Nutrition Information:
Calories per Serving: 462; Carbs: 24.5g; Protein: 33.7g; Fat: 26.6g

Portobello Mushroom Pizza

Serves: 4, Cooking Time: 12 minutes

Ingredients:
- ½ teaspoon red pepper flakes
- A handful of fresh basil, chopped
- 1 can black olives, chopped
- 1 medium onion, chopped
- 1 green pepper, chopped
- ¼ cup chopped roasted yellow peppers
- ½ cup prepared nut cheese, shredded
- 2 cups prepared gluten-free pizza sauce
- 8 Portobello mushrooms, cleaned and stems removed

Directions for Cooking:

1) Preheat the oven toaster.
2) Take a baking sheet and grease it. Set aside.
3) Place the Portobello mushroom cap-side down and spoon 2 tablespoon of packaged pizza sauce on the underside of each cap. Add nut cheese and top with the remaining ingredients.
4) Broil for 12 minutes or until the toppings are wilted.

Nutrition Information:
Calories per Serving: 578; Carbs: 73.0g; Protein: 24.4g; Fat: 22.4g

Provolone Over Herbed Portobello Mushrooms

Serves: 2 , Cooking Time: 10 minutes

Ingredients:
- ¼ cup grated provolone cheese
- 1 tsp minced garlic
- ¼ tsp dried rosemary
- 1 tbsp brown sugar
- ½ cup balsamic vinegar
- 2 Portobello mushrooms, stemmed and wiped clean

Directions for Cooking:
1) In oven, position rack 4-inches away from the top and preheat broiler.
2) Prepare a baking dish by spraying with cooking spray lightly.
3) Stemless, place mushroom gill side up.
4) Mix well garlic, rosemary, brown sugar and vinegar in a small bowl.
5) Drizzle over mushrooms equally.
6) Marinate for at least 5 minutes before popping into the oven and broiling for 4 minutes per side or until tender.
7) Once cooked, remove from oven, sprinkle cheese, return to broiler and broil for a minute or two or until cheese melts.
8) Remove from oven and serve right away.

Nutrition Information:
Calories per Serving: 168; Carbs: 21.5g; Protein: 8.6g; Fat: 5.1g

Ratatouille Grilled Style

Serves: 4, Cooking Time: 20 minutes

Ingredients:

- 2 tbsp walnuts, toasted and chopped
- 2 tbsp apple cider
- 2 tbsp extra virgin olive oil
- 2 medium yellow squash, cut into ¼" rounds
- 1 large zucchini, cut into ¼" rounds
- 1 large zucchini, cut into ¼" rounds
- 1 large Portobello mushroom cap, cut into ¼" slices
- 1 medium eggplant, cut into ¼" rounds
- 1 red bell pepper, quartered, stems and seeds removed
- 1 large red onion, cut into ¼" slices

Directions for Cooking:

1) Preheat grill to medium high and lightly grease grill pan with cooking spray.
2) Place all sliced veggies in grill pan and drizzle with olive oil. Toss well to coat.
3) Place in grill and grill for ten minutes. Toss vegetables to ensure even heating and continue grilling for another 10 minutes.
4) Toss vegetables and check if lightly charred and cooked through. If needed, grill some more to desired doneness.
5) Transfer grilled veggies into salad bowl, add walnuts and zero belly dressing. Toss to combine well, serve and enjoy.

Nutrition Information:

Calories per Serving: 212; Carbs: 27.6g; Protein: 7.4g; Fat: 10.6g

Ratatouille Pasta Style

Serves: 4 , Cooking Time: 25 minutes

Ingredients:

- freshly ground black pepper
- ½ cup shredded fresh basil leaves
- 1 tsp salt
- 4 plum tomatoes, coarsely chopped
- 1 red bell pepper, julienned
- 1 small zucchini, spiralized
- 1 small eggplant, spiralized
- 1 small bay leaf
- 4 garlic cloves, peeled and minced
- 1 onion, sliced thinly
- 3 tbsp olive oil

Directions for Cooking:

1) Place a large nonstick saucepan on medium slow fire and heat oil.
2) Add bay leaf, garlic and onion. Sauté until onions are translucent and soft.
3) Add eggplant and cook for 7 minutes while occasionally stirring.
4) Add salt, tomatoes, red bell pepper and zucchini then increase fire to medium high. Continue cooking until veggies are tender around 5 to 7 minutes.
5) Turn off fire and add pepper and basil. Stir to mix.
6) Serve and enjoy.

Nutrition Information:

Calories per Serving: 175; Carbs: 21.1g; Protein: 2.0g; Fat: 10.5g

Red Lentil Soup

Serves: 6, Cooking Time: 25 minutes

Ingredients:

- 1 (14 ounce) can diced tomatoes
- 1 1/2 cups dried red lentils
- 1 medium onion, diced
- 1 tablespoon ground cumin
- 1 tablespoon olive oil
- 1 teaspoon ground coriander
- 2 tablespoons lemon juice, or to taste
- 4 garlic cloves, minced
- 5 cups vegetable broth
- Fresh chopped cilantro or parsley, for serving
- Harissa paste, to taste (optional)

Directions for Cooking:

1) Place a pot on medium-high fire and heat for 2 minutes.

2) Add oil and heat for 2 minutes. Add onion and sauté for 5 minutes or until soft.
3) Stir in coriander, cumin, and garlic for a minute.
4) Add tomatoes, broth, and lentils. Mix well.
5) Simmer uncovered for 20 minutes until lentils are soft.

6) Turn off fire and stir in harissa and lemon juice.
7) Season with pepper and salt.
8) Serve and enjoy.

Nutrition Information:
Calories per Serving: 235; Carbs: 33.8g; Protein: 13.4g; Fats: 3.2g

Refreshing Greek Salad

Serves: 8 , Cooking Time: 0 minutes
Ingredients:
- ½ red onion, sliced
- 1/3 cup diced oil packed dried tomatoes, oil drained and reserved
- 3 cups diced roma tomatoes
- 1 cup black olives, pitted and sliced
- 1 ½ cups crumbled feta cheese
- 3 cucumbers, seeded and ribbon cut

Directions for Cooking:

1) Mix thoroughly the red onion, 2 tbsp of reserved sun-dried tomato oil, sundried tomatoes, roma tomatoes, olives, feta cheese and cucumbers in a large salad bowl.
2) Serve and enjoy.

Nutrition Information:
Calories per Serving: 123; Carbs: 7.1g; Protein: 5.3g; Fat: 8.6g

Roasted and Curried Cauliflower

Serves: 6, Cooking Time: 50 minutes
Ingredients:
- 1 lime (juiced)
- 1 medium head of cauliflower
- 1 tsp cayenne pepper
- 1 tsp sea salt
- 1 tsp smoked paprika
- 1 ½ cups full fat Greek yogurt
- ½ tsp black pepper
- 2 tbsp yellow curry powder
- 2 tsp lime zest

Topping Ingredients:
- 1 clove garlic
- 1 tbsp cilantro
- 1/2 cup pine nuts
- 1/4 cup olive oil
- 1/4 cup sun-dried tomatoes (packed in oil, drained)
- 2 tbsp feta cheese (crumbled)

Directions for Cooking:
1) Line a baking sheet with parchment paper and preheat the oven to 375 degrees F.

2) Mix well lime zest, curry, black pepper, yogurt, paprika, sea salt, and lime in a bowl. Rub all over the cauliflower.
3) Place cauliflower on the prepared pan and po in the oven. Bake until crispy and golden, about 45 minutes.
4) Meanwhile, make the topping ingredients by pulsing sun dried tomatoes, half of pine nits, and garlic in a food processor. Process until chunky.
5) Transfer mixture in a bowl and fold in remaining topping ingredients.
6) One cauliflower is done, remove from the oven and let it cool enough to handle. Break into bite sized pieces and drizzle topping ingredients over it.
7) Serve and enjoy.

Nutrition Information:
Calories per serving: 384; Protein: 15.0g; Carbs: 13.5g; Fat: 30.0g

Roasted Asparagus with Red Bell Peppers

Serves: 6, Cooking Time: 13 minutes

Ingredients:

- 3 tablespoons olive oil
- 4 cloves of garlic, minced
- 1-pound fresh asparagus spears, trimmed
- 2 large red bell peppers, seeded and julienned
- ½ teaspoon thyme
- 5 tablespoons water
- Salt and pepper to taste

Directions for Cooking:

1) Place olive oil in a pot and heat for 2 minutes.
2) Stir in garlic and cook for a minute.
3) Stir in remaining ingredients and cook for 10 minutes or until crisp tender.

Nutrition Information:

Calories per serving: 99; Carbs: 5.8g; Protein: 2.4g; Fat: 8.2g

Roasted Brussels Sprouts And Pecans

Serves: 7, Cooking Time: minutes

Ingredients:

- 1 ½ pounds fresh Brussels sprouts
- 4 tablespoons olive oil
- 4 cloves of garlic, minced
- 3 tablespoons water
- Salt and pepper to taste
- ½ cup chopped pecans

Directions for Cooking:

1) Place all ingredients in the Instant Pot.
2) Combine all ingredients until well combined.
3) Close the lid and make sure that the steam release vent is set to "Venting."
4) Press the "Slow Cook" button and adjust the cooking time to 3 hours.
5) Sprinkle with a dash of lemon juice if desired.

Nutrition Information:

Calories per serving: 161; Carbs:10.2g; Protein: 4.1g; Fat: 13.1g

Stir Fried Eggplant

Serves: 2 , Cooking Time: 30 minutes

Ingredients:

- 1 tsp cornstarch + 2 tbsp water, mixed
- 1 tsp brown sugar
- 2 tbsp oyster sauce
- 1 tbsp fish sauce
- 2 tbsp soy sauce
- ½ cup fresh basil
- 2 tbsp oil
- ¼ cup water
- 2 cups Chinese eggplant, spiral
- 1 red chili
- 6 cloves garlic, minced
- ½ purple onion, sliced thinly
- 1 3-oz package medium firm tofu, cut into slivers

Directions for Cooking:

1) Prepare sauce by mixing cornstarch and water in a small bowl. In another bowl mix brown sugar, oyster sauce and fish sauce and set aside.
2) On medium-high fire, place a large nonstick saucepan and heat 2 tbsp oil. Sauté chili, garlic and onion for 4 minutes. Add tofu, stir fry for 4 minutes.
3) Add eggplant noodles and stir fry for 10 minutes. If pan dries up, add water in small amounts to moisten pan and cook noodles.
4) Pour in sauce and mix well. Once simmering, slowly add cornstarch mixer while continuing to mix vigorously. Once sauce thickens add fresh basil and cook for a minute.
5) Remove from fire, transfer to a serving plate and enjoy.

Nutrition Information:

Calories per Serving: 369; Carbs: 28.4g; Protein: 11.4g; Fat: 25.3g

Roasted Root Veggies

Serves: 6, Cooking Time: 1 hour and 30 minutes

Ingredients:

- 2 tbsp olive oil
- 1 head garlic, cloves separated and peeled
- 1 large turnip, peeled and cut into ½-inch pieces
- 1 medium sized red onion, cut into ½-inch pieces
- 1 ½ lbs. beets, trimmed but not peeled, scrubbed and cut into ½-inch pieces
- 1 ½ lbs. Yukon gold potatoes, unpeeled, cut into ½-inch pieces
- 2 ½ lbs. butternut squash, peeled, seeded, cut into ½-inch pieces

Directions for Cooking:

1) Grease 2 rimmed and large baking sheets. Preheat oven to 425 degrees F.
2) In a large bowl, mix all ingredients thoroughly.
3) Into the two baking sheets, evenly divide the root vegetables, spread in one layer.
4) Season generously with pepper and salt.
5) Pop into the oven and roast for 1 hour and 15 minute or until golden brown and tender.
6) Remove from oven and let it cool for at least 15 minutes before serving.

Nutrition Information:

Calories per Serving: 298; Carbs: 61.1g; Protein: 7.4g; Fat: 5.0g

Roasted Vegetables and Zucchini Pasta

Serves: 2, Cooking Time: 7 minutes

Ingredients:

- ¼ cup raw pine nuts
- 4 cups leftover vegetables
- 2 garlic cloves, minced
- 1 tbsp extra virgin olive oil
- 4 medium zucchinis, cut into long strips resembling noodles

Directions for Cooking:

1) Heat oil in a large skillet over medium heat and sauté the garlic for 2 minutes.
2) Add the leftover vegetables and place the zucchini noodles on top. Let it cook for five minutes. Garnish with pine nuts.

Nutrition Information:

Calories per Serving: 288; Carbs: 23.6g; Protein: 8.2g; Fat: 19.2g

Savoy Cabbage with Coconut Cream Sauce

Serves: 6, Cooking Time: minutes

Ingredients:

- 3 tablespoons olive oil
- 1 onion, chopped
- 4 cloves of garlic, minced
- 1 head savoy cabbage, chopped finely
- 2 cups bone broth
- 1 cup coconut milk, freshly squeezed
- 1 bay leaf
- Salt and pepper to taste
- 2 tablespoons chopped parsley

Directions for Cooking:

1) Heat oil in a pot for 2 minutes.
2) Stir in the onions, bay leaf, and garlic until fragrant, around 3 minutes.
3) Add the rest of the ingredients, except for the parsley and mix well.
4) Cover pot, bring to a boil, and let it simmer for 5 minutes or until cabbage is tender to taste.
5) Stir in parsley and serve.

Nutrition Information:

Calories per serving: 195; Carbs: 12.3g; Protein: 2.7g; Fat: 19.7g

Slow Cooked Olive Oil Mushrooms

Serves: 4, Cooking Time: 10 minutes

Ingredients:
- 2 tablespoons olive oil
- 3 cloves of garlic, minced
- 16 ounces fresh brown mushrooms, sliced
- 7 ounces fresh shiitake mushrooms, sliced
- A dash of thyme
- Salt and pepper to taste

Directions for Cooking:

1) Heat the oil in a pot.
2) Sauté the garlic until fragrant, around 1 minute.
3) Stir in the rest of the ingredients and cook until soft, around 9 minutes.

Nutrition Information:
Calories per serving: 192; Carbs:12.7g; Protein: 3.8g; Fat: 15.5g

Steamed Squash Chowder

Serves: 4, Cooking Time: 40 minutes

Ingredients:
- 3 cups chicken broth
- 1 tsp chili powder
- ½ tsp cumin
- 1 ½ tsp salt
- 2 tsp cinnamon
- 3 tbsp olive oil
- 2 carrots, chopped
- 1 small yellow onion, chopped
- 1 green apple, sliced and cored
- 1 large butternut squash, peeled, seeded, and chopped to ½-inch cubes

Directions for Cooking:
1) In a large pot on medium-high fire, heat oil.
2) Once oil is hot, sauté onions for 5 minutes or until soft and translucent.
3) Add chili powder, cumin, salt, and cinnamon. Sauté for half a minute.
4) Add chopped squash and apples.
5) Sauté for 10 minutes while stirring once in a while.
6) Add broth, cover and cook on medium fire for twenty minutes or until apples and squash are tender.
7) With an immersion blender, puree chowder. Adjust consistency by adding more water.
8) Add more salt or pepper depending on desire.
9) Serve and enjoy.

Nutrition Information:
Calories per Serving: 228; Carbs: 17.9g; Protein: 2.2g; Fat: 18.0g

Steamed Zucchini-Paprika

Serves: 4, Cooking Time: minutes

Ingredients:
- 4 tablespoons olive oil
- 3 cloves of garlic, minced
- 1 onion, chopped
- 3 medium-sized zucchinis, sliced thinly
- A dash of paprika
- Salt and pepper to taste

Directions for Cooking:
1) Place all ingredients in the Instant Pot.
2) Give a good stir to combine all ingredients.
3) Close the lid and make sure that the steam release valve is set to "Venting."
4) Press the "Slow Cook" button and adjust the cooking time to 4 hours.
5) Halfway through the cooking time, open the lid and give a good stir to brown the other side.

Nutrition Information:
Calories per serving: 93; Carbs: 3.1g; Protein: 0.6g; Fat: 10.2g

Stir Fried Brussels Sprouts and Carrots

Serves: 6, Cooking Time: 15 minutes
Ingredients:
- 1 tbsp cider vinegar
- 1/3 cup water
- 1 lb. Brussels sprouts, halved lengthwise
- 1 lb. carrots cut diagonally into ½-inch thick lengths
- 3 tbsp olive oil
- 2 tbsp chopped shallot
- ½ tsp pepper
- ¾ tsp salt

Directions for Cooking:
1) On medium-high fire, place a nonstick medium fry pan and heat 2 tbsp oil
2) Add shallots and cook until softened, around one to two minutes while occasionally stirring.
3) Add pepper salt, Brussels sprouts and carrots. Stir fry until vegetables starts to brown on the edges, around 3 to 4 minutes.
4) Add water, cook and cover.
5) After 5 to 8 minutes, or when veggies are already soft, add remaining oil.
6) If needed season with more pepper and salt to taste.
7) Turn off fire, transfer to a platter, serve and enjoy.

Nutrition Information:
Calories per Serving: 98; Carbs: 13.9g; Protein: 3.5g; Fat: 4.2g

Stir Fried Bok Choy

Serves: 4, Cooking Time: 13 minutes
Ingredients:
- 3 tablespoons olive oil
- 4 cloves of garlic, minced
- 1 onion, chopped
- 2 heads bok choy, rinsed and chopped
- 2 teaspoons coconut aminos
- Salt and pepper to taste
- 2 tablespoons sesame oil
- 2 tablespoons sesame seeds, toasted

Directions for Cooking:
1) Heat the oil in a pot for 2 minutes.
2) Sauté the garlic and onions until fragrant, around 3 minutes.
3) Stir in the bok choy, coconut aminos, salt and pepper.
4) Cover pan and cook for 5 minutes.
5) Stir and continue cooking for another 3 minutes.
6) Drizzle with sesame oil and sesame seeds on top before serving.

Nutrition Information:
Calories per serving: 358; Carbs: 5.2g; Protein: 21.5g; Fat: 28.4g

Summer Vegetables

Serves: 6, Cooking Time: 1 hour and 40 minutes
Ingredients:
- 1 tsp dried marjoram
- 1/3 cup Parmesan cheese
- 1 small eggplant, sliced into ¼-inch thick circles
- 1 small summer squash, peeled and sliced diagonally into ¼-inch thickness
- 3 large tomatoes, sliced into ¼-inch thick circles
- ½ cup dry white wine
- ½ tsp freshly ground pepper, divided
- ½ tsp salt, divided
- 5 cloves garlic, sliced thinly
- 2 cups leeks, sliced thinly
- 4 tbsp extra virgin olive oil, divided

Directions for Cooking:
1) On medium fire, place a large nonstick saucepan and heat 2 tbsp oil.

2) Sauté garlic and leeks for 6 minutes or until garlic is starting to brown. Season with pepper and salt, ¼ tsp each.
3) Pour in wine and cook for another minute. Transfer to a 2-quart baking dish.
4) In baking dish, layer in alternating pattern the eggplant, summer squash, and tomatoes. Do this until dish is covered with vegetables. If there are excess vegetables, store for future use.
5) Season with remaining pepper and salt. Drizzle with remaining olive oil and pop in a preheated 425 degrees F oven.
6) Bake for 75 minutes. Remove from oven and top with marjoram and cheese.
7) Return to oven and bake for 15 minutes more or until veggies are soft and edges are browned.
8) Allow to cool for at least 5 minutes before serving.

Nutrition Information:
Calories per Serving: 150; Carbs: 11.8g; Protein: 3.3g; Fat: 10.8g

Summer Veggies in Instant Pot

Serves: 6, Cooking Time: 7 minutes
Ingredients:
- 2 cups okra, sliced
- 1 cup grape tomatoes
- 1 cup mushroom, sliced
- 1 ½ cups onion, sliced
- 2 cups bell pepper, sliced
- 2 ½ cups zucchini, sliced
- 2 tablespoons basil, chopped
- 1 tablespoon thyme, chopped
- ½ cups balsamic vinegar
- ½ cups olive oil
- Salt and pepper

Directions for Cooking:
1) Place all ingredients in the Instant Pot.
2) Stir the contents and close the lid.
3) Close the lid and press the Manual button.
4) Adjust the cooking time to 7 minutes.
5) Do quick pressure release.
6) Once cooled, evenly divide into serving size, keep in your preferred container, and refrigerate until ready to eat.

Nutrition Information:
Calories per serving:233; Carbs: 7g; Protein: 3g; Fat: 18g

Sumptuous Tomato Soup

Serves: 2, Cooking Time: 30 minutes
Ingredients:
- Pepper and salt to taste
- 2 tbsp tomato paste
- 1 ½ cups vegetable broth
- 1 tbsp chopped parsley
- 1 tbsp olive oil
- 5 garlic cloves
- ½ medium yellow onion
- 4 large ripe tomatoes

Directions for Cooking:
1) Preheat oven to 350 degrees F.
2) Chop onion and tomatoes into thin wedges. Place on a rimmed baking sheet. Season with parsley, pepper, salt, and olive oil. Toss to combine well. Hide the garlic cloves inside tomatoes to keep it from burning.
3) Pop in the oven and bake for 30 minutes.
4) On medium pot, bring vegetable stock to a simmer. Add tomato paste.
5) Pour baked tomato mixture into pot. Continue simmering for another 10 minutes.
6) With an immersion blender, puree soup.
7) Adjust salt and pepper to taste before serving.

Nutrition Information:
Calories per Serving: 179; Carbs: 26.7g; Protein: 5.2g; Fat: 7.7g

Superfast Cajun Asparagus

Serves: 3; Calories: 84;, Cooking Time: 8 minutes

Ingredients:

- 1 teaspoon Cajun seasoning
- 1-pound asparagus
- 1 tsp Olive oil

Directions for Cooking:

1) Snap the asparagus and make sure that you use the tender part of the vegetable.
2) Place a large skillet on stovetop and heat on high for a minute.
3) Then grease skillet with cooking spray and spread asparagus in one layer.
4) Cover skillet and continue cooking on high for 5 to eight minutes.
5) Halfway through cooking time, stir skillet and then cover and continue to cook.
6) Once done cooking, transfer to plates, serve, and enjoy!

Nutrition Information:

Calories per Serving: 81; Carbs: 0g; Protein: 0g; Fat: 9g

Sweet and Nutritious Pumpkin Soup

Serves: 8, Cooking Time: 40 minutes

Ingredients:

- 1 tsp chopped fresh parsley
- ½ cup half and half
- ½ tsp chopped fresh thyme
- 1 tsp salt
- 4 cups pumpkin puree
- 6 cups vegetable stock, divided
- 1 clove garlic, minced
- 1 1-inch piece gingerroot, peeled and minced
- 1 cup chopped onion

Directions for Cooking:

1) On medium-high fire, place a heavy bottomed pot and for 5 minutes heat ½ cup vegetable stock, ginger, garlic and onions or until veggies are tender.
2) Add remaining stock and cook for 30 minutes.
3) Season with thyme and salt.
4) With an immersion blender, puree soup until smooth.
5) Turn off fire and mix in half and half.
6) Transfer pumpkin soup into 8 bowls, garnish with parsley, serve and enjoy.

Nutrition Information:

Calories per Serving: 58; Carbs: 6.6g; Protein: 5.1g; Fat: 1.7g

Sweet Potato Puree

Serves: 6, Cooking Time: 15 minutes

Ingredients:

- 2 pounds sweet potatoes, peeled
- 1 ½ cups water
- 5 Medjool dates, pitted and chopped

Directions for Cooking:

1) Place all ingredients in a pot.
2) Close the lid and allow to boil for 15 minutes until the potatoes are soft.
3) Drain the potatoes and place in a food processor together with the dates.
4) Pulse until smooth.
5) Place in individual containers.
6) Put a label and store in the fridge.
7) Allow to thaw at room temperature before heating in the microwave oven.

Nutrition Information:

Calories per serving: 619; Carbs: 97.8g; Protein: 4.8g; Fat: 24.3g; Fiber: 14.7g

Sweet Potato Soup

Serves: 4, Cooking Time: 30 minutes

Ingredients:

- Pepper and salt to taste
- 2 tbsp thyme leaves
- Juice of half a lemon
- 1 tsp ground cumin
- 2 cups mashed sweet potato
- 4 cups chicken stock
- 4 bell pepper, diced
- 1 onion, diced
- 1 tbsp olive oil

Directions for Cooking:

1) On medium low fire, place a heavy bottomed pot and heat olive oil.
2) Sauté peppers and onions for 5 minutes or until slightly soft.
3) Meanwhile, in a blender puree mashed sweet potatoes with 2 cups chicken stock. Pour into pot.
4) Add cumin and remaining chicken stock. Cover and bring to a boil.
5) Lower fire to a simmer and cook for 20 minutes or until peppers are tender.
6) Season with pepper, salt, thyme and lemon juice.
7) Serve while hot.

Nutrition Information:
Calories per Serving: 112; Carbs: 17.5g; Protein: 3.5g; Fat: 4.6g

Sweet Potatoes Oven Fried

Serves: 7, Cooking Time: 30 minutes

Ingredients:

- 1 small garlic clove, minced
- 1 tsp grated orange rind
- 1 tbsp fresh parsley, chopped finely
- ¼ tsp pepper
- ¼ tsp salt
- 1 tbsp olive oil
- 4 medium sweet potatoes, peeled and sliced to ¼-inch thickness

Directions for Cooking:

1) In a large bowl mix well pepper, salt, olive oil and sweet potatoes.
2) In a greased baking sheet, in a single layer arrange sweet potatoes.
3) Pop in a preheated 400 degrees F oven and bake for 15 minutes, turnover potato slices and return to oven. Bake for another 15 minutes or until tender.
4) Meanwhile, mix well in a small bowl garlic, orange rind and parsley, sprinkle over cooked potato slices and serve.
5) You can store baked sweet potatoes in a lidded container and just microwave whenever you want to eat it. Do consume within 3 days.

Nutrition Information:
Calories per Serving: 176; Carbs: 36.6g; Protein: 2.5g; Fat: 2.5g

Tasty Avocado Sauce over Zoodles

Serves: 2, Cooking Time: 0 minutes

Ingredients:

- 1 zucchini peeled and spiralized into noodles
- 4 tbsp pine nuts
- 2 tbsp lemon juice
- 1 avocado peeled and pitted
- 12 sliced cherry tomatoes
- 1/3 cup water
- 1 1/4 cup basil
- Pepper and salt to taste

Directions for Cooking:

1) Make the sauce in a blender by adding pine nuts, lemon juice, avocado, water, and basil. Pulse until smooth and creamy. Season with pepper and salt to taste. Mix well.
2) Place zoodles in salad bowl. Pour over avocado sauce and toss well to coat.
3) Add cherry tomatoes, serve, and enjoy.

Nutrition Information:
Calories per serving: 313; Protein: 6.8g; Carbs: 18.7g; Fat: 26.8g

Tomato Basil Cauliflower Rice

Serves: 4, Cooking Time: 10 minutes
Ingredients:

- Salt and pepper to taste
- Dried parsley for garnish
- ¼ cup tomato paste
- ½ teaspoon garlic, minced
- ½ teaspoon onion powder
- ½ teaspoon marjoram
- 1 ½ teaspoon dried basil
- 1 teaspoon dried oregano
- 1 large head of cauliflower
- 1 teaspoon oil

Directions for Cooking:

1) Cut the cauliflower into florets and place in the food processor.
2) Pulse until it has a coarse consistency similar with rice. Set aside.
3) In a skillet, heat the oil and sauté the garlic and onion for three minutes. Add the rest of the ingredients. Cook for 8 minutes.

Nutrition Information:
Calories per Serving: 106; Carbs: 15.1g; Protein: 3.3g; Fat: 5.0g

Vegan Sesame Tofu and Eggplants

Serves: 4, Cooking Time: minutes
Ingredients:

- 5 tablespoons olive oil
- 1-pound firm tofu, sliced
- 3 tablespoons rice vinegar
- 2 teaspoons Swerve sweetener
- 2 whole eggplants, sliced
- ¼ cup soy sauce
- Salt and pepper to taste
- 4 tablespoons toasted sesame oil
- ¼ cup sesame seeds
- 1 cup fresh cilantro, chopped

Directions for Cooking:

1) Heat the oil in a pan for 2 minutes.
2) Pan fry the tofu for 3 minutes on each side.
3) Stir in the rice vinegar, sweetener, eggplants, and soy sauce. Season with salt and pepper to taste.
4) Cover and cook for 5 minutes on medium fire. Stir and continue cooking for another 5 minutes.
5) Toss in the sesame oil, sesame seeds, and cilantro.
6) Serve and enjoy.

Nutrition Information:
Calories per serving: 616; Carbs: 27.4g; Protein: 23.9g; Fat: 49.2g

Vegetable Soup Moroccan Style

Serves: 6, Calories per Recipe: 260
Ingredients:

- ½ tsp pepper
- 1 tsp salt
- 2 oz whole wheat orzo
- 1 large zucchini, peeled and cut into ¼-insh cubes
- 8 sprigs fresh cilantro, plus more leaves for garnish
- 12 sprigs flat leaf parsley, plus more for garnish
- A pinch of saffron threads
- 2 stalks celery leaves included, sliced thinly
- 2 carrots, diced
- 2 small turnips, peeled and diced
- 1 14-oz can diced tomatoes
- 6 cups water
- 1 lb. lamb stew meat, trimmed and cut into ½-inch cubes
- 2 tsp ground turmeric
- 1 medium onion, diced finely
- 2 tbsp extra virgin olive oil

Directions for Cooking:

1) On medium-high fire, place a large Dutch oven and heat oil.
2) Add turmeric and onion, stir fry for two minutes.
3) Add meat and sauté for 5 minutes.

4) Add saffron, celery, carrots, turnips, tomatoes and juice, and water.
5) With a kitchen string, tie cilantro and parsley sprigs together and into pot.
6) Cover and bring to a boil. Once boiling reduce fire to a simmer and continue to cook for 45 to 50 minutes or until meat is tender.
7) Once meat is tender, stir in zucchini. Cover and cook for 8 minutes.
8) Add orzo; cook for 10 minutes or until soft.
9) Remove and discard cilantro and parsley sprigs.
10) Season with pepper and salt.
11) Transfer to a serving bowl and garnish with cilantro and parsley leaves before serving.

Nutrition Information:
Calories per Serving: 268; Carbs: 12.9g; Protein: 28.1g; Fat: 11.7g

Vegetarian Coconut Curry

Serves: 4, Cooking Time: minutes
Ingredients:
- 4 tablespoons olive oil
- 1 medium onion, chopped
- 1 teaspoon minced garlic
- 1 teaspoon minced ginger
- 1 cup broccoli florets
- 2 cups fresh spinach leaves
- 2 teaspoons fish sauce
- 1 tablespoon garam masala
- ½ cup coconut milk
- Salt and pepper to taste

Directions for Cooking:
1) Heat oil in a pot.
2) Sauté the onion and garlic until fragrant, around 3 minutes.
3) Stir in the rest of the ingredients, except for spinach leaves.
4) Season with salt and pepper to taste.
5) Cover and cook on medium fire for 5 minutes.
6) Stir and add spinach leaves. Cover and cook for another 2 minutes.
7) Turn off fire and let it sit for two more minutes before serving.

Nutrition Information:
Calories per serving: 210; Carbs: 6.5g; Protein: 2.1g; Fat: 20.9g

Zucchini Pasta with Mango-Kiwi Sauce

Serves: 2 , Cooking Time: 0 minutes
Ingredients:
- 1 tsp dried herbs – optional
- ½ Cup Raw Kale leaves, shredded
- 2 small dried figs
- 3 medjool dates
- 4 medium kiwis
- 2 big mangos, seed discarded
- 2 cup zucchini, spiralized
- ¼ cup roasted cashew

Directions for Cooking:
1) On a salad bowl, place kale then topped with zucchini noodles and sprinkle with dried herbs. Set aside.
2) In a food processor, grind to a powder the cashews. Add figs, dates, kiwis and mangoes then puree to a smooth consistency.
3) Pour over zucchini pasta, serve and enjoy.

Nutrition Information:
Calories per Serving: 530; Carbs: 95.4g; Protein: 8.0g; Fat: 18.5g

Veggie Jamaican Stew

Serves: 4, Cooking Time: 30 minutes
Ingredients:
- 1 tbsp cilantro, chopped
- 1 tsp salt
- 1 tsp pepper
- 1 tbsp lime juice
- 2 cups collard greens, sliced
- 3 cups carrots, cut into bite-sized chunks
- ½ yellow plantain, cut into bite-sized pieces
- 1 cup okra, cut into ½" pieces

- 2 cups potatoes, cut into bite-sized cubes
- 2 cups taro, cut into bite sized cubes
- 2 cups pumpkin, cut into bite sized cubes
- 2 cups water
- 2 cups coconut milk
- 2 bay leaves
- 3 green onions, white bottom removed
- ½ tsp dried thyme
- ½ tsp ground allspice
- 4 garlic cloves, minced
- 1 onion, chopped
- 1 tbsp olive oil

Directions for Cooking:
1) On medium fire, place a stockpot and heat oil. Sauté onions for 4 minutes or until translucent and soft. Add thyme, all spice and garlic. Sauté for a minute.

2) Pour in water and coconut milk and bring to a simmer. Add bay leaves and green onions.
3) Once simmering, slow fire to keep broth at a simmer and add taro and pumpkin. Cook for 5 minutes.
4) Add potatoes and cook for three minutes.
5) Add carrots, plantain and okra. Mix and cook for five minutes.
6) Then remove and fish for thyme sprigs, bay leaves and green onions and discard.
7) Add collard greens and cook for four minutes or until bright green and darker in color.
8) Turn off fire, add pepper, salt and lime juice to taste. Once it tastes good, mix well, transfer to a serving bowl, serve and enjoy.

Nutrition Information:
Calories per Serving: 531; Carbs: 59.7g; Protein: 8.3g; Fat: 32.7g

Veggie Lo Mein

Serves: 4, Cooking Time: 6 minutes
Ingredients:
- 2 tablespoons olive oil
- 5 cloves of garlic, minced
- 2-inch knob of ginger, grated
- 8 ounces mushrooms, sliced
- ½ pounds zucchini, spiralized
- 1 carrot, julienned
- 1 spring green onions, chopped
- 3 tablespoons coconut aminos
- Salt and pepper to taste
- 1 tablespoon sesame oil

Directions for Cooking:
1) Heat the oil in a skillet and sauté the garlic and ginger until fragrant.

2) Stir in the mushrooms, zucchini, carrot, and green onions.
3) Season with coconut aminos, salt and pepper.
4) Close the lid and allow to simmer for 5 minutes.
5) Drizzle with sesame oil last.
6) Place in individual containers.
7) Put a label and store in the fridge.
8) Allow to thaw at room temperature before heating in the microwave oven.

Nutrition Information:
Calories per serving:288; Carbs: 48.7g; Protein: 7.6g; Fat: 11g; Fiber: 7.9g

Veggie Ramen Miso Soup

Serves: 1 , Cooking Time: 20 minutes
Ingredients:
- 2 tsp thinly sliced green onion
- A pinch of salt
- ½ tsp shoyu
- 2 tbsp mellow white miso
- 1 cup zucchini, cut into angel hair spirals
- ½ cup thinly sliced cremini mushrooms
- ½ medium carrot, cut into angel hair spirals
- 1/2 cup baby spinach leaves – optional
- 2 ¼ cups water

- ½ box of medium firm tofu, cut into ¼-inch cubes
- 1 hardboiled egg

Directions for Cooking:
1) In a small bowl, mix ¼ cup of water and miso. Set aside.
2) In a small saucepan on medium-high fire, bring to a boil 2 cups water, mushrooms, tofu and carrots. Add salt, shoyu and miso mixture.

Allow to boil for 5 minutes. Remove from fire and add green onion, zucchini and baby spinach leaves if using.
3) Let soup stand for 5 minutes before transferring to individual bowls.

4) Garnish with ½ of hardboiled egg per bowl, serve and enjoy.

Nutrition Information:
Calories per serving: 335; Carbs: 19.0g; Protein: 30.6g; Fat: 17.6g

Yummy Cauliflower Fritters

Serves: 6, Cooking Time: 15 minutes
Ingredients:
- 1 large cauliflower head, cut into florets
- 2 eggs, beaten
- ½ teaspoon turmeric
- ½ teaspoon salt
- ¼ teaspoon black pepper
- 6 tablespoons olive oil

Directions for Cooking:
1) Place the cauliflower florets in a pot with water.
2) Bring to a boil and drain once cooked.
3) Place the cauliflower, eggs, turmeric, salt, and pepper into the food processor.
4) Pulse until the mixture becomes coarse.

5) Transfer into a bowl. Using your hands, form six small flattened balls and place in the fridge for at least 1 hour until the mixture hardens.
6) Heat the oil in a skillet and fry the cauliflower patties for 3 minutes on each side
7) Place in individual containers.
8) Put a label and store in the fridge.
9) Allow to thaw at room temperature before heating in the microwave oven.

Nutrition Information:
Calories per serving:157; Carbs: 2.8g; Protein: 3.9g; Fat: 15.3g; Fiber:0.9g

Zucchini Garlic Fries

Serves: 6, Cooking Time: 20 minutes
Ingredients:
- ¼ teaspoon garlic powder
- ½ cup almond flour
- 2 large egg whites, beaten
- 3 medium zucchinis, sliced into fry sticks
- Salt and pepper to taste

Directions for Cooking:
1) Preheat oven to 400 degrees F.

2) Mix all ingredients in a bowl until the zucchini fries are well coated.
3) Place fries on cookie sheet and spread evenly.
4) Put in oven and cook for 20 minutes.
5) Halfway through cooking time, stir fries.

Nutrition Information:
Calories per serving: 11; Carbs: 1.1g; Protein: 1.5g; Fat: 0.1g

Chapter 5 Pasta, Rice and Grains Recipes

Amazingly Good Parsley Tabbouleh

Serves: 4, Cooking Time: 15 minutes
Ingredients:

- ¼ cup chopped fresh mint
- ¼ cup lemon juice
- ¼ tsp salt
- ½ cup bulgur
- ½ tsp minced garlic
- 1 cup water
- 1 small cucumber, peeled, seeded and diced
- 2 cups finely chopped flat-leaf parsley
- 2 tbsp extra virgin olive oil
- 2 tomatoes, diced
- 4 scallions, thinly sliced
- Pepper to taste

Directions for Cooking:

1) Cook bulgur according to package instructions. Drain and set aside to cool for at least 15 minutes.
2) In a small bowl, mix pepper, salt, garlic, oil, and lemon juice.
3) Transfer bulgur into a large salad bowl and mix in scallions, cucumber, tomatoes, mint, and parsley.
4) Pour in dressing and toss well to coat.
5) Place bowl in ref until chilled before serving.

Nutrition Information:
Calories per Serving: 134.8; Carbs: 13g; Protein: 7.2g; Fat: 6g

Artichokes, Olives & Tuna Pasta

Serves: 4, Cooking Time: 15 minutes
Ingredients:

- ¼ cup chopped fresh basil
- ¼ cup chopped green olives
- ¼ tsp freshly ground pepper
- ½ cup white wine
- ½ tsp salt, divided
- 1 10-oz package frozen artichoke hearts, thawed and squeezed dry
- 2 cups grape tomatoes, halved
- 2 tbsp lemon juice
- 2 tsp chopped fresh rosemary
- 2 tsp freshly grated lemon zest
- 3 cloves garlic, minced
- 4 tbsp extra virgin olive oil, divided
- 6-oz whole wheat penne pasta
- 8-oz tuna steak, cut into 3 pieces

Directions for Cooking:

1) Cook penne pasta according to package instructions. Drain and set aside.
2) Preheat grill to medium high.
3) In bowl, toss and mix ¼ tsp pepper, ¼ tsp salt, 1 tsp rosemary, lemon zest, 1 tbsp oil and tuna pieces.
4) Grill tuna for 3 minutes per side. Allow to cool and flake into bite sized pieces.
5) On medium fire, place a large nonstick saucepan and heat 3 tbsp oil.
6) Sauté remaining rosemary, garlic olives, and artichoke hearts for 4 minutes
7) Add wine and tomatoes, bring to a boil and cook for 3 minutes while stirring once in a while.
8) Add remaining salt, lemon juice, tuna pieces and pasta. Cook until heated through.
9) To serve, garnish with basil and enjoy.

Nutrition Information:
Calories per Serving: 127.6; Carbs: 13g; Protein: 7.2g; Fat: 5.2g

Baked Parmesan and Eggplant Pasta

Serves: 8, Cooking Time: 50 minutes

Ingredients:

- ½ tsp dried basil
- ½ cup grated Parmesan cheese, divided
- 8-oz mozzarella cheese, shredded and divided
- 6 cups spaghetti sauce
- 2 cups Italian seasoned breadcrumbs
- ½ lb. ground beef
- 6 cups eggplant, spiralized
- 1 tbsp olive oil

Directions for Cooking:

1) Grease a 9x13 baking dish and preheat oven to 350 degrees F.
2) On medium-high fire, place a nonstick large saucepan and heat oil. Sauté ground beef until cooked around 8 minutes. Pour in spaghetti sauce and cook until heated through.
3) Scoop out two cups of spaghetti meat sauce and set aside.
4) Add eggplant spirals in saucepan and mix well.
5) Scoop out half of eggplant spaghetti into baking dish, top with half of mozzarella cheese and cover with breadcrumbs. Top again with the remaining spaghetti, mozzarella and Parmesan cheese.
6) Pop into oven and bake until tops are golden brown around 35 minutes.
7) Remove from oven and evenly slice into 8 pieces.
8) Serve and enjoy while warm.

Nutrition Information:

Calories per Serving: 297; Carbs: 26.6g; Protein: 22.9g; Fat: 11.1g

Bell Peppers 'n Tomato-Chickpea Rice

Serves: 4, Cooking Time: 35 minutes

Ingredients:

- 2 tablespoons olive oil
- 1/2 chopped red bell pepper
- 1/2 chopped green bell pepper
- 1/2 chopped yellow pepper
- 1/2 chopped red pepper
- 1 medium onion, chopped
- 1 clove garlic, minced
- 2 cups cooked jasmine rice
- 1 teaspoon tomato paste
- 1 cup chickpeas
- salt to taste
- 1/2 teaspoon paprika
- 1 small tomato, chopped
- Parsley for garnish

Directions for Cooking:

1) In a large mixing bowl, whisk well olive oil, garlic, tomato paste, and paprika. Season with salt generously.
2) Mix in rice and toss well to coat in the dressing.
3) Add remaining ingredients and toss well to mix.
4) Let salad rest to allow flavors to mix for 15 minutes.
5) Toss one more time and adjust salt to taste if needed.
6) Garnish with parsley and serve.

Nutrition Information:

Calories per serving: 490; Carbs: 93.0g; Protein: 10.0g; Fat: 8.0g

Belly-Filling Cajun Rice & Chicken

Serves: 6, Cooking Time: 20 minutes

Ingredients:

- 1 tablespoon oil
- 1 onion, diced
- 3 cloves of garlic, minced
- 1-pound chicken breasts, sliced
- 1 tablespoon Cajun seasoning
- 1 tablespoon tomato paste
- 2 cups chicken broth
- 1 ½ cups white rice, rinsed

- 1 bell pepper, chopped

Directions for Cooking:
1) Press the Sauté on the Instant Pot and pour the oil.
2) Sauté the onion and garlic until fragrant.
3) Stir in the chicken breasts and season with Cajun seasoning.
4) Continue cooking for 3 minutes.
5) Add the tomato paste and chicken broth. Dissolve the tomato paste before adding the rice and bell pepper.
6) Close the lid and press the rice button.
7) Once done cooking, do a natural release for 10 minutes.
8) Then, do a quick release.
9) Once cooled, evenly divide into serving size, keep in your preferred container, and refrigerate until ready to eat.

Nutrition Information:
Calories per serving: 337; Carbohydrates: 44.3g; Protein: 26.1g; Fat: 5.0g

Black Beans and Quinoa

Serves: 6, Cooking Time: 30 minutes
Ingredients:
- ½ cup chopped cilantro
- 2 15-oz cans black beans, rinsed and drained
- 1 cup frozen corn kernels
- Pepper and salt to taste
- ¼ tsp cayenne pepper
- 1 tsp ground cumin
- 1 ½ cups vegetable broth
- ¾ cup quinoa
- 3 cloves garlic, chopped
- 1 onion, chopped
- 1 tsp vegetable oil

Directions for Cooking:
1) On medium fire, place a saucepan and heat oil.
2) Add garlic and onions. Sauté for 5 minutes or until onions are soft.
3) Add quinoa. Pour vegetable broth and bring to a boil while increasing fire.
4) As you wait for broth to boil, season quinoa mixture with pepper, salt, cayenne pepper, and cumin.
5) Once boiling, reduce fire to a simmer, cover and simmer around 20 minutes or until liquid is fully absorbed.
6) Once liquid is fully absorbed, stir in black beans and frozen corn. Continue cooking until heated through, around 5 minutes.
7) To serve, add cilantro, toss well to mix, and enjoy.

Nutrition Information:
Calories per serving: 262; Carbs: 47.1g; Protein: 13.0g; Fat: 2.9g

Blue Cheese and Grains Salad

Serves: 4, Cooking Time: 40 minutes
Ingredients:
- ¼ cup thinly sliced scallions
- ½ cup millet, rinsed
- ½ cup quinoa, rinsed
- 1 ½ tsp olive oil
- 1 Bartlett pear, cored and diced
- 1/8 tsp ground black pepper
- 2 cloves garlic, minced
- 2 oz blue cheese
- 2 tbsp fresh lemon juice
- 2 tsp dried rosemary
- 4 4-oz boneless, skinless chicken breasts
- 6 oz baby spinach
- olive oil cooking spray

Dressing Ingredients:
- ¼ cup fresh raspberries
- 1 tbsp pure maple syrup
- 1 tsp fresh thyme leaf
- 2 tbsp grainy mustard
- 6 tbsp balsamic vinegar

Directions for Cooking:
1) Bring millet, quinoa, and 2 ¼ cups water on a small saucepan to a boil. Once boiling, slow fire to a simmer and stir once. Cover and cook until water is fully absorbed and grains are soft around 15 minutes. Turn off fire, fluff grains with a fork and set aside to cool a bit.

2) Arrange one oven rack to highest position and preheat broiler. Line a baking sheet with foil, and grease with cooking spray.
3) Whisk well pepper, oil, rosemary, lemon juice and garlic. Rub onto chicken.
4) Place chicken on prepared pan, pop into the broiler and broil until juices run clear and no longer pin inside around 12 minutes.
5) Meanwhile, make the dressing by combining all ingredients in a blender. Blend until smooth.
6) Remove chicken from oven, cool slightly before cutting into strips, against the grain.
7) To assemble, place grains in a large salad bowl. Add in dressing and spinach, toss to mix well.
8) Add scallions and pear, mix gently and evenly divide into four plates. Top each salad with cheese and chicken.
9) Serve and enjoy.

Nutrition Information:
Calories per Serving: 530.4; Carbs: 77g; Protein: 21.4g; Fat: 15.2g

Breakfast Salad from Grains and Fruits

Serves: 6 , Cooking Time: 20 minutes
Ingredients:
- ¼ tsp salt
- ¾ cup bulgur
- ¾ cup quick cooking brown rice
- 1 8-oz low fat vanilla yogurt
- 1 cup raisins
- 1 Granny Smith apple
- 1 orange
- 1 Red delicious apple
- 3 cups water

Directions for Cooking:
1) On high fire, place a large pot and bring water to a boil.
2) Add bulgur and rice. Lower fire to a simmer and cook for ten minutes while covered.
3) Turn off fire, set aside for 2 minutes while covered.
4) In baking sheet, transfer and evenly spread grains to cool.
5) Meanwhile, peel oranges and cut into sections. Chop and core apples.
6) Once grains are cool, transfer to a large serving bowl along with fruits.
7) Add yogurt and mix well to coat.
8) Serve and enjoy.

Nutrition Information:
Calories per Serving: 48.6; Carbs: 23.9g; Protein: 3.7g; Fat: 1.1g

Brown Rice Pilaf with Butternut Squash

Serves: 8, Cooking Time: 50 minutes
Ingredients:
- Pepper to taste
- A pinch of cinnamon
- 1 tsp salt
- 2 tbsp chopped fresh oregano
- ½ cup chopped fennel fronds
- ½ cup white wine
- 1 ¾ cups water + 2 tbsp, divided
- 1 cup instant or parboiled brown rice
- 1 tbsp tomato paste
- 1 garlic clove, minced
- 1 large onion, finely chopped
- 3 tbsp extra virgin olive oil
- 2 lbs. butternut squash, peeled, halved and seeded

Directions for Cooking:
1) In a large hole grater, grate squash.
2) On medium low fire, place a large nonstick skillet and heat oil for 2 minutes.
3) Add garlic and onions. Sauté for 8 minutes or until lightly colored and soft.
4) Add 2 tbsp water and tomato paste. Stir well to combine and cook for 3 minutes.
5) Add rice, mix well to coat in mixture and cook for 5 minutes while stirring frequently.
6) If needed, add squash in batches until it has wilted so that you can cover pan.
7) Add remaining water and increase fire to medium high.

8) Add wine, cover and boil. Once boiling, lower fire to a simmer and cook for 20 to 25 minutes or until liquid is fully absorbed.

9) Stir in pepper, cinnamon, salt, oregano, and fennel fronds.

10) Turn off fire, cover and let it stand for 5 minutes before serving.

Nutrition Information:
Calories per Serving: 147; Carbs: 22.1g; Protein: 2.3g; Fat: 5.5g

Butternut Squash, Quinoa & Apple Salad

Serves: 6, Cooking Time: 40 minutes
Ingredients:

- 3 cups of peeled and diced butternut squash
- 3 Tbs olive oil, divided
- ½ tsp salt
- ¼ tsp black pepper
- 1 onion, diced
- 2 garlic cloves, minced
- 1 cup cooked quinoa
- ¼ cup dried cranberries
- ½ cup chopped pecans, toasted
- ½ tsp salt
- ¼ tsp black pepper
- ½ vanilla bean, pinch of seeds*
- 1 tsp ground cinnamon
- 1 medium apple, peeled and chopped
- 3 tbsp maple syrup
- 2 tbsp apple cider vinegar

Directions for Cooking:

1) Roast the squash. In shallow glass baking dish, toss the squash with 1 Tbs oil and sprinkle with salt and pepper. Either bake in oven with at 350 for approximately 30-40 minutes, or microwave for 5-8 minutes, until softened.

2) In skillet over medium heat, sauté the onions and garlic in 1 Tbs olive oil until onions and garlic have softened. Add the chopped apple.

3) Combine the cooked quinoa, toasted pecans, dried cranberries, apple cider vinegar, maple syrup, 1 Tbs olive oil, vanilla beans, and cinnamon in bowl and mix well.

4) Once squash is roasted, in the large skillet combine all the ingredients until heated thoroughly.

5) Serve warm.

Nutrition Information:
Calories per serving: 246; Carbs: 31.3g; Protein: 3.2g; Fat: 13.5g

Cinnamon Quinoa Bars

Serves: 4, Cooking Time: 30 minutes
Ingredients:

- 2 ½ cups cooked quinoa
- 4 large eggs
- 1/3 cup unsweetened almond milk
- 1/3 cup pure maple syrup
- Seeds from ½ whole vanilla bean pod or 1 tbsp vanilla extract
- 1 ½ tbsp cinnamon
- 1/4 tsp salt

Directions for Cooking:

1) Preheat oven to 375 degrees F.
2) Combine all ingredients into large bowl and mix well.
3) In an 8 x 8 Baking pan, cover with parchment paper.

4) Pour batter evenly into baking dish.
5) Bake for 25-30 minutes or until it has set. It should not wiggle when you lightly shake the pan because the eggs are fully cooked.
6) Remove as quickly as possible from pan and parchment paper onto cooling rack.
7) Cut into 4 pieces.
8) Enjoy on its own, with a small spread of almond or nut butter or wait until it cools to enjoy the next morning.

Nutrition Information:
Calories per serving: 285; Carbs: 46.2g; Protein: 8.5g; Fat: 7.4g

Chicken and Sweet Potato Stir Fry

Serves: 6`, Cooking Time: minutes

Ingredients:
- ¼ tsp salt
- ½ cups quinoa, rinsed and drained
- 1 clove garlic, minced
- 1 cup frozen peas
- 1 cup water
- 1 jalapeno chili pepper, chopped
- 1 medium onion, chopped
- 1 medium-sized red bell pepper, chopped
- 1 tsp cumin, ground
- 1/8 tsp black pepper
- 12oz boneless chicken
- 1med sweet potatoes, cubed
- 3 tbsp fresh cilantro, chopped
- 4 tsp canola oil

Directions for Cooking:
1) Bring to a boil water and quinoa over medium heat. Simmer until the quinoa has absorbed the water.
2) In a small saucepan, put the sweet potatoes and enough water to cover the potatoes. Bring to a boil. Drain the potatoes and discard the water.
3) In a skillet, add the chicken and cook until brown. Transfer to a bowl.
4) Using the same skillet, heat 2 tablespoon of oil and sauté the onions and jalapeno pepper for one minute.
5) Add the bell pepper, cumin and garlic. Cook for three minutes until the vegetables have softened.
6) Add the peas and chicken. Cook for two minutes before adding the sweet potato and quinoa.
7) Stir cilantro and add salt and pepper to taste.
8) Serve and enjoy.

Nutrition Information:
Calories per Serving: 187.6; Carbs: 18g; Protein: 16.3g; Fat: 5.6g

Chicken Pasta Parmesan

Serves: 1, Cooking Time: 20 minutes

Ingredients:
- ¼ cup prepared marinara sauce
- ½ cup cooked whole wheat spaghetti
- 1 oz reduced fat mozzarella cheese, grated
- 1 tbsp olive oil
- 2 tbsp seasoned dry breadcrumbs
- 4 oz skinless chicken breast

Directions for Cooking:
1) On medium-high fire, place an ovenproof skillet and heat oil.
2) Pan fry chicken for 3 to 5 minutes per side or until cooked through.
3) Pour marinara sauce, stir and continue cooking for 3 minutes.
4) Turn off fire, add mozzarella and breadcrumbs on top.
5) Pop into a preheated broiler on high and broil for 10 minutes or until breadcrumbs are browned and mozzarella is melted.
6) Remove from broiler, serve and enjoy.

Nutrition Information:
Calories per Serving: 529; Carbs: 34.4g; Protein: 38g; Fat: 26.6g

Citrus Quinoa & Chickpea Salad

Serves: 4, Cooking Time: 0 minutes

Ingredients:
- 2 cups cooked quinoa
- 1 can chickpeas, drained & rinsed
- 1 ripe avocado, diced
- 1 red bell pepper, diced
- 1/2 red onion, diced
- 1/4 cup lime juice
- 1/2 tbsp garlic powder
- 1/2 tbsp paprika
- 1/4-1/2 cup chopped cilantro
- 1 tbsp chopped jalapenos
- Sea salt to taste

Directions for Cooking:

1) Add all ingredients in a large bowl and mix well.
2) Enjoy right away or refrigerate for later.

Nutrition Information:
Calories per serving: 300; Carbs: 43.5g; Protein: 10.3g; Fat: 10.9g

Cranberry and Roasted Squash Delight

Serves: 8, Cooking Time: 60 minutes
Ingredients:
- ¼ cup chopped walnuts
- ¼ tsp thyme
- ½ tbsp chopped Italian parsley
- 1 cup diced onion
- 1 cup fresh cranberries
- 1 small orange, peeled and segmented
- 2 tsp canola oil, divided
- 4 cups cooked wild rice
- 4 cups diced winter squash, peeled and cut into ½-inch cubes
- Pepper to taste

Directions for Cooking:
1) Grease roasting pan with cooking spray and preheat oven to 400 degrees F.
2) In prepped roasting pan place squash cubes, add a teaspoon of oil and toss to coat. Place in oven and roast until lightly browned, around 40 minutes.
3) On medium-high fire, place a nonstick fry pan and heat remaining oil. Once hot, add onions and sauté until lightly browned and tender, around 5 minutes.
4) Add cranberries and continue stir frying for a minute.
5) Add remaining ingredients into pan and cook until heated through around four to five minutes.
6) Best served warm.

Nutrition Information:
Calories per Serving: 166.2; Protein: 4.8g; Carbs: 29.1g; Fat: 3.4g

Creamy Alfredo Fettuccine

Serves: 4, Cooking Time: 25 minutes
Ingredients:
- Grated parmesan cheese
- ½ cup freshly grated parmesan cheese
- 1/8 tsp freshly ground black pepper
- ½ tsp salt
- 1 cup whipping cream
- 2 tbsp butter
- 8 oz dried fettuccine, cooked and drained

Directions for Cooking:
1) On medium-high fire, place a big fry pan and heat butter.
2) Add pepper, salt and cream and gently boil for three to five minutes.
3) Once thickened, turn off fire and quickly stir in ½ cup of parmesan cheese. Toss in pasta, mix well.
4) Top with another batch of parmesan cheese and serve.

Nutrition Information:
Calories per Serving: 202; Carbs: 21.1g; Protein: 7.9g; Fat: 10.2g

Creamy Artichoke Lasagna

Serves: 8, Cooking Time: 70 minutes
Ingredients:
- 1 cup shredded mozzarella cheese
- 2 cups light cream
- ¼ cup all-purpose flour
- 1 cup vegetable broth
- ¾ tsp salt
- 1 egg
- 1 cup snipped fresh basil
- 1 cup finely shredded Parmesan cheese
- 1 15-oz carton ricotta cheese
- 4 cloves garlic, minced
- ½ cup pine nuts
- 3 tbsp olive oil

- 9 dried lasagna noodles, cooked, rinsed in cold water and drained
- 15 fresh baby artichokes
- ¼ cup lemon juice
- 3 cups water

Directions for Cooking:
1) Prepare in a medium bowl lemon juice and water. Put aside. Slice off artichoke base and remove yellowed outer leaves and cut into quarters. Immediately soak sliced artichokes in prepared liquid and drain after a minute.
2) Over medium fire, place a big saucepan with 2 tbsp oil and fry half of garlic, pine nuts and artichokes. Stir frequently and cook until artichokes are soft around ten minutes. Turn off fire and transfer mixture to a big bowl and quickly stir in salt, egg, ½ cup of basil, ½ cup of parmesan cheese and ricotta cheese. Mix thoroughly.
3) In a small bowl mix flour and broth. In same pan, add 1 tbsp oil and fry remaining garlic for half a minute. Add light cream and flour mixture. Stir constantly and cook until thickened. Remove from fire and stir in ½ cup of basil.
4) In a separate bowl mix ½ cup parmesan and mozzarella cheese.
5) Assemble the lasagna by layering the following in a greased rectangular glass dish: lasagna, 1/3 of artichoke mixture, 1/3 of sauce, sprinkle with the dried cheeses and repeat layering procedure until all ingredients are used up.
6) For forty minutes, bake lasagna in a pre-heated oven of 350 degrees F. Remove lasagna from oven and before serving, let it stand for fifteen minutes.

Nutrition Information:
Calories per Serving: 425; Carbs: 41.4g; Protein: 21.3g; Fat: 19.8g

Cucumber and Tomato Salad

Serves: 4, Cooking Time: 0 minutes
Ingredients:
- Ground pepper to taste
- Salt to taste
- 1 tbsp fresh lemon juice
- 1 onion, chopped
- 1 cucumber, peeled and diced
- 2 tomatoes, chopped
- 4 cups spinach

Directions for Cooking:

1) In a salad bowl, mix onions, cucumbers and tomatoes.
2) Season with pepper and salt to taste.
3) Add lemon juice and mix well.
4) Add spinach, toss to coat, serve and enjoy.

Nutrition Information:
Calories per Serving: 70.3; Fat: 0.3g; Protein: 1.3g; Carbohydrates: 7.1g

Cucumber Salad with Rice and Asparagus

Serves: 6, Cooking Time: 21 minutes
Ingredients:
- 4 heads butter lettuce
- ¼ cup chopped fresh dill
- 2 ½ tbsp Vegetable oil
- ½ tsp dry mustard
- 1 tbsp white wine vinegar
- 1 tbsp sugae2 tbsp Dijon mustard
- 3 green onions, chopped
- 1 ½ cups English cucumber, peeled, seeded and chopped
- 1 lb. thin asparagus spears, trimmed and cut into 1-inch

- 1 cup long grain white rice
- 1 ¾ cups water

Directions for Cooking:
1) Bring to a boil 1 ¾ cups water in a medium saucepan. Add rice and bring again to a boil. Once boiling, reduce fire to low. Continue cooking around 20 minutes or until water is fully absorbed and rice is tender. Turn of fire and fluff rice with a fork and transfer to a bowl to cool.

2) For 1 minute, cook asparagus in boiling and salted water. Drain and rinse asparagus and cut into 1-inch long pieces.
3) Mix rice, green onions, cucumber and asparagus thoroughly. Cover and chill
4) In a separate medium bowl, stir thoroughly chopped dill, oil, dry mustard, vinegar, sugar and mustard. Cover and chill.

5) Mix dressing and salad and season with pepper and salt to taste.
6) Then, in a large bowl lined with lettuce, transfer the rice salad and garnish with sprigs of dill. Serve and enjoy.

Nutrition Information:
Calories per serving: 220; Carbs: 34.7g; Protein: 5.8g; Fat: 6.4g

Delicious Quinoa Bowl

Serves: 4, Cooking Time: 35 minutes
Ingredients:
- 1 avocado (sliced)
- 1 cup canned chickpeas (drained and rinsed)
- 1/2 cup hummus
- 1/4 red onion (finely chopped)
- 1/4 teaspoon salt
- 2 cups cherry tomatoes (multicoloured, quartered)
- 2 tablespoons cider vinegar
- 2 tablespoons extra virgin olive oil
- 2 teaspoons oregano (dried Greek)
- 2/3 cup crumbled feta
- 2/3 cup quinoa (rinsed)
- 3 mini cucumbers (chopped)
- 8 kalamata olives (pitted)

Directions for Cooking:

1) Mix 1 1/3 cups water and quinoa in a saucepan.
2) Bring to a boil and reduce to a simmer.
3) Cover and cook for 15 min, until quinoa is tender.
4) Turn off fire and let stand for 5 min.
5) Fluff with a fork, then stir in chickpeas.
6) Mix salt, oregano, oil vinegar, onion, tomatoes, and cucumbers in a bowl.
7) Evenly divide quinoa into 4 bowls. Top with the cucumber mixture. Garnish evenly with hummus, olives, feta, avocado, and any leftover dressing.

Nutrition Information:
Calories per Serving: 215; Carbs: 34.1g; Protein: 10.7g; Fat: 4.0g

Escarole and Cannellini Beans on Pasta

Serves: 8, Cooking Time: 25 minutes
Ingredients:
- Pepper and salt to taste
- 1 can 14.5-oz diced tomatoes with garlic and onion, drained
- 1 can 15.5-oz cannellini beans, with liquid
- 1 head escarole chopped
- 1 package 16-oz dry penne pasta

Directions for Cooking:
1) Cook pasta according to package instructions, then drain and rinse under cold running water.

2) On medium-high fire, place skillet and cook diced tomatoes, cannellini beans with liquid and escarole.
3) Season with pepper and salt and cook until boiling.
4) Remove from fire and mix pasta.
5) Serve and enjoy.

Nutrition Information:
Calories per Serving: 310; Carbs: 60.1g; Protein: 13.7g; Fat: 2.0g

Filling Macaroni Soup

Serves: 6, Cooking Time: 45 minutes

Ingredients:

- 1 cup of minced beef or chicken or a combination of both
- 1 cup carrots, diced
- 1 cup milk
- ½ medium onion, sliced thinly
- 3 garlic cloves, minced
- Salt and pepper to taste
- 2 cups broth (chicken, vegetable or beef)
- ½ tbsp olive oil
- 1 cup uncooked whole wheat pasta like macaroni, shells, even angel hair broken to pieces
- 1 cup water

Directions for Cooking:

1) In a heavy bottomed pot on medium-high fire heat oil.
2) Add garlic and sauté for a minute or two until fragrant but not browned.
3) Add onions and sauté for 3 minutes or until soft and translucent.
4) Add a cup of minced meat. You can also use whatever leftover frozen meat you have.
5) Sauté the meat well until cooked around 8 minutes. While sautéing, season meat with pepper and salt.
6) Add water and broth and bring to a boil.
7) Once boiling, add pasta. I use any leftover pasta that I have in the pantry. If all you have left is spaghetti, lasagna, angel hair or fettuccine, just break them into pieces—around 1-inch in length before adding to the pot.
8) Slow fire to a simmer and cook while covered until pasta is soft.
9) Halfway through cooking the pasta, around 8 minutes I add the carrots.
10) Once the pasta is soft, turn off fire and add milk.
11) Mix well and season to taste again if needed.
12) Serve and enjoy.

Nutrition Information:

Calories per Serving: 125; Carbs: 11.4g; Protein: 10.1g; Fat: 4.3g

Fresh Basil and Sun-dried Tomato Quinoa Bowl

Serves: 4, Cooking Time: 35 minutes

Ingredients:

- 2 cups quinoa (cooked, about 1 cup uncooked)
- 1 red bell pepper (chopped)
- 1/2 cucumber (chopped)
- 1 cup chickpeas
- 1/2 red onion (small, finely chopped)
- 1/2 cup kalamata olives (cut in half)
- 1/4 cup sundried tomatoes (finely chopped)
- 1/3 cup fresh basil (finely chopped)
- 1/4 cup crumbled feta cheese
- 2 tablespoons lemon juice
- 1 tablespoon white wine vinegar
- 1/3 cup olive oil
- 1 tablespoon Dijon mustard
- 1 teaspoon maple syrup
- 1/2 teaspoon dried oregano
- 1/2 teaspoon garlic powder
- 1/4 teaspoon ground cumin
- Salt and pepper to taste

Directions for Cooking:

1) Mix 1 1/3 cups water and quinoa in a saucepan.
2) Bring to a boil and reduce to a simmer.
3) Cover and cook for 15 min, until quinoa is tender.
4) Turn off fire and let stand for 5 min.
5) Fluff with a fork, then stir in chickpeas.
6) Mix salt, oregano, oil vinegar, onion, tomatoes, and cucumbers in a bowl.
7) Evenly divide quinoa into 4 bowls. Top with the cucumber mixture. Garnish evenly with hummus, olives, feta, avocado, and any leftover dressing.

Nutrition Information:

Calories per serving: 361; Carbs: 47.0g; Protein: 12.0g; Fat: 14.0g

Fresh Herbs and Clams Linguine

Serves: 4, Cooking Time: 10 minutes

Ingredients:

- ½ tsp freshly ground black pepper
- ¾ tsp salt
- 2 tbsp butter
- 1.5 lbs. littleneck clams
- ½ cup white wine
- 4 garlic cloves, sliced
- ¼ tsp crushed red pepper
- 2 cups vertically sliced red onion
- 2 tbsp olive oil
- 2 tsp grated lemon zest
- 1 tbsp chopped fresh oregano
- 1/3 cup parsley leaves
- 8-oz linguine, cooked and drained

Directions for Cooking:

1) Chop finely lemon rind, oregano and parsley. Set aside.
2) On medium-high fire, place a nonstick fry pan with olive oil and fry for four minutes garlic, red pepper and onion.
3) Add clams and wine and cook until shells have opened, around five minutes. Throw any unopened clam.
4) Transfer mixture into a large serving bowl. Add pepper, salt, butter and pasta. Toss to mix well. Serve with parsley garnish.

Nutrition Information:

Calories per Serving: 507; Carbs: 53.9g; Protein: 34.2g; Fat: 16.8g

Fruity Asparagus-Quinoa Salad

Serves: 8, Cooking Time: 25 minutes

Salad Ingredients:

- ¼ cup chopped pecans, toasted
- ½ cup finely chopped white onion
- ½ jalapeno pepper, diced
- ½ lb. asparagus, sliced to 2-inch lengths, steamed and chilled
- ½ tsp kosher salt
- 1 cup fresh orange sections
- 1 cup uncooked quinoa
- 1 tsp olive oil
- 2 cups water
- 2 tbsp minced red onion
- 5 dates, pitted and chopped

Dressing Ingredients:

- ¼ tsp ground black pepper
- ¼ tsp kosher salt
- 1 garlic clove, minced
- 1 tbsp olive oil
- 2 tbsp chopped fresh mint
- 2 tbsp fresh lemon juice
- Mint sprigs – optional

Directions for Cooking:

1) Wash and rub with your hands the quinoa in a bowl at least three times, discarding water each and every time.
2) On medium-high fire, place a large nonstick fry pan and heat 1 tsp olive oil. For two minutes, sauté onions before adding quinoa and sautéing for another five minutes.
3) Add ½ tsp salt and 2 cups water and bring to a boil. Lower fire to a simmer, cover and cook for 15 minutes. Turn off fire and let stand until water is absorbed.
4) Add pepper, asparagus, dates, pecans and orange sections into a salad bowl. Add cooked quinoa, toss to mix well.
5) In a small bowl, whisk mint, garlic, black pepper, salt, olive oil and lemon juice to create the dressing.
6) Pour dressing over salad, serve and enjoy.

Nutrition Information:

Calories per Serving: 172.7; Fat: 6.3g; Protein: 4.3g; Carbohydrates: 24.7g

Garlic Avocado-Pesto and Zucchini Pasta

Serves: 2, Cooking Time: 0 minutes

Ingredients:

- salt and pepper to taste
- 1 tbsp pine nuts
- 1 tbsp cashew nuts
- 1 lemon juice
- 4 cloves garlic, minced
- 1 small ripe avocado
- 2 cups zucchini, spiral
- 2 tbsp olive oil
- 2 tbsp grated Pecorino Cheese
- ½ cup packed fresh basil leaves

Directions for Cooking:

1) In a food processor grind pine nuts and cashew nuts to a fine powder.
2) Add basil leaves, cheese, olive oil, ripe avocado, garlic, lemon juice, salt and pepper to taste and process until you have a smooth mixture.
3) Arrange zucchini pasta on two plates and top evenly with the Avocado pesto mixture.
4) Serve and enjoy.

Nutrition Information:

Calories per Serving: 353; Carbs: 17.0g; Protein: 5.5g; Fat: 31.9g

Garlicky Peas and Clams on Veggie Spiral

Serves: 4, Cooking Time: 15 minutes

Ingredients:

- 2 tbsp chopped fresh basil
- ½ cup pre-shredded Parmesan cheese
- 1 cup frozen green peas
- ¼ tsp crushed red pepper
- ¼ cup dry white wine
- 1 cup organic vegetable broth
- 3 cans chopped clams, clams and juice separated
- 1 ½ tsp bottled minced garlic
- 2 tbsp olive oil
- 6 cups zucchini, spiral

Directions for Cooking:

1) Bring a pot of water to a rolling boil and blanch zucchini for 4 minutes on high fire. Drain and let stand for a couple of minutes to continue cooking.
2) On medium-high fire, add a large nonstick saucepan and heat oil. Add and sauté for a minute the garlic. Pour in wine, broth and clam juice.
3) Once liquid is boiling, low fire to a simmer and add pepper. Continue cooking and stirring for 5 minutes.
4) Add peas and clams, cook until heated through or around two minutes.
5) Toss in zucchini, mix well. Cook until heated through.
6) Add basil and cheese, toss to mix well then remove from fire.
7) Transfer equally to four serving bowls and enjoy.

Nutrition Information:

Calories per Serving: 210; Carbs: 24.0g; Protein: 8.5g; Fat: 9.2g

Gorgonzola and Chicken Pasta

Serves: 8, Cooking Time: 40 minutes

Ingredients:

- 12 oz pastas, cooked and drained
- ¼ cup snipped fresh Italian parsley
- 2/3 cup Parmesan cheese
- 1 cup crumbled Gorgonzola cheese
- 2 cups whipping cream
- 8 oz stemmed fresh cremini or shiitake mushrooms
- 3 tbsp olive oil
- ½ tsp ground pepper
- ½ tsp salt
- 1 ½ lbs. skinless chicken breast, cut into ½-inch slices

Directions for Cooking:

1) Season chicken breasts with ¼ tsp pepper and ¼ tsp salt.
2) On medium-high fire, place a nonstick pan with 1 tbsp oil and stir fry half of the chicken until cooked and lightly browned, around 5 minutes per side. Transfer chicken to a clean dish and repeat procedure to remaining batch of uncooked chicken.
3) In same pan, add a tablespoon of oil and stir fry mushroom until liquid is evaporated and mushrooms are soft, around eight minutes. Stir occasionally.
4) Add chicken back to the mushrooms along with cream and simmer for three minutes. Then add the remaining pepper and salt, parmesan cheese and ½ cup of Gorgonzola cheese. Cook until mixture is uniform. Turn off fire.
5) Add pasta into the mixture, tossing to combine. Transfer to serving dish and garnish with remaining Gorgonzola cheese and serve.

Nutrition Information:
Calories per Serving: 358; Carbs: 23.1g; Protein: 27.7g; Fat: 17.1g

Greek Couscous Salad and Herbed Lamb Chops

Serves: 4, Cooking Time: 30 minutes
Ingredients:
- ¼ tsp salt
- ½ cup crumbled feta
- ½ cup whole wheat couscous
- 1 cup water
- 1 medium cucumber, peeled and chopped
- 1 tbsp finely chopped fresh parsley
- 1 tbsp minced garlic
- 2 ½ lbs. lamb loin chops, trimmed of fat
- 2 medium tomatoes, chopped
- 2 tbsp finely chopped fresh dill
- 2 tsp extra virgin olive oil
- 3 tbsp lemon juice

Directions for Cooking:
1) On medium saucepan, add water and bring to a boil.
2) Ibn a small bowl, mix salt, parsley, and garlic. Rub onto lamb chops.
3) On medium-high fire, place a large nonstick saucepan and heat oil.
4) Pan fry lamb chops for 5 minutes per side or to desired doneness. Once done, turn off fire and keep warm.
5) On saucepan of boiling water, add couscous. Once boiling, lower fire to a simmer, cover and cook for two minutes.
6) After two minutes, turn off fire, cover and let it stand for 5 minutes.
7) Fluff couscous with a fork and place into a medium bowl.
8) Add dill, lemon juice, feta, cucumber, and tomatoes in bowl of couscous and toss well to combine.
9) Serve lamb chops with a side of couscous and enjoy.

Nutrition Information:
Calories per Serving: 524.1; Carbs: 12.3g; Protein: 61.8g; Fat: 25.3g

Grilled Veggie and Pasta with Marinara Sauce

Serves: 4, Cooking Time: 30 minutes
Ingredients:
- 8 oz whole wheat spaghetti
- 1 sweet onion, sliced into ¼-inch wide rounds
- 1 zucchini, sliced lengthwise
- 1 yellow summer squash, sliced lengthwise
- 2 red peppers, sliced into chunks
- 1/8 tsp freshly ground black pepper
- ½ tsp dried oregano
- 1 tsp sugar
- 1 tbsp chopped fresh basil or 1 tsp dried basil
- 2 tbsp chopped onion
- ½ tsp minced garlic
- salt
- 10 large fresh tomatoes, peeled and diced
- 2 tbsp extra virgin olive oil, divided

Directions for Cooking:
1) Make the marinara sauce by heating on medium-high fire a tablespoon of oil in a large fry pan.
2) Sauté black pepper, oregano, sugar, basil, onions, garlic, salt and tomatoes. Once

simmering, lower fire and allow to simmer for 30 minutes or until sauce has thickened.

3) Meanwhile, preheat broiler and grease baking pan with cooking spray.

4) Add sweet onion, zucchini, squash and red peppers in baking pan and brush with oil. Broil for 5 to 8 minutes or until vegetables are tender. Remove from oven and transfer veggies into a bowl.

5) Bring a large pot of water to a boil. Once boiling, add pasta and cook following manufacturer's instructions. Once al dente, drain and divide equally into 4 plates.

6) To serve, equally divide marinara sauce on to pasta, top with grilled veggies and enjoy.

Nutrition Information:
Calories per Serving:256 ; Carbs: 41.9g; Protein: 8.3g; Fat: 6.2g

Instant Pot Quinoa Pilaf

Serves: 10, Cooking Time: 20 minutes
Ingredients:
- 3 tablespoons butter
- 2 tablespoons onion, chopped
- 1 tablespoon garlic, minced
- 2 tablespoons chopped celery
- 2 cups quinoa, rinsed
- 2 cups chicken broth
- ¾ teaspoon garlic powder
- ¼ teaspoon paprika
- Salt and pepper to taste
- 1 tablespoon parsley, chopped

Directions for Cooking:
1) Press the Sauté button on the Instant Pot.
2) Melt the butter and sauté the onion, garlic, and celery until fragrant.

3) Add the quinoa, chicken broth, garlic, powder, and paprika.
4) Season with salt and pepper to taste.
5) Close the lid and press the Manual button.
6) Adjust the cooking time to 15 minutes
7) Do natural pressure release.
8) Garnish with parsley.
9) Once cooled, evenly divide into serving size, keep in your preferred container, and refrigerate until ready to eat.

Nutrition Information:
Calories per serving: 237; Carbohydrates: 23.3g; Protein: 15.4g; Fat: 8.9g

Kasha with Onions and Mushrooms

Serves: 4, Cooking Time: 40 minutes
Ingredients:
- ½ tsp pepper
- ½ tsp rubbed sage
- ¾ cup carrot juice
- 1 cup water
- 1 cup whole grain kasha
- 1 tbsp olive oil
- 12oz shiitake mushrooms
- 2 large onions, thinly sliced
- 2 tsp sugar
- Salt to taste

Directions for Cooking:
1) In a large skillet, heat oil over medium-high heat and add onions and sugar. Cook until the onions are brown.

2) Add the sage, mushrooms and pepper stir constantly until the mushrooms are tender. Set aside.
3) In the same skillet, place kasha and cook over medium heat. Stir constantly until lightly toasted.
4) Combine carrot juice, water and salt in a saucepan and bring to a boil over medium heat.
5) Add kasha and cook until tender.
6) Fluff with fork and transfer the contents to the skillet with the onion and sugar mixture.
7) Toss until well combined.
8) Serve and enjoy.

Nutrition Information:
Calories per Serving: 254.5; Carbs: 46.8 g; Protein: 6.7g; Fat: 4.5g

Kefta Styled Beef Patties with Cucumber Salad

Serves: 4, Cooking Time: 10 minutes

Ingredients:

- 2 pcs of 6-inch pita, quartered
- ½ tsp freshly ground black pepper
- 1 tbsp fresh lemon juice
- ½ cup plain Greek yogurt, fat-free
- 2 cups thinly sliced English cucumber
- ½ tsp ground cinnamon
- ½ tsp salt
- 1 tsp ground cumin
- 2 tsp ground coriander
- 1 tbsp peeled and chopped ginger
- ¼ cup cilantro, fresh
- ¼ cup plus 2 tbsp fresh parsley, chopped and divided
- 1 lb. ground sirloin

Directions for Cooking:

1) On medium-high fire, preheat a grill pan coated with cooking spray.
2) In a medium bowl, mix together cinnamon, salt, cumin, coriander, ginger, cilantro, parsley and beef. Then divide the mixture equally into four parts and shaping each portion into a patty ½ inch thick.
3) Then place patties on pan cooking each side for three minutes or until desired doneness is achieved.
4) In a separate bowl, toss together vinegar and cucumber.
5) In a small bowl, whisk together pepper, juice, 2 tbsp parsley and yogurt.
6) Serve each patty on a plate with ½ cup cucumber mixture and 2 tbsp of the yogurt sauce.

Nutrition Information:
Calories per serving: 313; Carbs: 11.7g; Protein: 33.9g; Fat: 14.1g

Lemon Asparagus Risotto

Serves: 5, Cooking Time: 6 minutes

Ingredients:

- 1 tablespoons olive oil
- 1 shallot, chopped
- 1 clove of garlic, minced
- 1 ½ cup Arborio rice
- 1/3 cup white wine
- 3 cups vegetable broth
- 1 teaspoon lemon zest
- 2 teaspoon thyme leaves
- Salt and pepper to taste
- 1 bunch asparagus spears, trimmed
- 1 tablespoons butter
- 2 tablespoons parmesan cheese, grated

Directions for Cooking:

1) Heat olive oil in a pot for 2 minutes.
2) Sauté the shallot and garlic until fragrant, around 2 minutes.
3) Add the Arborio rice and stir for 2 minutes before adding the white wine.
4) Pour in the vegetable broth. Season with salt and pepper to taste.
5) Stir in the lemon zest and thyme leaves.
6) Cover and cook on medium fire for 15 minutes.
7) Stir in the asparagus spears and allow to simmer for 3 minutes.
8) Add the butter and sprinkle with parmesan cheese.
9) Turn off fire and let it sit covered for 10 minutes.

Nutrition Information:
Calories per serving: 179; Carbohydrates: 21.4g; Protein:5.7g; Fat: 12.9g

Lime-Cilantro Rice Chipotle Style

Serves: 10, Cooking Time: 17 minutes

Ingredients:

- 1 can vegetable broth
- ¾ cup water
- 2 tablespoons canola oil
- 3 tablespoons juice of lime juice
- 2 cups long grain white rice, rinsed
- Zest of 1 lime
- ½ cup cilantro, chopped
- ½ teaspoon salt

Instructions
1) Place everything in the pot and give a good stir.
2) Give a good stir and close the lid.
3) Seal off the vent.
4) Press the Rice button and adjust the cooking time to 17 minutes.
5) Do natural pressure release.
6) Fluff the rice before serving.
7) Once cooled, evenly divide into serving size, keep in your preferred container, and refrigerate until ready to eat.

Nutrition Information:
Calories per serving: 166; Carbohydrates: 31.2g; Protein:2.7 g; Fat: 3.1g

Lipsmacking Chicken Tetrazzini

Serves: 8, Cooking Time: 3 hours
Ingredients:
- Toasted French bread slices
- ¾ cup thinly sliced green onion
- 2/3 cup grated parmesan cheese
- 10 oz dried spaghetti or linguine, cooked and drained
- ¼ tsp ground nutmeg
- ¼ tsp ground black pepper
- 2 tbsp dry sherry
- ¼ cup chicken broth or water
- 1 16oz jar of Alfredo pasta sauce
- 2 4.5oz jars of sliced mushrooms, drained
- 2.5 lbs. skinless chicken breasts cut into ½ inch slices

Directions for Cooking:
1) In a slow cooker, mix mushrooms and chicken.
2) In a bowl, mix well nutmeg, pepper, sherry, broth and alfredo sauce before pouring over chicken and mushrooms.
3) Set on high heat, cover and cook for two to three hours.
4) Once chicken is cooked, pour over pasta, garnish with green onion and serve with French bread on the side.

Nutrition Information:
Calories per Serving: 505; Carbs: 24.7g; Protein: 35.1g; Fat: 30.2g

Mediterranean Diet Pasta with Mussels

Serves: 4, Cooking Time: 20 minutes
Ingredients:
- 1 tbsp finely grated lemon zest
- ¼ cup chopped fresh parsley
- Freshly ground pepper to taste
- ¼ tsp salt
- Big pinch of crushed red pepper
- ¾ cup dry white wine
- 2 lbs. mussels, cleaned
- Big pinch of saffron threads soaked in 2 tbsp of water
- 1 can of 15 oz crushed tomatoes with basil
- 2 large cloves garlic, chopped
- ¼ cup extra virgin olive oil
- 8 oz whole wheat linguine or spaghetti

Directions for Cooking:
1) Cook your pasta following the package label, drain and set aside while covering it to keep it warm.
2) On medium heat, place a large pan and heat oil. Sauté for two to three minutes the garlic and add the saffron plus liquid and the crushed tomatoes. Let it simmer for five minutes.
3) On high heat and in a different pot, boil the wine and mussels for four to six minutes or until it opens. Then transfer the mussels into a clean bowl while disposing of the unopened ones.
4) Then, with a sieve strain the mussel soup into the tomato sauce, add the red pepper and continue for a minute to simmer the sauce. Lastly, season with pepper and salt.
5) Then transfer half of the sauce into the pasta bowl and toss to mix. Then ladle the pasta into 4 medium sized serving bowls, top with mussels, remaining sauce, lemon zest and parsley in that order before serving.

Nutrition Information:
Calories per Serving: 402; Carbs: 26.0g; Protein: 35.0g; Fat: 17.5g

Mediterranean Style Roasted Vegetables with Polenta

Serves: 6 , Cooking Time: 35 minutes

Ingredients:
- 2 tsp oregano
- 110 ripe olives, chopped
- 6 dry-packed sun-dried tomatoes, soaked in water to rehydrate, drained and chopped
- 2 plum or Roma tomatoes, sliced
- 10-oz frozen spinach, thawed
- ¼ tsp cracked black pepper
- 2 tsp trans-free margarine
- 1 ½ cups coarse polenta
- 6 cups water
- 2 tbsp + 1 tsp extra virgin olive oil
- 1 sweet red pepper, seeded, cored and cut into chunks
- 6 medium mushrooms, sliced
- 1 small green zucchini, cut into ¼-inch slices
- 1 small yellow zucchini, cut into ¼-inch slices
- 1 small eggplant, peeled and cut into ¼-inch slices

Directions for Cooking:
1) Grease a baking sheet and a 12-inch circle baking dish, position oven rack 4-inches away from heat source and preheat broiler.
2) With 1 tbsp olive oil, brush red pepper, mushrooms, zucchini and eggplant. Place in prepared baking sheet in a single layer. Pop in the broiler and broil under low setting.
3) Turn and brush again with oil the veggies after 5 minutes. Continue broiling until veggies are slightly browned and tender.
4) Wash and drain spinach. Set aside.
5) Preheat oven to 350 degrees F.
6) Bring water to a boil in a medium saucepan.
7) Whisk in polenta and lower fire to a simmer. For 5 minutes, cook and stir.
8) Once polenta no longer sticks to pan, add 1/8 tsp pepper and margarine. Mix well and turn off fire.
9) Evenly spread polenta on base of prepped baking dish. Brush tops with olive oil and for ten minutes bake in the oven.
10) When done, remove polenta from oven and keep warm.
11) With paper towels remove excess water from spinach. Layer spinach on top of polenta followed by sliced tomatoes, olives, sun-dried tomatoes, and roasted veggies. Season with remaining pepper and bake for another 10 minutes.
12) Remove from oven, cut into equal servings and enjoy.

Nutrition Information:
Calories per Serving: 282.5; Carbs: 34.6g; Protein: 6.1g; Fat: 13.3g

Mexican Baked Beans and Rice

Serves: 6 , Cooking Time: 45 minutes

Ingredients:
- 1 ½ cups cooked brown rice
- 1 15-oz can no-salt added black beans, drained and rinsed
- 1 cup chopped poblano pepper
- 1 cup chopped red bell pepper
- 1 cup frozen yellow corn
- 1 cup shredded reduced fat Monterey Jack cheese
- 1 lb. skinless, boneless chicken breast cut into bite sized pieces
- 1 tbsp chili powder
- 1 tbsp cumin
- 2 14.5-oz cans no salt added tomatoes, diced or crushed
- 4 garlic cloves, crushed

Directions for Cooking:
1) With cooking spray, grease a 3-quart shallow casserole and preheat oven to 400 degrees F.
2) Spread cooked brown rice in bottom of casserole.
3) Layer chicken on top of brown rice.
4) Mix well garlic, seasonings, peppers, corn, beans and tomatoes in a medium bowl.
5) Evenly spread bean mixture on top of chicken.
6) Sprinkle cheese on top of beans and pop into the oven.
7) Bake for 45 minutes, remove from oven and serve.

Nutrition Information:
Calories per Serving: 238.9; Carbs: 15.2g; Protein: 26.3g; Fat: 8.1g

Mexican Quinoa Bake

Serves: 4, Cooking Time: 40 minutes

Ingredients:

- 3 cups sweet potato, peeled, diced very small (about 1 large sweet potato)
- 2 cups cooked quinoa
- 1 cup shredded sharp cheddar cheese
- 2 Tbs chili powder
- T Tbs paprika
- 1 1/4 cup salsa of your choice
- 1 red bell pepper, diced
- 1 large carrot, diced
- 3 Tbs canned green chiles
- 1 small onion, diced
- 3 garlic cloves, minced
- 2 cups cooked black beans

Directions for Cooking:

1) Preheat oven to 400 degrees F.
2) Dice, chop, measure and prep all ingredients.
3) Combine all ingredients in one big bowl and toss ingredients well.
4) Spray a 9 X 13-inch pan with cooking spray and pour all ingredients in.
5) Bake for 35-40 minutes or until sweet potato pieces are slightly mushy, cheese is melted and items are heated all the way through.
6) Let sit for about 5 minutes, scoop into bowls and enjoy!

Nutrition Information:

Calories per serving: 414; Carbs: 56.6g; Protein: 22.0g; Fat: 13.0g

Nutty and Fruity Amaranth Porridge

Serves: 2, Cooking Time: 30 minutes

Ingredients:

- ¼ cup pumpkin seeds
- ½ cup blueberries
- 1 medium pear, chopped
- 1 tbsp raw honey
- 1 tsp cinnamon
- 2 cups filtered water
- 2/3 cups whole-grain amaranth

Directions for Cooking:

1) In a nonstick pan with cover, boil water and amaranth. Slow fire to a simmer and continue cooking until liquid is absorbed completely, around 25-30 minutes.
2) Turn off fire.
3) Mix in cinnamon, honey and pumpkin seeds. Mix well.
4) Pour equally into two bowls.
5) Garnish with pear and blueberries.
6) Serve and enjoy.

Nutrition Information:

Calories per Serving: 393.4; Carbs: 68.5g; Protein: 10.5g; Fat: 8.6g

Orange, Dates and Asparagus on Quinoa Salad

Serves: 8, Cooking Time: 25 minutes

Ingredients:

- ¼ cup chopped pecans, toasted
- ½ cup white onion, finely chopped
- ½ jalapeno pepper, diced
- ½ lb. asparagus, sliced into 2-inch lengths, steamed and chilled
- ½ tsp salt
- 1 cup fresh orange sections
- 1 cup uncooked quinoa
- 1 tsp olive oil
- 2 cups water
- 2 tbsp minced red onion
- 5 dates, pitted and chopped

Dressing Ingredients:

- ¼ tsp freshly ground black pepper
- ¼ tsp salt
- 1 garlic clove, minced
- 1 tbsp extra virgin olive oil
- 2 tbsp chopped fresh mint
- 2 tbsp fresh lemon juice
- Mint sprigs – optional

Directions for Cooking:

1) On medium-high fire, place a large nonstick pan and heat 1 tsp oil.
2) Add white onion and sauté for two minutes.
3) Add quinoa and for 5 minutes sauté it.
4) Add salt and water. Bring to a boil, once boiling, slow fire to a simmer and cook for 15 minutes while covered.
5) Turn off fire and leave for 15 minutes, to let quinoa absorb the remaining water.
6) Transfer quinoa to a large salad bowl. Add jalapeno pepper, asparagus, dates, red onion, pecans and oranges. Toss to combine.
7) Make the dressing by mixing garlic, pepper, salt, olive oil and lemon juice in a small bowl.
8) Pour dressing into quinoa salad along with chopped mint, mix well.
9) If desired, garnish with mint sprigs before serving.

Nutrition Information:
Calories per Serving: 265.2; Carbs: 28.3g; Protein: 14.6g; Fat: 10.4g

Pasta and Tuna Salad

Serves: 4, Cooking Time: 12 minutes
Ingredients:
- ¼ cup mayonnaise
- ¼ cup sliced carrots
- ½ cup chopped zucchini
- 2 cups whole wheat macaroni, uncooked
- 1/3 cup diced onion
- 2 5-oz cans low-sodium tuna, water pack

Directions for Cooking:
1) In a pot of boiling water, cook macaroni according to manufacturer's instructions.
2) Drain macaroni, run under cold tap water until cool and set aside.
3) Drain and discard tuna liquid.
4) Place tuna in a salad bowl.
5) Add zucchini, carrots, drained macaroni and onion. Toss to mix.
6) Add mayonnaise and mix well.
7) Serve and enjoy.

Nutrition Information:
Calories per Serving: 168.2; Carbs: 24.6g; Protein: 5.3g; Fat: 5.4g

Pasta Primavera without Cream

Serves: 6, Cooking Time: 30 minutes
Ingredients:
- ½ cup grated Romano cheese
- 3 tbsp balsamic vinegar
- 1/3 cup chopped fresh parsley
- 1/3 cup chopped fresh basil
- 2 tsp lemon zest
- 2 cloves garlic, sliced thinly
- ¼ large yellow onion, sliced thinly
- 1 tbsp butter
- 1 tbsp Italian seasoning
- ¼ tsp coarsely ground black pepper
- ¼ tsp salt
- ¼ cup olive oil, divided
- 5 spears asparagus, trimmed and cut into 1-inch pieces
- 1 cup fresh green beans, trimmed and cut into 1-inch pieces
- ½ pint grape tomatoes
- ½ red bell pepper, julienned
- 1 carrot, julienned
- 1 zucchini, chopped
- 1 package 12-oz penne pasta

Directions for Cooking:
1) Cook pasta according to manufacturer's instructions, drain and rinse in running cold water.
2) Line baking sheet with aluminum foil and preheat oven to 450 degrees F.
3) Mix thoroughly together in a bowl Italian seasoning, lemon juice, pepper, salt, 2 tbsp olive oil, asparagus, green beans, tomatoes, red bell pepper, carrot, zucchini and squash.
4) Arrange veggies in baking sheet and bake until tender for 15 minutes. Remove from oven.

5) In a large skillet, heat butter and stir fry garlic and onion until soft.
6) Add balsamic vinegar, parsley, basil, lemon zest and pasta. Continue cooking until heated through while gently tossing around the pasta.
7) Remove from fire and transfer to a large serving bowl and mix in the roasted veggies.
8) Serve and enjoy.

Nutrition Information:
Calories per Serving: 406; Carbs: 54.4g; Protein: 15.4g; Fat: 13.6g

Pasta Shells Stuffed with Feta

Serves: 10, Cooking Time: 40 minutes
Ingredients:
- Cooking spray
- 20 jumbo pasta shells, cooked and drained
- 2 garlic cloves, minced
- 5 oz frozen chopped spinach, thawed, drained and squeezed dry
- 1 9oz package frozen artichoke hearts, thawed and chopped
- ¼ tsp freshly ground black pepper
- ½ cup fat-free cream cheese softened
- 1 cup crumbled feta cheese
- 1 cup shredded provolone cheese, divided
- 1 8oz can no salt added tomato sauce
- 1 28oz can fire roasted crushed tomatoes with added puree
- ¼ cup chopped pepperoncini peppers
- 1 tsp dried oregano

Directions for Cooking:
1) On medium fire, place a medium fry pan and for 12 minutes cook tomato sauce, crushed tomatoes, peppers and oregano. Put aside.
2) In a medium bowl, mix garlic, spinach, artichoke, black pepper, cream cheese, feta cheese and ½ cup provolone. Evenly stuff these to the cooked pasta shells.
3) Grease a rectangular glass dish and arrange all the pasta shells within. Cover with tomato mixture and top with provolone.
4) Bake for 25 minutes in a preheated 375 degrees F oven.

Nutrition Information:
Calories per Serving: 284; Carbs: 38.5g; Protein: 15.9g; Fat: 8.3g

Pasta Shells Stuffed with Scampi

Serves: 10, Cooking Time: 45 minutes
Ingredients:
- 1/3 cup grated fresh Parmigiano-Reggiano cheese
- 3 cups lower-sodium marinara sauce, divided
- Cooking spray
- 1 tbsp potato starch
- 1 lb. medium shrimp, peeled, deveined and chopped coarsely
- 1/3 cup chopped fresh basil
- ¼ tsp ground red pepper
- ¼ cup reduced fat milk
- ½ cup 1/3-less fat cream cheese
- 2 tbsp minced garlic
- ½ cup chopped shallots
- 1 ½ tbsp Olive oil
- 20 jumbo pasta shells, cooked and drained

Directions for Cooking:
1) On medium fire, place a nonstick fry pan with oil and fry for four minutes the shallots while occasionally mixing. Stir in garlic and cook for another minute.
2) In a bowl, place shrimp and sprinkle with potato starch and set aside.
3) Add pepper, milk and cream cheese while stirring constantly and cooking until cheese is melted and well mixed. Remove from fire and quickly stir in shrimp and basil.
4) In a greased rectangular glass dish, pour a cup of marinara sauce and spread evenly. Then equally stuff the pasta shells with the shrimp mixture and arrange the shells in the glass dish. Pour remaining marinara sauce on top of shells and garnish with cheese.
5) Place the dish in a preheated 400 degrees F oven and cook for 30 minutes.

Nutrition Information:
Calories per Serving: 270; Carbs: 35.2g; Protein: 14.7g; Fat: 7.6g

Pastitsio an Italian Dish

Serves: 8, Cooking Time: 30 minutes

Ingredients:

- 2 tbsp chopped fresh flat leaf parsley
- ¾ cup shredded mozzarella cheese
- 1 3oz package of fat-free cream cheese
- ½ cup 1/3 less fat cream cheese
- 1 can 14.5-oz of diced tomatoes, drained
- 2 cups fat-free milk
- 1 tbsp all-purpose flour
- ¾ tsp kosher salt
- 5 garlic cloves, minced
- 1 ½ cups chopped onion
- 1 tbsp olive oil
- 1 lb. ground sirloin
- Cooking spray
- 8 oz penne, cooked and drained

Directions for Cooking:

1) On medium-high fire, place a big nonstick saucepan and for five minutes sauté beef. Keep on stirring to break up the pieces of ground meat. Once cooked, remove from pan and drain fat.

2) Using same pan, heat oil and fry onions until soft around four minutes while occasionally stirring.

3) Add garlic and continue cooking for another minute while constantly stirring.

4) Stir in beef and flour, cook for another minute. Mix constantly.

5) Add the fat-free cream cheese, less fat cream cheese, tomatoes and milk. Cook until mixture is smooth and heated. Toss in pasta and mix well.

6) Transfer pasta into a greased rectangular glass dish and top with mozzarella. Cook in a preheated broiler for four minutes. Remove from broiler and garnish with parsley before serving.

Nutrition Information:

Calories per Serving: 263; Carbs: 17.8g; Protein: 24.1g; Fat: 10.6g

Pesto Pasta and Shrimps

Serves: 4, Cooking Time: 15 minutes

Ingredients:

- ¼ cup pesto, divided
- ¼ cup shaved Parmesan Cheese
- 1 ¼ lbs. large shrimp, peeled and deveined
- 1 cup halved grape tomatoes
- 4-oz angel hair pasta, cooked, rinsed and drained

Directions for Cooking:

1) On medium-high fire, place a nonstick large fry pan and grease with cooking spray.

2) Add tomatoes, pesto and shrimp. Cook for 15 minutes or until shrimps are opaque, while covered.

3) Stir in cooked pasta and cook until heated through.

4) Transfer to a serving plate and garnish with Parmesan cheese.

Nutrition Information:

Calories per Serving: 319; Carbs: 23.6g; Protein: 31.4g; Fat: 11g

Pecorino Pasta with Sausage and Fresh Tomato

Serves: 4, Cooking Time: 20 minutes

Ingredients:

- ¼ cup torn fresh basil leaves
- 1/8 tsp black pepper
- ¼ tsp salt
- 6 tbsp grated fresh pecorino Romano cheese, divided
- 1 ¼ lbs. tomatoes, chopped

- 2 tsp minced garlic
- 1 cup vertically sliced onions
- 2 tsp olive oil
- 8 oz sweet Italian sausage
- 8 oz uncooked penne, cooked and drained

Directions for Cooking:

1) On medium-high fire, place a nonstick fry pan with oil and cook for five minutes onion and sausage. Stir constantly to break sausage into pieces.
2) Stir in garlic and continue cooking for two minutes more.
3) Add tomatoes and cook for another two minutes.
4) Remove pan from fire, season with pepper and salt. Mix well.
5) Stir in 2 tbsp cheese and pasta. Toss well.
6) Transfer to a serving dish, garnish with basil and remaining cheese before serving.

Nutrition Information:
Calories per Serving: 376; Carbs: 50.8g; Protein: 17.8g; Fat: 11.6g

Prosciutto e Faggioli

Serves: 4, Cooking Time: 15 minutes
Ingredients:
- 12 oz pasta, cooked and drained
- Pepper and salt to taste
- 3 tbsp snipped fresh chives
- 3 cups arugula or watercress leaves, loosely packed
- ½ cup chicken broth, warm
- 1 tbsp Herbed garlic butter
- ½ cup shredded pecorino Toscano
- 4 oz prosciutto, cut into bite sizes
- 2 cups cherry tomatoes, halved
- 1 can of 19oz white kidney beans, rinsed and drained

Directions for Cooking:

1) Heat over medium low fire herbed garlic butter, cheese, prosciutto, tomatoes and beans in a big saucepan for 2 minutes.
2) Once mixture is simmering, stir constantly to melt cheese while gradually stirring in the broth.
3) Once cheese is fully melted and incorporated, add chives, arugula, pepper and salt.
4) Turn off the fire and toss in the cooked pasta. Serve and enjoy.

Nutrition Information:
Calories per Serving: 452; Carbs: 57.9g; Protein: 30.64g; Fat: 11.7g

Quinoa & Black Bean Stuffed Sweet Potatoes

Serves: 8, Cooking Time: 60 minutes
Ingredients:
- 4 sweet potatoes
- ½ onion, diced
- 1 garlic glove, crushed and diced
- ½ large bell pepper diced (about 2/3 cups)
- Handful of diced cilantro
- ½ cup cooked quinoa
- ½ cup black beans
- 1 tbsp olive oil
- 1 tbsp chili powder
- ½ tbsp cumin
- ½ tbsp paprika
- ½ tbsp oregano
- 2 tbsp lime juice
- 2 tbsp honey
- Sprinkle salt
- 1 cup shredded cheddar cheese
- Chopped spring onions, for garnish (optional)

Directions for Cooking:

1) Preheat oven to 400 degrees F.
2) Wash and scrub outside of potatoes. Poke with fork a few times and then place on parchment paper on cookie sheet. Bake for 40-45 minutes or until it is cooked.
3) While potatoes are baking, sauté onions, garlic, olive oil and spices in a pan on the stove until onions are translucent and soft.
4) In the last 10 minutes while the potatoes are cooking, in a large bowl combine the onion mixture with the beans, quinoa, honey, lime juice, cilantro and ½ cup cheese. Mix well.
5) When potatoes are cooked, remove from oven and let cool slightly. When cool to touch, cut in half (hot dog style) and scoop out most of the insides. Leave a thin ring of potato so that it will hold its shape. You can save the sweet potato guts for another recipe, such as my veggie burgers (recipe posted below).

6) Fill with bean and quinoa mixture. Top with remaining cheddar cheese.
7) (If making this a freezer meal, stop here. Individually wrap potato skins in plastic wrap and place on flat surface to freeze. Once frozen, place all potatoes in large zip lock container or Tupperware.)

8) Return to oven for an additional 10 minutes or until cheese is melted.

Nutrition Information:
Calories per serving: 243; Carbs: 37.6g; Protein: 8.5g; Fat: 7.3g

Puttanesca Style Bucatini

Serves: 4, Cooking Time: 40 minutes
Ingredients:

- 1 tbsp capers, rinsed
- 1 tsp coarsely chopped fresh oregano
- 1 tsp finely chopped garlic
- 1/8 tsp salt
- 12-oz bucatini pasta
- 2 cups coarsely chopped canned no-salt-added whole peeled tomatoes with their juice
- 3 tbsp extra virgin olive oil, divided
- 4 anchovy fillets, chopped
- 8 black Kalamata olives, pitted and sliced into slivers

Directions for Cooking:
1) Cook bucatini pasta according to package directions. Drain, keep warm, and set aside.

2) On medium fire, place a large nonstick saucepan and heat 2 tbsp oil.
3) Sauté anchovies until it starts to disintegrate.
4) Add garlic and sauté for 15 seconds.
5) Add tomatoes, sauté for 15 to 20 minutes or until no longer watery. Season with 1/8 tsp salt.
6) Add oregano, capers, and olives.
7) Add pasta, sautéing until heated through.
8) To serve, drizzle pasta with remaining olive oil and enjoy.

Nutrition Information:
Calories per Serving: 207.4; Carbs: 31g; Protein: 5.1g; Fat: 7g

Quinoa Buffalo Bites

Serves: 4, Cooking Time: 15 minutes
Ingredients:

- 2 cups cooked quinoa
- 1 cup shredded mozzarella
- 1/2 cup buffalo sauce
- 1/4 cup +1 Tbsp flour
- 1 egg
- 1/4 cup chopped cilantro
- 1 small onion, diced

Directions for Cooking:
1) Preheat oven to 350 degrees F.

2) Mix all ingredients in large bowl.
3) Press mixture into greased mini muffin tins.
4) Bake for approximately 15 minutes or until bites are golden.
5) Enjoy on its own or with blue cheese or ranch dip.

Nutrition Information:
Calories per serving: 212; Carbs: 30.6g; Protein: 15.9g; Fat: 3.0g

Quinoa and Three Beans Recipe

Serves: 8, Cooking Time: 35 minutes
Ingredients:

- 1 cup grape tomatoes, sliced in half
- 1 cup quinoa
- 1 cup seedless cucumber, chopped
- 1 red bell pepper, seeds removed and chopped
- 1 tablespoon balsamic vinegar

- 1 yellow bell pepper, seeds removed and chopped
- 1/2-pound green beans, trimmed and snapped into 2-inch pieces
- 1/3 cup pitted kalamata olives, cut in half

- 1/4 cup chopped fresh basil
- 1/4 cup diced red onion
- 1/4 cup feta cheese crumbles
- 1/4 cup olive oil
- 1/4 teaspoon dried basil
- 1/4 teaspoon dried oregano
- 15 ounces garbanzo beans, drained and rinsed
- 15 ounces white beans, drained and rinsed
- 2 cups water
- 2 garlic cloves, smashed
- kosher salt and freshly ground black pepper to taste

Directions for Cooking:
1) Bring water and quinoa to a boil in a medium saucepan. Cover, reduce heat to low, and cook until quinoa is tender, around 15 minutes.
2) Remove from heat and let stand for 5 minutes, covered.

3) Remove lid and fluff with a fork. Transfer to a large salad bowl.
4) Meanwhile. Bring a large pot of salted water to a boil and blanch the green beans for two minutes. Drain and place in a bowl of ice water. Drain well.
5) Add the fresh basil, olives, feta cheese, red onion, tomatoes, cucumbers, peppers, white beans, garbanzo beans, and green beans in bowl of quinoa.
6) In a small bowl, whisk together the pepper, salt, oregano, dried basil, balsamic, and olive oil. Pour dressing over the salad and gently toss salad until coated with dressing.
7) Season with additional salt and pepper if needed.
8) Serve and enjoy.

Nutrition Information:
Calories per serving: 249; Carbs: 31.0g; Protein: 8.0g; Fat: 10.0g

Red Quinoa Peach Porridge

Serves: 1, Cooking Time: 30 minutes
Ingredients:
- ¼ cup old fashioned rolled oats
- ¼ cup red quinoa
- ½ cup milk
- 1 ½ cups water
- 2 peaches, peeled and sliced

Directions for Cooking:
1) On a small saucepan, place the peaches and quinoa. Add water and cook for 30 minutes.

2) Add the oatmeal and milk last and cook until the oats become tender.
3) Stir occasionally to avoid the porridge from sticking on the bottom of the pan.

Nutrition Information:
Calories per Serving: 456.6; Carbs: 77.3g; Protein: 16.6g; Fat: 9g

Raisins, Nuts and Beef on Hashweh Rice

Serves: 8, Cooking Time: 50 minutes
Ingredients:
- ½ cup dark raisins, soaked in 2 cups water for an hour
- 1/3 cup slivered almonds, toasted and soaked in 2 cups water overnight
- 1/3 cup pine nuts, toasted and soaked in 2 cups water overnight
- ½ cup fresh parsley leaves, roughly chopped
- Pepper and salt to taste
- ¾ tsp ground cinnamon, divided
- ¾ tsp cloves, divided
- 1 tsp garlic powder
- 1 ¾ tsp allspice, divided

- 1 lb. lean ground beef or lean ground lamb
- 1 small red onion, finely chopped
- Olive oil
- 1 ½ cups medium grain rice

Directions for Cooking:
1) For 15 to 20 minutes, soak rice in cold water. You will know that soaking is enough when you can snap a grain of rice easily between your thumb and index finger. Once soaking is done, drain rice well.
2) Meanwhile, drain pine nuts, almonds and raisins for at least a minute and transfer to one bowl. Set aside.

3) On a heavy cooking pot on medium-high fire, heat 1 tbsp olive oil.

4) Once oil is hot, add red onions. Sauté for a minute before adding ground meat and sauté for another minute.

5) Season ground meat with pepper, salt, ½ tsp ground cinnamon, ½ tsp ground cloves, 1 tsp garlic powder, and 1 ¼ tsp allspice.

6) Sauté ground meat for 10 minutes or until browned and cooked fully. Drain fat.

7) In same pot with cooked ground meat, add rice on top of meat.

8) Season with a bit of pepper and salt. Add remaining cinnamon, ground cloves, and allspice. Do not mix.

9) Add 1 tbsp olive oil and 2 ½ cups of water. Bring to a boil and once boiling, lower fire to a simmer. Cook while covered until liquid is fully absorbed, around 20 to 25 minutes.

10) Turn of fire.

11) To serve, place a large serving platter that fully covers the mouth of the pot. Place platter upside down on mouth of pot, and invert pot. The inside of the pot should now rest on the platter with the rice on bottom of plate and ground meat on top of it.

12) Garnish the top of the meat with raisins, almonds, pine nuts, and parsley.

13) Serve and enjoy.

Nutrition Information:
Calories per serving: 357; Carbs: 39.0g; Protein: 16.7g; Fat: 15.9g

Raw Tomato Sauce & Brie on Linguine

Serves: 4, Cooking Time: 12 minutes
Ingredients:
- ¼ cup grated low-fat Parmesan cheese
- ½ cup loosely packed fresh basil leaves, torn
- 12 oz whole wheat linguine
- 2 cups loosely packed baby arugula
- 2 green onions, green parts only, sliced thinly
- 2 tbsp balsamic vinegar
- 2 tbsp extra virgin olive oil
- 3 large vine-ripened tomatoes
- 3 oz low-fat Brie cheese, cubed, rind removed and discarded
- 3 tbsp toasted pine nuts
- Pepper and salt to taste

Directions for Cooking:

1) Toss together pepper, salt, vinegar, oil, onions, Parmesan, basil, arugula, Brie and tomatoes in a large bowl and set aside.

2) Cook linguine following package instructions. Reserve 1 cup of pasta cooking water after linguine is cooked. Drain and discard the rest of the pasta. Do not run under cold water, instead immediately add into bowl of salad. Let it stand for a minute without mixing.

3) Add ¼ cup of reserved pasta water into bowl to make a creamy sauce. Add more pasta water if desired. Toss to mix well.

4) Serve and enjoy.

Nutrition Information:
Calories per Serving: 274.7; Carbs: 30.9g; Protein: 14.6g; Fat: 10.3g

Red Wine Risotto

Serves: 8, Cooking Time: 25 minutes
Ingredients:
- Pepper to taste
- 1 cup finely shredded Parmigian-Reggiano cheese, divided
- 2 tsp tomato paste
- 1 ¾ cups dry red wine
- ¼ tsp salt
- 1 ½ cups Italian 'risotto' rice
- 2 cloves garlic, minced
- 1 medium onion, freshly chopped
- 2 tbsp extra-virgin olive oil
- 4 ½ cups reduced sodium beef broth

Directions for Cooking:

1) On medium-high fire, bring to a simmer broth in a medium fry pan. Lower fire so broth is steaming but not simmering.

2) On medium low heat, place a Dutch oven and heat oil.
3) Sauté onions for 5 minutes. Add garlic and cook for 2 minutes.
4) Add rice, mix well, and season with salt.
5) Into rice, add a generous splash of wine and ½ cup of broth.
6) Lower fire to a gentle simmer, cook until liquid is fully absorbed while stirring rice every once in a while.
7) Add another splash of wine and ½ cup of broth. Stirring once in a while.
8) Add tomato paste and stir to mix well.
9) Continue cooking and adding wine and broth until broth is used up.
10) Once done cooking, turn off fire and stir in pepper and ¾ cup cheese.
11) To serve, sprinkle with remaining cheese and enjoy.

Nutrition Information:
Calories per Serving: 231; Carbs: 33.9g; Protein: 7.9g; Fat: 5.7g

Rice & Currant Salad Mediterranean Style

Serves: 4, Cooking Time: 50 minutes
Ingredients:
- 1 cup basmati rice
- salt
- 2 1/2 Tablespoons lemon juice
- 1 teaspoon grated orange zest
- 2 Tablespoons fresh orange juice
- 1/4 cup olive oil
- 1/2 teaspoon cinnamon
- Salt and pepper to taste
- 4 chopped green onions
- 1/2 cup dried currants
- 3/4 cup shelled pistachios or almonds
- 1/4 cup chopped fresh parsley

Directions for Cooking:
1) Place a nonstick pot on medium-high fire and add rice. Toast rice until opaque and starts to smell, around 10 minutes.
2) Add 4 quarts of boiling water to pot and 2 tsp salt. Boil until tender, around 8 minutes uncovered.
3) Drain the rice and spread out on a lined cookie sheet to cool completely.
4) In a large salad bowl, whisk well the oil, juices and spices. Add salt and pepper to taste.
5) Add half of the green onions, half of parsley, currants, and nuts.
6) Toss with the cooled rice and let stand for at least 20 minutes.
7) If needed adjust seasoning with pepper and salt.
8) Garnish with remaining parsley and green onions.

Nutrition Information:
Calories per serving: 450; Carbs: 50.0g; Protein: 9.0g; Fat: 24.0g

Ricotta and Spinach Ravioli

Serves: 2, Cooking Time: 15 minutes
Ingredients:
- 1 cup chicken stock
- 1 cup frozen spinach, thawed
- 1 batch pasta dough

Filling Ingredients:
- 3 tbsp heavy cream
- 1 cup ricotta
- 1 ¾ cups baby spinach
- 1 small onion, finely chopped
- 2 tbsp butter

Directions for Cooking:
1) Create the filling: In a fry pan, sauté onion and butter around five minutes. Add the baby spinach leaves and continue simmering for another four minutes. Remove from fire, drain liquid and mince the onion and leaves. Then combine with 2 tbsp cream and the ricotta ensuring that it is well combined. Add pepper and salt to taste.
2) With your pasta dough, divide it into four balls. Roll out one ball to ¼ inch thick rectangular spread. Cut a 1 ½ inch by 3-inch

rectangles. Place filling on the middle of the rectangles, around 1 tablespoonful and brush filling with cold water. Fold the rectangles in half, ensuring that no air is trapped within and seal using a cookie cutter. Use up all the filling.

3) Create Pasta Sauce: Until smooth, puree chicken stock and spinach. Pour into heated fry pan and for two minutes cook it. Add 1 tbsp cream and season with pepper and salt.

Continue cooking for a minute and turn of fire.

4) Cook the raviolis by submerging in a boiling pot of water with salt. Cook until al dente then drain. Then quickly transfer the cooked ravioli into the fry pan of pasta sauce, toss to mix and serve.

Nutrition Information:
Calories per Serving: 443; Carbs: 12.3g; Protein: 18.8g; Fat: 36.8g

Roasted Red Peppers and Shrimp Pasta

Serves: 6, Cooking Time: 10 minutes
Ingredients:
- 12 oz pasta, cooked and drained
- 1 cup finely shredded Parmesan Cheese
- ¼ cup snipped fresh basil
- ½ cup whipping cream
- ½ cup dry white wine
- 1 12oz jar roasted red sweet peppers, drained and chopped
- ¼ tsp crushed red pepper
- 6 cloves garlic, minced
- 1/3 cup finely chopped onion
- 2 tbsp olive oil
- ¼ cup almond oil
- 1 ½ lbs. fresh, peeled, deveined, rinsed and drained medium shrimps

Directions for Cooking:

1) On medium-high fire, heat almond oil in a big fry pan and add garlic and onions. Stir fry until onions are soft, around two minutes. Add crushed red pepper and shrimps, sauté for another two minutes before adding wine and roasted peppers.

2) Allow mixture to boil before lowering heat to low fire and for two minutes, let the mixture simmer uncovered. Stirring occasionally, add cream once shrimps are cooked and simmer for a minute.

3) Add basil and remove from fire. Toss in the pasta and mix gently. Transfer to serving plates and top with cheese.

Nutrition Information:
Calories per Serving: 418; Carbs: 26.9g; Protein: 37.1g; Fat: 18.8g

Shrimp, Lemon and Basil Pasta

Serves: 4, Cooking Time: 25 minutes
Ingredients:
- 2 cups baby spinach
- ½ tsp salt
- 2 tbsp fresh lemon juice
- 2 tbsp extra virgin olive oil
- 3 tbsp drained capers
- ¼ cup chopped fresh basil
- 1 lb. peeled and deveined large shrimp
- 8 oz uncooked spaghetti
- 3 quarts water

Directions for Cooking:

1) In a pot, bring to boil 3 quarts water. Add the pasta and allow to boil for another eight mins before adding the shrimp and boiling for another three mins or until pasta is cooked.

2) Drain the pasta and transfer to a bowl. Add salt, lemon juice, olive oil, capers and basil while mixing well.

3) To serve, place baby spinach on plate around ½ cup and topped with ½ cup of pasta.

Nutrition Information:
Calories per Serving: 151; Carbs: 18.9g; Protein: 4.3g; Fat: 7.4g

Seafood and Veggie Pasta

Serves: 4, Cooking Time: 20 minutes

Ingredients:

- ¼ tsp pepper
- ¼ tsp salt
- 1 lb raw shelled shrimp
- 1 lemon, cut into wedges
- 1 tbsp olive oil
- 2 5-oz cans chopped clams, drained (reserve 2 tbsp clam juice)
- 2 tbsp dry white wine
- 4 cloves garlic, minced
- 4 cups zucchini, spiraled (use a veggie spiralizer)
- 4 tbsp Parmesan Cheese
- Chopped fresh parsley to garnish

Directions for Cooking:

1) Ready the zucchini and spiralize with a veggie spiralizer. Arrange 1 cup of zucchini noodle per bowl. Total of 4 bowls.
2) On medium fire, place a large nonstick saucepan and heat oil.
3) For a minute, sauté garlic. Add shrimp and cook for 3 minutes until opaque or cooked.
4) Add white wine, reserved clam juice and clams. Bring to a simmer and continue simmering for 2 minutes or until half of liquid has evaporated. Stir constantly.
5) Season with pepper and salt. And if needed add more to taste.
6) Remove from fire and evenly distribute seafood sauce to 4 bowls.
7) Top with a tablespoonful of Parmesan cheese per bowl, serve and enjoy.

Nutrition Information:

Calories per Serving: 324.9; Carbs: 12g; Protein: 43.8g; Fat: 11.3g

Tortellini Salad with Broccoli

Serves: 12, Cooking Time: 20 minutes

Ingredients:

- 1 red onion, chopped finely
- 1 cup sunflower seeds
- 1 cup raisins
- 3 heads fresh broccoli, cut into florets
- 2 tsp cider vinegar
- ½ cup sugar
- ½ cup mayonnaise
- 20-oz fresh cheese filled tortellini

Directions for Cooking:

1) In a large pot of boiling water, cook tortellini according to manufacturer's instructions. Drain and rinse with cold water and set aside.
2) Whisk vinegar, sugar and mayonnaise to create your salad dressing.
3) Mix together in a large bowl red onion, sunflower seeds, raisins, tortellini and broccoli. Pour dressing and toss to coat.
4) Serve and enjoy.

Nutrition Information:

Calories per Serving: 272; Carbs: 38.7g; Protein: 5.0g; Fat: 8.1g

Stuffed Tomatoes with Green Chili

Serves: 6, Cooking Time: 55 minutes

Ingredients:

- 4 oz Colby-Jack shredded cheese
- ¼ cup water
- 1 cup uncooked quinoa
- 6 large ripe tomatoes
- ¼ tsp freshly ground black pepper
- ¾ tsp ground cumin
- 1 tsp salt, divided
- 1 tbsp fresh lime juice
- 1 tbsp olive oil
- 1 tbsp chopped fresh oregano
- 1 cup chopped onion
- 2 cups fresh corn kernels
- 2 poblano chilies

Directions for Cooking:

1) Preheat broiler to high.
2) Slice lengthwise the chilies and press on a baking sheet lined with foil. Broil for 8 minutes. Remove from oven and let cool for 10 minutes. Peel the chilies and chop coarsely and place in medium sized bowl.
3) Place onion and corn in baking sheet and broil for ten minutes. Stir two times while broiling. Remove from oven and mix in with chopped chilies.
4) Add black pepper, cumin, ¼ tsp salt, lime juice, oil and oregano. Mix well.
5) Cut off the tops of tomatoes and set aside. Leave the tomato shell intact as you scoop out the tomato pulp.
6) Drain tomato pulp as you press down with a spoon. Reserve 1 ¼ cups of tomato pulp liquid and discard the rest. Invert the tomato shells on a wire rack for 30 mins and then wipe the insides dry with a paper towel.
7) Season with ½ tsp salt the tomato pulp.
8) On a sieve over a bowl, place quinoa. Add water until it covers quinoa. Rub quinoa grains for 30 seconds together with hands; rinse and drain. Repeat this procedure two times and drain well at the end.
9) In medium saucepan bring to a boil remaining salt, ¼ cup water, quinoa and tomato liquid.
10) Once boiling, reduce heat and simmer for 15 minutes or until liquid is fully absorbed. Remove from heat and fluff quinoa with fork. Transfer and mix well the quinoa with the corn mixture.
11) Spoon ¾ cup of the quinoa-corn mixture into the tomato shells, top with cheese and cover with the tomato top. Bake in a preheated 350 degrees F oven for 15 minutes and then broil high for another 1.5 minutes.

Nutrition Information:
Calories per serving: 276; Carbs: 46.3g; Protein: 13.4g; Fat: 4.1g

Seafood Paella with Couscous

Serves: 4, Cooking Time: 15 minutes
Ingredients:
- ½ cup whole wheat couscous
- 4 oz small shrimp, peeled and deveined
- 4 oz bay scallops, tough muscle removed
- ¼ cup vegetable broth
- 1 cup freshly diced tomatoes and juice
- Pinch of crumbled saffron threads
- ¼ tsp freshly ground pepper
- ¼ tsp salt
- ½ tsp fennel seed
- ½ tsp dried thyme
- 1 clove garlic, minced
- 1 medium onion, chopped
- 2 tsp extra virgin olive oil

Directions for Cooking:
1) Put on medium fire a large saucepan and add oil. Stir in the onion and sauté for three minutes before adding: saffron, pepper, salt, fennel seed, thyme, and garlic. Continue to sauté for another minute.
2) Then add the broth and tomatoes and let boil. Once boiling, reduce the fire, cover and continue to cook for another 2 minutes.
3) Add the scallops and increase fire to medium and stir occasionally and cook for two minutes. Add the shrimp and wait for two minutes more before adding the couscous. Then remove from fire, cover and set aside for five minutes before carefully mixing.

Nutrition Information:
Calories per Serving: 117; Carbs: 11.7g; Protein: 11.5g; Fat: 3.1g

Shrimp Paella Made with Quinoa

Serves: 7, Cooking Time: 40 minutes

Ingredients:

- 1 lb. large shrimp, peeled, deveined and thawed
- 1 tsp seafood seasoning
- 1 cup frozen green peas
- 1 red bell pepper, cored, seeded & membrane removed, sliced into ½" strips
- ½ cup sliced sun-dried tomatoes, packed in olive oil
- Salt to taste
- ½ tsp black pepper
- ½ tsp Spanish paprika
- ½ tsp saffron threads (optional turmeric)
- 1 bay leaf
- ¼ tsp crushed red pepper flakes
- 3 cups chicken broth, fat-free, low sodium
- 1 ½ cups dry quinoa, rinse well
- 1 tbsp olive oil
- 2 cloves garlic, minced
- 1 yellow onion, diced

Directions for Cooking:

1) Season shrimps with seafood seasoning and a pinch of salt. Toss to mix well and refrigerate until ready to use.
2) Prepare and wash quinoa. Set aside.
3) On medium low fire, place a large nonstick skillet and heat oil. Add onions and for 5 minutes sauté until soft and tender.
4) Add paprika, saffron (or turmeric), bay leaves, red pepper flakes, chicken broth and quinoa. Season with salt and pepper.
5) Cover skillet and bring to a boil. Once boiling, lower fire to a simmer and cook until all liquid is absorbed, around ten minutes.
6) Add shrimp, peas and sun-dried tomatoes. For 5 minutes, cover and cook.
7) Once done, turn off fire and for ten minutes allow paella to set while still covered.
8) To serve, remove bay leaf and enjoy with a squeeze of lemon if desired.

Nutrition Information:
Calories per Serving: 324.4; Protein: 22g; Carbs: 33g; Fat: 11.6g

Simple Penne Anti-Pasto

Serves: 4, Cooking Time: 15 minutes

Ingredients:

- ¼ cup pine nuts, toasted
- ½ cup grated Parmigiano-Reggiano cheese, divided
- 8oz penne pasta, cooked and drained
- 1 6oz jar drained, sliced, marinated and quartered artichoke hearts
- 1 7 oz jar drained and chopped sun-dried tomato halves packed in oil
- 3 oz chopped prosciutto
- 1/3 cup pesto
- ½ cup pitted and chopped Kalamata olives
- 1 medium red bell pepper

Directions for Cooking:

1) Slice bell pepper, discard membranes, seeds and stem. On a foiled lined baking sheet, place bell pepper halves, press down by hand and broil in oven for eight minutes. Remove from oven, put in a sealed bag for 5 minutes before peeling and chopping.
2) Place chopped bell pepper in a bowl and mix in artichokes, tomatoes, prosciutto, pesto and olives.
3) Toss in ¼ cup cheese and pasta. Transfer to a serving dish and garnish with ¼ cup cheese and pine nuts. Serve and enjoy!

Nutrition Information:
Calories per Serving: 606; Carbs: 70.3g; Protein: 27.2g; Fat: 27.6g

Spaghetti in Lemon Avocado White Sauce

Serves: 6, Cooking Time: 30 minutes
Ingredients:
* Freshly ground black pepper
* Zest and juice of 1 lemon
* 1 avocado, pitted and peeled
* 1-pound spaghetti
* Salt
* 1 tbsp Olive oil
* 8 oz small shrimp, shelled and deveined
* ¼ cup dry white wine
* 1 large onion, finely sliced

Directions for Cooking:
1) Let a big pot of water boil. Once boiling add the spaghetti or pasta and cook following manufacturer's instructions until al dente. Drain and set aside.
2) In a large fry pan, over medium fire sauté wine and onions for ten minutes or until onions are translucent and soft.
3) Add the shrimps into the fry pan and increase fire to high while constantly sautéing until shrimps are cooked around five minutes. Turn the fire off. Season with salt and add the oil right away. Then quickly toss in the cooked pasta, mix well.
4) In a blender, until smooth, puree the lemon juice and avocado. Pour into the fry pan of pasta, combine well. Garnish with pepper and lemon zest then serve.

Nutrition Information:
Calories per Serving: 206; Carbs: 26.3g; Protein: 10.2g; Fat: 8.0g

Spanish Rice Casserole with Cheesy Beef

Serves: 2, Cooking Time: 32 minutes
Ingredients:
* 2 tablespoons chopped green bell pepper
* 1/4 teaspoon Worcestershire sauce
* 1/4 teaspoon ground cumin
* 1/4 cup shredded Cheddar cheese
* 1/4 cup finely chopped onion
* 1/4 cup chile sauce
* 1/3 cup uncooked long grain rice
* 1/2-pound lean ground beef
* 1/2 teaspoon salt
* 1/2 teaspoon brown sugar
* 1/2 pinch ground black pepper
* 1/2 cup water
* 1/2 (14.5 ounce) can canned tomatoes
* 1 tablespoon chopped fresh cilantro

Directions for Cooking:
1) Place a nonstick saucepan on medium fire and brown beef for 10 minutes while crumbling beef. Discard fat.
2) Stir in pepper, Worcestershire sauce, cumin, brown sugar, salt, chile sauce, rice, water, tomatoes, green bell pepper, and onion. Mix well and cook for 10 minutes until blended and a bit tender.
3) Transfer to an ovenproof casserole and press down firmly. Sprinkle cheese on top and cook for 7 minutes at 400 degrees F preheated oven. Broil for 3 minutes until top is lightly browned.
4) Serve and enjoy with chopped cilantro.

Nutrition Information:
Calories per serving: 460; Carbohydrates: 35.8g; Protein: 37.8g; Fat: 17.9g

Squash and Eggplant Casserole

Serves: 2, Cooking Time: 45 minutes
Vegetable Ingredients:
* ½ cup dry white wine
* 1 eggplant, halved and cut to 1-inch slices
* 1 large onion, cut into wedges
* 1 red bell pepper, seeded and cut to julienned strips
* 1 small butternut squash, cut into 1-inch slices
* 1 tbsp olive oil

- 12 baby corn
- 2 cups low sodium vegetable broth
- Salt and pepper to taste

Polenta Ingredients:
- ¼ cup parmesan cheese, grated
- 1 cup instant polenta
- 2 tbsp fresh oregano, chopped

Topping Ingredients:
- 1 garlic clove, chopped
- 2 tbsp slivered almonds
- 5 tbsp parsley, chopped
- Grated zest of 1 lemon

Directions for Cooking:
1) Preheat the oven to 350 degrees Fahrenheit.
2) In a casserole, heat the oil and add the onion wedges and baby corn. Sauté over medium-high heat for five minutes. Stir occasionally to prevent the onions and baby corn from sticking at the bottom of the pan.
3) Add the butternut squash to the casserole and toss the vegetables. Add the eggplants and the red pepper.
4) Cover the vegetables and cook over low to medium heat.
5) Cook for about ten minutes before adding the wine. Let the wine sizzle before stirring in the broth. Bring to a boil and cook in the oven for 30 minutes.
6) While the casserole is cooking inside the oven, make the topping by spreading the slivered almonds on a baking tray and toasting under the grill until they are lightly browned.
7) Place the toasted almonds in a small bowl and mix the remaining ingredients for the toppings.
8) Prepare the polenta. In a large saucepan, bring 3 cups of water to boil over high heat.
9) Add the polenta and continue whisking until it absorbs all the water.
10) Reduce the heat to medium until the polenta is thick. Add the parmesan cheese and oregano.
11) Serve the polenta on plates and add the casserole on top. Sprinkle the toppings on top.

Nutrition Information:
Calories per Serving: 579.3; Carbs: 79.2g; Protein: 22.2g; Fat: 19.3g

Tasty Lasagna Rolls

Serves: 6, Cooking Time: 20 minutes

Ingredients:
- ¼ tsp crushed red pepper
- ¼ tsp salt
- ½ cup shredded mozzarella cheese
- ½ cups parmesan cheese, shredded
- 1 14-oz package tofu, cubed
- 1 25-oz can of low-sodium marinara sauce
- 1 tbsp extra virgin olive oil
- 12 whole wheat lasagna noodles
- 2 tbsp Kalamata olives, chopped
- 3 cloves minced garlic
- 3 cups spinach, chopped

Directions for Cooking:
1) Put enough water on a large pot and cook the lasagna noodles according to package instructions. Drain, rinse and set aside until ready to use.
2) In a large skillet, sauté garlic over medium heat for 20 seconds. Add the tofu and spinach and cook until the spinach wilts. Transfer this mixture in a bowl and add parmesan olives, salt, red pepper and 2/3 cup of the marinara sauce.
3) In a pan, spread a cup of marinara sauce on the bottom. To make the rolls, place noodle on a surface and spread ¼ cup of the tofu filling. Roll up and place it on the pan with the marinara sauce. Do this procedure until all lasagna noodles are rolled.
4) Place the pan over high heat and bring to a simmer. Reduce the heat to medium and let it cook for three more minutes. Sprinkle mozzarella cheese and let the cheese melt for two minutes. Serve hot.

Nutrition Information:
Calories per Serving: 304; Carbs: 39.2g; Protein: 23g; Fat: 19.2g

Tasty Mushroom Bolognese

Serves: 6, Cooking Time: 65 minutes
Ingredients:

- ¼ cup chopped fresh parsley
- 1.5 oz Parmigiano-reggiano cheese, grated
- 1 tbsp kosher salt
- 10-oz whole wheat spaghetti, cooked and drained
- ¼ cup milk
- 1 14-oz can whole peeled tomatoes
- ½ cup white wine
- 2 tbsp tomato paste
- 1 tbsp minced garlic
- 8 cups finely chopped cremini mushrooms
- ½ lb. ground pork
- ½ tsp freshly ground black pepper, divided
- ¾ tsp kosher salt, divided
- 2 ½ cups chopped onion
- 1 tbsp olive oil
- 1 cup boiling water
- ½-oz dried porcini mushrooms

Directions for Cooking:

1) Let porcini stand in a boiling bowl of water for twenty minutes, drain (reserve liquid), rinse and chop. Set aside.
2) On medium-high fire, place a Dutch oven with olive oil and cook for ten minutes cook pork, ¼ tsp pepper, ¼ tsp salt and onions. Constantly mix to break ground pork pieces.
3) Stir in ¼ tsp pepper, ¼ tsp salt, garlic and cremini mushrooms. Continue cooking until liquid has evaporated, around fifteen minutes.
4) Stirring constantly, add porcini and sauté for a minute.
5) Stir in wine, porcini liquid, tomatoes and tomato paste. Let it simmer for forty minutes. Stir occasionally. Pour milk and cook for another two minutes before removing from fire.
6) Stir in pasta and transfer to a serving dish. Garnish with parsley and cheese before serving.

Nutrition Information:
Calories per Serving: 358; Carbs: 32.8g; Protein: 21.1g; Fat: 15.4g

Veggie Pasta with Shrimp, Basil and Lemon

Serves: 4, Cooking Time: 5 minutes
Ingredients:

- 2 cups baby spinach
- ½ tsp salt
- 2 tbsp fresh lemon juice
- 2 tbsp extra virgin olive oil
- 3 tbsp drained capers
- ¼ cup chopped fresh basil
- 1 lb. peeled and deveined large shrimp
- 4 cups zucchini, spirals

Directions for Cooking:

1) Bring a pot of water to a rolling boil and blanch zucchini and shrimp for 3 minutes or until desired softness is achieved. Remove from fire, drain and let stand for a minute while draining.
2) Meanwhile, in a large salad bowl, mix salt, lemon juice, olive oil, capers and basil.
3) Toss in zucchini and shrimps. Toss to mix well.
4) Evenly divide into 4 serving plates, top with ¼ cup of spinach, serve and enjoy.

Nutrition Information:
Calories per Serving: 51; Carbs: 4.4g; Protein: 1.8g; Fat: 3.4g

Veggies and Sun-Dried Tomato Alfredo

Serves: 4, Cooking Time: 30 minutes

Ingredients:
- 2 tsp finely shredded lemon peel
- ½ cup finely shredded Parmesan cheese
- 1 ¼ cups milk
- 2 tbsp all-purpose flour
- 8 fresh mushrooms, sliced
- 1 ½ cups fresh broccoli florets
- 4 oz fresh trimmed and quartered Brussels sprouts
- 4 oz trimmed fresh asparagus spears
- 1 tbsp olive oil
- 4 tbsp almond oil
- ½ cup chopped dried tomatoes
- 8 oz dried fettuccine

Directions for Cooking:
1) In a boiling pot of water, add fettuccine and cook following manufacturer's instructions. Two minutes before the pasta is cooked, add the dried tomatoes. Drain pasta and tomatoes and return to pot to keep warm. Set aside.
2) On medium-high fire, in a big fry pan with 1 tbsp almond oil, fry mushrooms, broccoli, Brussels sprouts and asparagus. Cook for eight minutes while covered, transfer to a plate and put aside.
3) Using same fry pan, add remaining almond oil and flour. Stirring vigorously, cook for a minute or until thickened. Add Parmesan cheese, milk and mix until cheese is melted around five minutes.
4) Toss in the pasta and mix. Transfer to serving dish. Garnish with Parmesan cheese and lemon peel before serving.

Nutrition Information:
Calories per Serving: 439; Carbs: 52.0g; Protein: 16.3g; Fat: 19.5g

Yangchow Chinese Style Fried Rice

Serves: 4, Cooking Time: 20 minutes

Ingredients:
- 4 cups cold cooked rice
- 1/2 cup peas
- 1 medium yellow onion, diced
- 5 tbsp olive oil
- 4 oz frozen medium shrimp, thawed, shelled, deveined and chopped finely
- 6 oz roast pork
- 3 large eggs
- Salt and freshly ground black pepper
- 1/2 tsp cornstarch

Directions for Cooking:
1) Combine the salt and ground black pepper and 1/2 tsp cornstarch, coat the shrimp with it. Chop the roasted pork. Beat the eggs and set aside.
2) Stir-fry the shrimp in a wok on high fire with 1 tbsp heated oil until pink, around 3 minutes. Set the shrimp aside and stir fry the roasted pork briefly. Remove both from the pan.
3) In the same pan, stir-fry the onion until soft, Stir the peas and cook until bright green. Remove both from pan.
4) Add 2 tbsp oil in the same pan, add the cooked rice. Stir and separate the individual grains. Add the beaten eggs, toss the rice. Add the roasted pork, shrimp, vegetables and onion. Toss everything together. Season with salt and pepper to taste.

Nutrition Information:
Calories per serving: 556; Carbs: 60.2g; Protein: 20.2g; Fat: 25.2g

Chapter 6 Breads, Flatbreads, Pizzas Recipes

Avocado and Spinach Breakfast Wrap

Serves: 4, Cooking Time: 10 minutes

Ingredients:

- ¼ tsp pepper
- ½ tsp salt
- 1 5-oz box or bag of baby spinach, chopped
- 1 avocado, sliced
- 4 egg whites
- 4 eggs
- 4 oz shredded pepper jack cheese
- 4 thin, whole wheat pita bread, 8-inch
- Hot sauce, optional
- Nonstick cooking spray

Directions for Cooking:

1) On medium-high fire, place a nonstick skillet greased with cooking spray.
2) Once hot, sauté spinach for 2 minutes or until wilted.
3) Meanwhile, in a small bowl whisk egg whites and eggs. Season with pepper and salt, whisk again. Pour into skillet and scramble. Cook for 3 to 4 minutes or to desired doneness.
4) Evenly divide egg into 4 equal portions and place in middle of pita bread and add 2 to 4 slices of avocadoes beside the egg and roll tortilla like a burrito.
5) Serve and enjoy with a side of hot sauce.

Nutrition Information:
Calories per Serving: 532; Carbs: 42.7g; Protein: 28.2g; Fat: 27.6g

Avocado and Tomato Sandwich

Serves: 4, Cooking Time: 0 minutes

Ingredients:

- 1 avocado, peeled and sliced into ¼-inch thick
- 1 large ripe tomato, thinly sliced
- 12 thin slices of cucumber
- 2 tbsp fat-free mayonnaise
- 4 large Romaine lettuce leaves
- 8 slices Manna Organic Ciao Chia Bread, toasted

Directions for Cooking:

1) On the 8 slices of bread, spread mayonnaise.
2) On 4 bread slices layer 1 lettuce leaf, 3 cucumber slices, ¼ avocado, and 1 tomato slice per bread. Top with remaining bread slices and cut diagonally in half before serving.

Nutrition Information:
Calories per Serving: 287.6; Carbs: 49.9g; Protein: 12.1g; Fat: 9.9g

Beef with Pesto Sandwich

Serves: 4, Cooking Time: 20 minutes

Ingredients:

- 4 slices mozzarella cheese
- ½ lb. thinly sliced roast beef deli
- ¼ cup basil pesto
- 2 tbsp olive oil
- 8 slices, ½-inch thick Italian bread

Directions for Cooking:

1) Spread the olive oil on one side of four of the bread slices, then top with pesto and evenly spread.
2) Top with beef, then cheese slices and cover with the bread slice.
3) Place on a Panini pan and grill until crispy. Serve and enjoy.

Nutrition Information:
Calories per Serving: 248; Carbs: 2.5g; Protein: 23.3g; Fat: 15.8g

Bread Dip and Topping Galore

Serves: 6, Cooking Time: 0 minutes

Ingredients:

- ¼ cup Balsamic Vinegar
- ¼ cup extra virgin olive oil
- ½ tbsp fresh basil, minced
- ½ tsp pepper
- ½ tsp salt
- 1 ½ tsp Italian seasoning
- 1 whole wheat French bread
- 2 cloves garlic minced
- 2 tbsp grated Parmesan Cheese or Asiago Cheese or combination
- 6 medium tomatoes, seeds discarded and cubed

Directions for Cooking:

1) In medium bowl, mix balsamic vinegar, olive oil, cheese, pepper, salt, Italian seasoning, and garlic. Mix well and set aside for at least 30 minutes.
2) In another medium bowl, place cubed tomatoes.
3) Slice the whole wheat French bread diagonally at least an inch thick and place on a serving platter.
4) Once the dip has been set aside for at least 30 minutes, add the fresh basil before serving.
5) To eat, you can add tomatoes on top of the bread and drizzle with the dip. You can also dip your bread on the dipping sauce. Either way you want to enjoy this delicious feast.
6) You can even prepare the dip ahead of time and can be a quick pick me up snack.

Nutrition Information:
Calories per Serving: 210; Fat: 10g; Protein: 6g; Carbs: 24g

Cheesy Mushroom Blend Panini

Serves: 4 , Cooking Time: 18 minutes

Ingredients:

- 1 garlic clove, halved
- Cooking spray
- 3 oz shaved Manchego cheese
- 8 slices 1-1/2-inch-thick sour dough bread
- 1 ½ tbsp. Sherry vinegar
- 1 package 8oz pre-sliced cremini mushrooms
- 2 packages 4 oz pre-sliced exotic mushroom blend (e.g. oyster, cremini and shiitake)
- ¼ tsp kosher salt
- ½ tsp ground black pepper
- 2 tsp minced fresh garlic
- 1 tbsp chopped fresh thyme
- ¼ cup minced shallots
- 1 tsp olive oil

Directions for Cooking:

1) On medium-high fire, heat oil in a skillet and sauté cremini mushrooms, exotic mushrooms, kosher salt, black pepper, fresh garlic, fresh thyme and minced shallots. Stir frequently and allow to cook until mushrooms are tender or for ten minutes. Pour in vinegar and continue cooking for 30-60 seconds more.
2) Evenly divide the mushroom mixture over 4 bread slices, top it with cheese and cover with remaining bread slices.
3) Grill in a Panini press until cheese is melted and bread is crisped and ridged.

Nutrition Information:
Calories per Serving: 259; Carbs: 22.2g; Protein: 10.3g; Fat: 14.4g

Cucumber, Chicken and Mango Wrap

Serves: 1, Cooking Time: 20 minutes

Ingredients:

- ½ of a medium cucumber cut lengthwise
- ½ of ripe mango
- 1 tbsp salad dressing of choice
- 1 whole wheat tortilla wrap
- 1-inch thick slice of chicken breast around 6-inch in length
- 2 tbsp oil for frying
- 2 tbsp whole wheat flour

- 2 to 4 lettuce leaves
- Salt and pepper to taste

Directions for Cooking:

1) Slice a chicken breast into 1-inch strips and just cook a total of 6-inch strips. That would be like two strips of chicken. Store remaining chicken for future use.
2) Season chicken with pepper and salt. Dredge in whole wheat flour.
3) On medium fire, place a small and nonstick fry pan and heat oil. Once oil is hot, add chicken strips and fry until golden brown around 5 minutes per side.
4) While chicken is cooking, place tortilla wraps in oven and cook for 3 to 5 minutes. Then remove from oven and place on a plate.
5) Slice cucumber lengthwise, use only ½ of it and store remaining cucumber. Peel cucumber cut into quarter and remove pith. Place the two slices of cucumber on the tortilla wrap, 1-inch away from the edge.
6) Slice mango and store the other half with seed. Peel the mango without seed, slice into strips and place on top of the cucumber on the tortilla wrap.
7) Once chicken is cooked, place chicken beside the cucumber in a line.
8) Add cucumber leaf, drizzle with salad dressing of choice.
9) Roll the tortilla wrap, serve and enjoy.

Nutrition Information:
Calories per Serving: 434; Fat: 10g; Protein: 21g; Carbohydrates: 65g

Feta, Beet & Hummus Wrap

Serves: 2, Cooking Time: 0 minutes
Ingredients:
- ½ cup peeled and grated beet
- ½ packed cup arugula, roughly chopped
- 2 6-inch sprouted or whole grain tortillas
- 2 tbsp feta
- 2 tbsp hummus

Directions for Cooking:
1) On each tortilla, leaving a 1 ½ inch border, spread 1 tbsp hummus.
2) Evenly sprinkle arugula, feta and beets.
3) Roll tortilla, by folding the sides of the tortilla on your left and right inward. Then holding the edge of the wrap near you, roll away from you.
4) Then cut tortilla diagonally in half.
5) Serve and enjoy.

Nutrition Information:
Calories per Serving: 53.5; Carbs: 33g; Protein: 5.2g; Fat: 2.3g

Fattoush Salad –Middle East Bread Salad

Serves: 6, Cooking Time: 15 minutes
Ingredients:
- 2 loaves pita bread
- 1 tbsp Extra Virgin Olive Oil
- 1/2 tsp sumac, more for later
- Salt and pepper
- 1 heart of Romaine lettuce, chopped
- 1 English cucumber, chopped
- 5 Roma tomatoes, chopped
- 5 green onions (both white and green parts), chopped
- 5 radishes, stems removed, thinly sliced
- 2 cups chopped fresh parsley leaves, stems removed
- 1 cup chopped fresh mint leaves

Dressing Ingredients:
- 1 1/2 lime, juice of
- 1/3 cup Extra Virgin Olive Oil
- Salt and pepper
- 1 tsp ground sumac
- 1/4 tsp ground cinnamon
- scant 1/4 tsp ground allspice

Directions for Cooking:
1) For 5 minutes toast the pita bread in the toaster oven. And then break the pita bread into pieces.
2) In a large pan on medium fire, heat 3 tbsp of olive oil in for 3 minutes. Add pita bread and fry until browned, around 4 minutes while tossing around.

3) Add salt, pepper and 1/2 tsp of sumac. Remove the pita chips from the heat and place on paper towels to drain.
4) Toss well the chopped lettuce, cucumber, tomatoes, green onions, sliced radish, mint leaves and parsley in a large salad bowl.
5) To make the lime vinaigrette, whisk together all ingredients in a small bowl.

6) Drizzle over salad and toss well to coat. Mix in the pita bread.
7) Serve and enjoy.
Nutrition Information:
Calories per Serving: 192; Carbs: 16.1g; Protein: 3.9g; Fats: 13.8g

Fruity and Cheesy Quesadilla

Serves: 1, Cooking Time: 15 minutes
Ingredients:
- ¼ cup hand grated jack cheese
- ½ cup finely chopped fresh mango
- 1 large whole-grain tortilla
- 1 tbsp chopped fresh cilantro
Directions for Cooking:
1) In a medium bowl, mix cilantro and mango.

2) Place mango mixture inside tortilla and top with cheese.
3) Pop in a preheated 350 degrees F oven and bake until cheese is melted completely around 10 to 15 minutes.
Nutrition Information:
Calories per Serving: 169; Fat: 9g; Protein: 7g; Carbohydrates: 15g

Garlic & Tomato Gluten Free Focaccia

Serves: 8, Cooking Time: 20 minutes
Ingredients:
- 1 egg
- ½ tsp lemon juice
- 1 tbsp honey
- 4 tbsp olive oil
- A pinch of sugar
- 1 ¼ cup warm water
- 1 tbsp active dry yeast
- 2 tsp rosemary, chopped
- 2 tsp thyme, chopped
- 2 tsp basil, chopped
- 2 cloves garlic, minced
- 1 ¼ tsp sea salt
- 2 tsp xanthan gum
- ½ cup millet flour
- 1 cup potato starch, not flour
- 1 cup sorghum flour
- Gluten free cornmeal for dusting
Directions for Cooking:
1) For 5 minutes, turn on the oven and then turn it off, while keeping oven door closed.

2) In a small bowl, mix warm water and pinch of sugar. Add yeast and swirl gently. Leave for 7 minutes.
3) In a large mixing bowl, whisk well herbs, garlic, salt, xanthan gum, starch, and flours.
4) Once yeast is done proofing, pour into bowl of flours. Whisk in egg, lemon juice, honey, and olive oil.
5) Mix thoroughly and place in a well-greased square pan, dusted with cornmeal.
6) Top with fresh garlic, more herbs, and sliced tomatoes.
7) Place in the warmed oven and let it rise for half an hour.
8) Turn on oven to 375 degrees F and after preheating time it for 20 minutes. Focaccia is done once tops are lightly browned.
9) Remove from oven and pan immediately and let it cool.
10) Best served when warm.
Nutrition Information:
Calories per Serving: 251; Carbs: 38.4g; Protein: 5.4g; Fat: 9.0g

Garlic-Rosemary Dinner Rolls

Serves: 8, Cooking Time: 20 minutes

Ingredients:

- 2 garlic cloves, minced
- 1 tsp dried crushed rosemary
- ½ tsp apple cider vinegar
- 2 tbsp olive oil
- 2 eggs
- 1 ¼ tsp salt
- 1 ¾ tsp xanthan gum
- ½ cup tapioca starch
- ¾ cup brown rice flour
- 1 cup sorghum flour
- 2 tsp dry active yeast
- 1 tbsp honey
- ¾ cup hot water

Directions for Cooking:

1) Mix well water and honey in a small bowl and add yeast. Leave it for exactly 7 minutes.
2) In a large bowl, mix the following with a paddle mixer: garlic, rosemary, salt, xanthan gum, sorghum flour, tapioca starch, and brown rice flour.
3) In a medium bowl, whisk well vinegar, olive oil, and eggs.
4) Into bowl of dry ingredients pour in vinegar and yeast mixture and mix well.
5) Grease a 12-muffin tin with cooking spray. Transfer dough evenly into 12 muffin tins and leave it 20 minutes to rise.
6) Then preheat oven to 375 degrees F and bake dinner rolls until tops are golden brown, around 17 to 19 minutes.
7) Remove dinner rolls from oven and muffin tins immediately and let it cool.
8) Best served when warm.

Nutrition Information:
Calories per Serving: 200; Carbs: 34.3g; Protein: 4.2g; Fat: 5.4g

Herbed Panini Fillet O'Fish

Serves: 4 , Cooking Time: 25 minutes

Ingredients:

- 4 slices thick sourdough bread
- 4 slices mozzarella cheese
- 1 portabella mushroom, sliced
- 1 small onion, sliced
- 6 tbsp oil
- 4 garlic and herb fish fillets

Directions for Cooking:

1) Prepare your fillets by adding salt, pepper and herbs (rosemary, thyme, parsley whatever you like). Then dredged in flour before deep frying in very hot oil. Once nicely browned, remove from oil and set aside.
2) On medium-high fire, sauté for five minutes the onions and mushroom in a skillet with 2 tbsp oil.
3) Prepare sourdough breads by layering the following over it: cheese, fish fillet, onion mixture and cheese again before covering with another bread slice.
4) Grill in your Panini press until cheese is melted and bread is crisped and ridged.

Nutrition Information:
Calories per Serving: 422; Carbs: 13.2g; Protein: 51.2g; Fat: 17.2g

Grilled Burgers with Mushrooms

Serves: 4, Cooking Time: 10 minutes

Ingredients:

- 2 Bibb lettuce, halved
- 4 slices red onion
- 4 slices tomato
- 4 whole wheat buns, toasted
- 2 tbsp olive oil
- ¼ tsp cayenne pepper, optional
- 1 garlic clove, minced
- 1 tbsp sugar
- ½ cup water
- 1/3 cup balsamic vinegar
- 4 large Portobello mushroom caps, around 5-inches in diameter

Directions for Cooking:
1) Remove stems from mushrooms and clean with a damp cloth. Transfer into a baking dish with gill-side up.
2) In a bowl, mix thoroughly olive oil, cayenne pepper, garlic, sugar, water and vinegar. Pour over mushrooms and marinate mushrooms in the ref for at least an hour.
3) Once the one hour is nearly up, preheat grill to medium-high fire and grease grill grate.
4) Grill mushrooms for five minutes per side or until tender. Baste mushrooms with marinade so it doesn't dry up.
5) To assemble, place ½ of bread bun on a plate, top with a slice of onion, mushroom, tomato and one lettuce leaf. Cover with the other top half of the bun. Repeat process with remaining ingredients, serve and enjoy.

Nutrition Information:
Calories per Serving: 244.1; Carbs: 32g; Protein: 8.1g; Fat: 9.3g

Grilled Sandwich with Goat Cheese

Serves: 4 , Cooking Time: 8 minutes
Ingredients:
- ½ cup soft goat cheese
- 4 Kaiser rolls 2-oz
- ¼ tsp freshly ground black pepper
- ¼ tsp salt
- 1/3 cup chopped basil
- Cooking spray
- 4 big Portobello mushroom caps
- 1 yellow bell pepper, cut in half and seeded
- 1 red bell pepper, cut in half and seeded
- 1 garlic clove, minced
- 1 tbsp olive oil
- ¼ cup balsamic vinegar

Directions for Cooking:
1) In a large bowl, mix garlic, olive oil and balsamic vinegar. Add mushroom and bell peppers. Gently mix to coat. Remove veggies from vinegar and discard vinegar mixture.
2) Coat with cooking spray a grill rack and the grill preheated to medium-high fire.
3) Place mushrooms and bell peppers on the grill and grill for 4 minutes per side. Remove from grill and let cool a bit.
4) Into thin strips, cut the bell peppers.
5) In a small bowl, combine black pepper, salt, basil and sliced bell peppers.
6) Horizontally, cut the Kaiser rolls and evenly spread cheese on the cut side. Arrange 1 Portobello per roll, top with 1/3 bell pepper mixture and cover with the other half of the roll.
7) Grill the rolls as you press down on them to create a Panini like line on the bread. Grill until bread is toasted.

Nutrition Information:
Calories per Serving: 317; Carbs: 41.7g; Protein: 14.0g; Fat: 10.5g

Halibut Sandwiches Mediterranean Style

Serves: 4 , Cooking Time: 23 minutes
Ingredients:
- 2 packed cups arugula or 2 oz.
- Grated zest of 1 large lemon
- 1 tbsp capers, drained and mashed
- 2 tbsp fresh flat leaf parsley, chopped
- ¼ cup fresh basil, chopped
- ¼ cup sun dried tomatoes, chopped
- ¼ cup reduced fat mayonnaise
- 1 garlic clove, halved
- 1 pc of 14 oz of ciabatta loaf bread with ends trimmed and split in half, horizontally
- 2 tbsp plus 1 tsp olive oil, divided
- Kosher salt and freshly ground pepper
- 2 pcs or 6 oz halibut fillets, skinned
- Cooking spray

Directions for Cooking:
1) Heat oven to 450 degrees F.
2) With cooking spray, coat a baking dish. Season halibut with a pinch of pepper and salt plus rub with a tsp of oil and place on baking dish. Then put in oven and bake until cooked or for ten to fifteen minutes. Remove from oven and let cool.

3) Get a slice of bread and coat with olive oil the sliced portions. Put in oven and cook until golden, around six to eight minutes. Remove from heat and rub garlic on the bread.
4) Combine the following in a medium bowl: lemon zest, capers, parsley, basil, sun dried tomatoes and mayonnaise. Then add the halibut, mashing with fork until flaked. Spread the mixture on one side of bread, add arugula and cover with the other bread half and serve.

Nutrition Information:
Calories per Serving: 125; Carbs: 8.0g; Protein: 3.9g; Fat: 9.2g

Italian Flat Bread Gluten-Free

Serves: 8, Cooking Time: 30 minutes
Ingredients:
- 1 tbsp apple cider
- 2 tbsp water
- ½ cup yogurt
- 2 tbsp olive oil
- 2 tbsp sugar
- 2 eggs
- 1 tsp xanthan gum
- ½ tsp salt
- 1 tsp baking soda
- 1 ½ tsp baking powder
- ½ cup potato starch, not potato flour
- ½ cup tapioca flour
- ¼ cup brown rice flour
- 1/3 cup sorghum flour

Directions for Cooking:
1) With parchment paper, line an 8 x 8-inch baking pan and grease parchment paper. Preheat oven to 375 degrees F.
2) Mix xanthan gum, salt, baking soda, baking powder, all flours, and starch in a large bowl.
3) Whisk well sugar and eggs in a medium bowl until creamed. Add vinegar, water, yogurt, and oil. Whisk thoroughly.
4) Pour in egg mixture into bowl of flours and mix well.
5) Transfer sticky dough into prepared pan and bake in the oven for 25 to 30 minutes.
6) If tops of bread start to brown a lot, cover top with foil and continue baking until done.
7) Remove from oven and pan right away and let it cool.
8) Best served when warm.

Nutrition Information:
Calories per Serving: 166; Carbs: 27.8g; Protein: 3.4g; Fat: 4.8g

Lemon Aioli and Swordfish Panini

Serves: 4 , Cooking Time: 25 minutes
Swordfish Panini Ingredients:
- 2 oz fresh arugula greens
- 1 loaf focaccia bread
- 2 cloves garlic minced
- 1 tbsp herbes de Provence
- Pepper and salt
- 4 pcs of 6oz swordfish fillet
- 1 ½ tbsp olive oil

Lemon Aioli Ingredients:
- ¼ tsp freshly ground black pepper
- ¼ tsp salt
- 1 clove garlic, minced
- 2 tbsp fresh lemon juice
- 1 lemon, zested
- 2/3 cup mayonnaise

Directions for Cooking:
1) In a small bowl, mix well all lemon Aioli ingredients and put aside.
2) Over medium-high fire, heat olive oil in skillet. Season with pepper, salt, minced garlic and herbs de Provence the swordfish. Then pan fry fish until golden brown on both sides, around 5 minutes per side.
3) Slice bread into four slices. Smear on the lemon aioli mixture on two bread slices, layer with arugula leaves and fried fish then cover with the remaining bread slices before grilling in a Panini press.
4) Grill until bread is crisped and ridged.

Nutrition Information:
Calories per Serving: 433; Carbs: 15.0g; Protein: 36.2g; Fat: 25.1g

Lemon, Buttered Shrimp Panini

Serves: 4 , Cooking Time: 10 minutes

Ingredients:
- 3 tbsp olive oil
- 1 baguette
- 1 tsp hot sauce
- 1 tbsp parsley
- 2 tbsp lemon juice
- 4 garlic cloves, minced
- 1 lb. shrimp peeled

Directions for Cooking:
1) Make a hollowed portion on your baguette.
2) Sauté the following on a skillet with oil, parsley, hot sauce, lemon juice and garlic. After a minute or two mix in the shrimps and sautéing for five minutes.
3) Scoop shrimps into baguette and grill in a Panini press until baguette is crisped and ridged.

Nutrition Information:
Calories per Serving: 262; Carbs: 14.1g; Protein: 26.1g; Fat: 10.8g

Mediterranean Baba Ghanoush

Serves: 4 , Cooking Time: 25 minutes

Ingredients:
- 1 bulb garlic
- 1 red bell pepper, halved and seeded
- 1 tbsp chopped fresh basil
- 1 tbsp olive oil
- 1 tsp black pepper
- 2 eggplants, sliced lengthwise
- 2 rounds of flatbread or pita
- Juice of 1 lemon

Directions for Cooking:
1) Grease grill grate with cooking spray and preheat grill to medium high.
2) Slice tops of garlic bulb and wrap in foil. Place in the cooler portion of the grill and roast for at least 20 minutes.
3) Place bell pepper and eggplant slices on the hottest part of grill.
4) Grill for at least two to three minutes each side.
5) Once bulbs are done, peel off skins of roasted garlic and place peeled garlic into food processor.
6) Add olive oil, pepper, basil, lemon juice, grilled red bell pepper and grilled eggplant.
7) Puree until smooth and transfer into a bowl.
8) Grill bread at least 30 seconds per side to warm.
9) Serve bread with the pureed dip and enjoy.

Nutrition Information:
Calories per Serving: 213.6; Carbs: 36.3g; Protein: 6.3g; Fat: 4.8g

Multi Grain & Gluten Free Dinner Rolls

Serves: 8, Cooking Time: 20 minutes

Ingredients:
- ½ tsp apple cider vinegar
- 3 tbsp olive oil
- 2 eggs
- 1 tsp baking powder
- 1 tsp salt
- 2 tsp xanthan gum
- ½ cup tapioca starch
- ¼ cup brown teff flour
- ¼ cup flax meal
- ¼ cup amaranth flour
- ¼ cup sorghum flour
- ¾ cup brown rice flour

Directions for Cooking:
1) Mix well water and honey in a small bowl and add yeast. Leave it for exactly 10 minutes.
2) In a large bowl, mix the following with a paddle mixer: baking powder, salt, xanthan gum, flax meal, sorghum flour, teff flour, tapioca starch, amaranth flour, and brown rice flour.
3) In a medium bowl, whisk well vinegar, olive oil, and eggs.

4) Into bowl of dry ingredients pour in vinegar and yeast mixture and mix well.
5) Grease a 12-muffin tin with cooking spray. Transfer dough evenly into 12 muffin tins and leave it for an hour to rise.
6) Then preheat oven to 375 degrees F and bake dinner rolls until tops are golden brown, around 20 minutes.
7) Remove dinner rolls from oven and muffin tins immediately and let it cool.
8) Best served when warm.

Nutrition Information:
Calories per Serving: 207; Carbs: 28.4g; Protein: 4.6g; Fat: 8.3g

Mushroom and Eggplant Vegan Panini

Serves: 4 , Cooking Time: 18 minutes

Ingredients:
- 4 thin slices Asiago Cheese
- 4 thin slices Swiss cheese
- ¼ cup fat-free ranch dressing
- 8 slices focaccia bread
- 2 tsp grated parmesan cheese
- 1 tsp onion powder
- 1 tsp garlic powder
- 4 slices ½-inch thick eggplant, peeled
- 1 cup fat-free balsamic vinaigrette
- 4 portobello mushroom caps
- 2 red bell peppers

Directions for Cooking:
1) Broil peppers in oven for five minutes or until its skin has blistered and blackened. Remove peppers and place in bowl while quickly covering with plastic wrap, let cool for twenty minutes before peeling off the skin and refrigerating overnight.
2) In a re-sealable bag, place mushrooms and vinaigrette and marinate in the ref for a night.
3) Next day, grill mushrooms while discarding marinade. While seasoning eggplant with onion and garlic powder then grill along with mushrooms until tender, around four to five minutes.
4) Remove mushrooms and eggplant from griller and top with parmesan.
5) On four slices of focaccia, smear ranch dressing evenly then layer: cheese, mushroom, roasted peppers and eggplant slices and cover with the remaining focaccia slices.
6) Grill in a Panini press until cheese has melted and bread is crisped and ridged.

Nutrition Information:
Calories per Serving: 574; Carbs: 77.1g; Protein: 29.6g; Fat: 19.9g

Panini with Chicken-Fontina

Serves: 2, Cooking Time: 45 minutes

Ingredients:
- ¼ Cup Arugula
- 2 oz sliced cooked chicken
- 3 oz fontina cheese thinly sliced
- 1 tbsp Dijon mustard
- 1 ciabatta roll
- ¼ cup water
- 1 tbsp + 1 tsp olive oil
- 1 large onion, diced

Directions for Cooking:
1) On medium low fire, place a skillet and heat 1 tbsp oil. Sauté onion and cook for 5 minutes. Pour in water while stirring and cooking continuously for 30 minutes until onion is golden brown and tender.
2) Slice bread roll lengthwise and spread the following on one bread half, on the cut side: mustard, caramelized onion, chicken, arugula and cheese. Cover with the remaining bread half.
3) Place the sandwich in a Panini maker and grill for 5 to 8 minutes or until cheese is melted and bread is ridged and crisped.

Nutrition Information:
Calories per Serving: 216; Carbs: 18.7g; Protein: 22.3g; Fat: 24.5g

Paleo Chocolate Banana Bread

Serves: 10, Cooking Time: 50 minutes

Ingredients:
- ¼ cup dark chocolate, chopped
- ½ cup almond butter
- ½ cup coconut flour, sifted
- ½ teaspoon cinnamon powder
- 1 teaspoon baking soda
- 1 teaspoon vanilla extract
- 4 bananas, mashed
- 4 eggs
- 4 tablespoon olive oil, melted
- A pinch of salt

Directions for Cooking:
1) Preheat the oven to 350 degrees F.
2) Grease an 8" x 8" square pan and set aside.
3) In a large bowl, mix together the eggs, banana, vanilla extract, almond butter and olive oil. Mix well until well combined.
4) Add the cinnamon powder, coconut flour, baking powder, baking soda and salt to the wet ingredients. Fold until well combined. Add in the chopped chocolates then fold the batter again.
5) Pour the batter into the greased pan. Spread evenly.
6) Bake in the oven for about 50 minutes or until a toothpick inserted in the center comes out clean.
7) Remove from the hot oven and cool in a wire rack for an hour.

Nutrition Information:
Calories per Serving: 150.3; Carbs: 13.9g; Protein: 3.2g; Fat: 9.1g

Panini and Eggplant Caponata

Serves: 4 , Cooking Time: 10 minutes

Ingredients:
- ¼ cup packed fresh basil leaves
- ¼ of a 7oz can of eggplant caponata
- 4 oz thinly sliced mozzarella
- 1 tbsp olive oil
- 1 ciabatta roll 6-7-inch length, horizontally split

Directions for Cooking:
1) Spread oil evenly on the sliced part of the ciabatta and layer on the following: cheese, caponata, basil leaves and cheese again before covering with another slice of ciabatta.
2) Then grill sandwich in a Panini press until cheese melts and bread gets crisped and ridged.

Nutrition Information:
Calories per Serving: 295; Carbs: 44.4g; Protein: 16.4g; Fat: 7.3g

Pesto, Avocado and Tomato Panini

Serves: 4 , Cooking Time: 10 minutes

Panini Ingredients:
- 2 tbsp extra virgin olive oil
- 8 oz fresh buffalo mozzarella cheese
- 2 vine-ripened tomatoes cut into ¼ inch thick slices
- 2 avocados, peeled, pitted, quartered and cut into thin strips
- 1 ciabatta loaf

Pesto Ingredients:
- Pepper and salt
- ½ lemon
- 1/3 cup extra virgin olive oil
- 1/3 cup parmesan cheese
- 1/3 cup pine nuts, toasted
- 1 ½ bunches fresh basil leaves
- 2 garlic cloves, peeled

Directions for Cooking:
1) To make the pesto, puree garlic in a food processor and transfer to a mortar and pestle and add in basil and smash into a coarse paste like consistency. Mix in the pine nuts and continue crushing. Once paste like, add the parmesan cheese and mix. Pour in olive oil

and blend thoroughly while adding lemon juice. Season with pepper and salt. Put aside.
2) Prepare Panini by slicing ciabatta loaf in three horizontal pieces. To prepare Panini, over bottom loaf slice layer the following: avocado, tomato, pepper, salt and mozzarella cheese. Then top with the middle ciabatta slice and repeat layering process again and cover with the topmost ciabatta bread slice.
3) Grill in a Panini press until cheese is melted and bred is crisped and ridged.

Nutrition Information:
Calories per Serving: 577; Carbs: 15.5g; Protein: 24.2g; Fat: 49.3g

Quinoa Pizza Muffins

Serves: 4 , Cooking Time: 30 minutes
Ingredients:
- 1 cup uncooked quinoa
- 2 large eggs
- ½ medium onion, diced
- 1 cup diced bell pepper
- 1 cup shredded mozzarella cheese
- 1 tbsp dried basil
- 1 tbsp dried oregano
- 2 tsp garlic powder
- 1/8 tsp salt
- 1 tsp crushed red peppers
- ½ cup roasted red pepper, chopped*
- Pizza Sauce, about 1-2 cups

Directions for Cooking:
1) Preheat oven to 350 degrees F.
2) Cook quinoa according to directions.
3) Combine all ingredients (except sauce) into bowl. Mix all ingredients well.
4) Scoop quinoa pizza mixture into muffin tin evenly. Makes 12 muffins.
5) Bake for 30 minutes until muffins turn golden in color and the edges are getting crispy.
6) Top with 1 or 2 tbsp pizza sauce and enjoy!

Nutrition Information:
Calories per Serving: 303; Carbs: 41.3g; Protein: 21.0g; Fat: 6.1g

Sandwich with Spinach and Tuna Salad

Serves: 4 , Cooking Time: 0 minutes
Ingredients:
- 1 cup fresh baby spinach
- 8 slices 100% whole wheat sandwich bread
- ¼ tsp freshly ground black pepper
- ½ tsp salt free seasoning blend
- Juice of one lemon
- 2 tbsp olive oil
- ½ tsp dill weed
- 2 ribs celery, diced

Directions for Cooking:
1) In a medium bowl, mix well dill weed, celery, onion, cucumber and tuna.

2) Add lemon juice and olive oil and mix thoroughly.
3) Season with pepper and salt-free seasoning blend.
4) To assemble sandwich, you can toast bread slices, on top of one bread slice layer ½ cup tuna salad, top with ¼ cup spinach and cover with another slice of bread.
5) Repeat procedure to remaining ingredients, serve and enjoy.

Nutrition Information:
Calories per Serving: 272.5; Carbs: 35.9g; Protein: 10.4g; Fat: 9.7g

Rosemary-Walnut Loaf Bread

Serves: 8, Cooking Time: 45 minutes
Ingredients:
- ½ cup chopped walnuts
- 4 tbsp fresh, chopped rosemary
- 1 1/3 cups lukewarm carbonated water
- 1 tbsp honey
- ½ cup extra virgin olive oil
- 1 tsp apple cider vinegar

- 3 eggs
- 5 tsp instant dry yeast granules
- 1 tsp salt
- 1 tbsp xanthan gum
- ¼ cup buttermilk powder
- 1 cup white rice flour
- 1 cup tapioca starch
- 1 cup arrowroot starch
- 1 ¼ cups all-purpose Bob's Red Mill gluten-free flour mix

Directions for Cooking:
1) In a large mixing bowl, whisk well eggs. Add 1 cup warm water, honey, olive oil, and vinegar.
2) While beating continuously, add the rest of the ingredients except for rosemary and walnuts.
3) Continue beating. If dough is too stiff, add a bit of warm water. Dough should be shaggy and thick.
4) Then add rosemary and walnuts continue kneading until evenly distributed.

5) Cover bowl of dough with a clean towel, place in a warm spot, and let it rise for 30 minutes.
6) Fifteen minutes into rising time, preheat oven to 400 degrees F.
7) Generously grease with olive oil a 2-quart Dutch oven and preheat inside oven without the lid.
8) Once dough is done rising, remove pot from oven, and place dough inside. With a wet spatula, spread top of dough evenly in pot.
9) Brush tops of bread with 2 tbsp of olive oil, cover Dutch oven and bake for 35 to 45 minutes.
10) Once bread is done, remove from oven. And gently remove bread from pot.
11) Allow bread to cool at least ten minutes before slicing.
12) Serve and enjoy.

Nutrition Information:
Calories per Serving: 424; Carbs: 56.8g; Protein: 7.0g; Fat: 19.0g

Sandwich with Hummus

Serves: 4 , Cooking Time: 0 minutes
Ingredients:
- 4 cups alfalfa sprouts
- 1 cup cucumber sliced 1/8 inch thick
- 4 red onion sliced ¼-inch thick
- 8 tomatoes sliced ¼-inch thick
- 2 cups shredded Bibb lettuce
- 12 slices 1-oz whole wheat bread
- 1 can 15.5-oz chickpeas, drained
- 2 garlic cloves, peeled
- ¼ tsp salt
- ½ tsp ground cumin
- 1 tbsp tahini
- 1 tbsp lemon juice
- 2 tbsp water

- 3 tbsp plain fat-free yogurt

Directions for Cooking:
1) In a food processor, blend chickpeas, garlic, salt, cumin, tahini, lemon juice, water and yogurt until smooth to create hummus.
2) On 1 slice of bread, spread 2 tbsp hummus, top with 1 onion slice, 2 tomato slices, ½ cup lettuce, another bread slice, 1 cup sprouts, ¼ cup cucumber and cover with another bread slice. Repeat procedure for the rest of the ingredients.

Nutrition Information:
Calories per Serving: 407; Carbs: 67.7g; Protein: 18.8 g; Fat: 6.8g

Sun-Dried Tomatoes Panini

Serves: 4, Cooking Time: 15 minutes
Ingredients:
- ½ cup shredded mozzarella cheese
- 8 slices country style Italian bread
- 1/8 tsp freshly ground black pepper
- Cooking spray
- 3/8 tsp salt, divided

- 1 6oz package fresh baby spinach
- 8 garlic cloves, thinly sliced
- 1/8 tsp crushed red pepper
- ¼ cup chopped drained oil packed sun-dried tomato

- 4 4oz chicken cutlets
- 1 tsp chopped rosemary
- 2 tbsp extra virgin olive oil, divided

Directions for Cooking:

1) In a re-sealable bag mix chicken, rosemary and 2 tsp olive oil. Allow to marinate for 30 minutes in the ref.
2) On medium-high fire, place a skillet and heat 4 tsp oil. Sauté for a minute garlic, red pepper and sun-dried tomato. Add 1/8 tsp salt and spinach and cook for a minute and put aside.

3) On a grill pan coated with cooking spray, grill chicken for three minutes per side. Season with black pepper and salt.
4) To assemble the sandwich, evenly layer the following on one bread slice: cheese, spinach mixture, and chicken cutlet. Cover with another bread slice.
5) Place sandwich in a Panini press and grill for around five minutes or until cheese is melted and bread is crisped and ridged.

Nutrition Information:
Calories per Serving: 369; Carbs: 25.7g; Protein: 42.7g; Fat: 10.1g

Sunflower Gluten Free Bread

Serves: 8, Cooking Time: 30 minutes

Ingredients:

- 1 tsp apple cider vinegar
- 3 tbsp olive oil
- 3 egg whites
- Extra seeds for sprinkling on top of loaf
- 1 ¼ tsp sea salt
- 2 ¾ tsp xanthan gum
- 2 tbsp hemp seeds
- 2 tbsp poppy seeds
- ¼ cup flax meal
- ¼ cup buckwheat flour
- ½ cup brown rice flour
- 1 cup tapioca starch
- 1 ½ cups sorghum flour
- 2 ½ tsp dry active yeast
- 1 tbsp honey
- 1 ¼ cup hot water

Directions for Cooking:

1) Mix honey and water in a small bowl. Add yeast and stir a bit and leave on for 7 minutes.
2) In a large mixing bowl, mix well salt, xanthan gum, hemp, poppy, flax meal, buckwheat flour, brown rice four, tapioca starch, and sorghum flour and beat with a paddle mixer.

3) In a medium bowl, beat well vinegar, oil, and eggs.
4) In bowl of dry ingredients, pour in bowl of egg mixture and yeast mixture and mix well until you have a smooth dough.
5) In a greased 10-inch cast iron skillet, transfer dough. Lightly wet hands with warm water and smoothen surface of dough until the surface is even. (A 9-inch cake pan will also do nicely if you don't have a cast iron skillet).
6) Sprinkle extra seeds on top of dough and leave dough in a warm corner for 45 to 60 minutes to rise.
7) Then pop risen dough in a 375 degrees F preheated oven until tops are golden brown, around 30 minutes.
8) Once done cooking, immediately remove dough from pan and let it cool a bit before slicing and serving.

Nutrition Information:
Calories per Serving: 291; Carbs: 49.1g; Protein: 6.0g; Fat: 8.5g

Tasty Crabby Panini

Serves: 4 , Cooking Time: 10 minutes

Ingredients:

- 1 tbsp Olive oil
- French bread split and sliced diagonally
- 1 lb. blue crab meat or shrimp or spiny lobster or stone crab
- ½ cup celery
- ¼ cup green onion chopped
- 1 tsp Worcestershire sauce
- 1 tsp lemon juice
- 1 tbsp Dijon mustard
- ½ cup light mayonnaise

Directions for Cooking:

1) In a medium bowl mix the following thoroughly: celery, onion, Worcestershire, lemon juice, mustard and mayonnaise. Season with pepper and salt. Then gently add in the almonds and crabs.
2) Spread olive oil on sliced sides of bread and smear with crab mixture before covering with another bread slice.
3) Grill sandwich in a Panini press until bread is crisped and ridged.

Nutrition Information:

Calories per Serving: 248; Carbs: 12.0g; Protein: 24.5g; Fat: 10.9g

Tuscan Bread Dipper

Serves: 8, Cooking Time: 0 minutes

Ingredients:

- ¼ cup balsamic vinegar
- ¼ cup extra virgin olive oil
- ¼ teaspoon salt
- ½ tbsp fresh basil, minced
- ½ teaspoon pepper
- 1 ½ teaspoon Italian seasoning
- 2 cloves garlic minced
- 8 pieces Food for Life Brown Rice English Muffins

Directions for Cooking:

1) In a small bowl mix well all ingredients except for bread. Allow herbs to steep in olive oil-balsamic vinegar mixture for at least 30 minutes.
2) To serve, toast bread, cut each muffin in half and serve with balsamic vinegar dip.

Nutrition Information:

Calories per Serving: 168.5; Carbs: 27.7g; Protein: 5.2g; Fat: 4.1g

Chapter 7 Salad Recipes

A Refreshing Detox Salad

Serves: 4, Cooking Time: 0 minutes
Ingredients:
- 1 large apple, diced
- 1 large beet, coarsely grated
- 1 large carrot, coarsely grated
- 1 tbsp chia seeds
- 2 tbsp almonds, chopped
- 2 tbsp lemon juice
- 2 tbsp pumpkin seed oil
- 4 cups mixed greens

Directions for Cooking:

1) In a medium salad bowl, except for mixed greens, combine all ingredients thoroughly.
2) Into 4 salad plates, divide the mixed greens.
3) Evenly top mixed greens with the salad bowl mixture.
4) Serve and enjoy.

Nutrition Information:
Calories per serving: 136.4; Protein: 1.93g; Carbs: 14.4g; Fat: 7.9g

Amazingly Fresh Carrot Salad

Serves: 4 , Cook Time: 0 minutes
Ingredients:
- ¼ tsp chipotle powder
- 1 bunch scallions, sliced
- 1 cup cherry tomatoes, halved
- 1 large avocado, diced
- 1 tbsp chili powder
- 1 tbsp lemon juice
- 2 tbsp olive oil
- 3 tbsp lime juice
- 4 cups carrots, spiralized
- salt to taste

Directions for Cooking:

1) In a salad bowl, mix and arrange avocado, cherry tomatoes, scallions and spiralized carrots. Set aside.
2) In a small bowl, whisk salt, chipotle powder, chili powder, olive oil, lemon juice and lime juice thoroughly.
3) Pour dressing over noodle salad. Toss to coat well.
4) Serve and enjoy at room temperature.

Nutrition Information:
Calories per Serving: 243.6; Fat: 14.8g; Protein: 3g; Carbs: 24.6g

Arugula with Blueberries 'n Almonds

Serves: 2, Cooking Time: 0 minutes
Ingredients:
- ½ cup slivered almonds
- ½ cup blueberries, fresh
- 1 ripe red pear, sliced
- 1 shallot, minced
- 1 tsp minced garlic
- 1 tsp whole grain mustard
- 2 tbsp fresh lemon juice
- 3 tbsp extra virgin olive oil
- 6 cups arugula

Directions for Cooking:

1) In a big mixing bowl, mix garlic, olive oil, lemon juice and mustard.
2) Once thoroughly mixed, add remaining ingredients.
3) Toss to coat.
4) Equally divide into two bowls, serve and enjoy.

Nutrition Information:
Calories per serving: 530.4; Protein: 6.1g; Carbs: 39.2g; Fat: 38.8g

Anchovy and Orange Salad

Serves: 4, Cooking Time: 0 minutes
Ingredients:

- 1 small red onion, sliced into thin rounds
- 1 tbsp fresh lemon juice
- 1/8 tsp pepper or more to taste
- 16 oil cure Kalamata olives
- 2 tsp finely minced fennel fronds for garnish
- 3 tbsp extra virgin olive oil
- 4 small oranges, preferably blood oranges
- 6 anchovy fillets

Directions for Cooking:

1) With a paring knife, peel oranges including the membrane that surrounds it.
2) In a plate, slice oranges into thin circles and allow plate to catch the orange juices.
3) On serving plate, arrange orange slices on a layer.
4) Sprinkle oranges with onion, followed by olives and then anchovy fillets.
5) Drizzle with oil, lemon juice and orange juice.
6) Sprinkle with pepper.
7) Allow salad to stand for 30 minutes at room temperature to allow the flavors to develop.
8) To serve, garnish with fennel fronds and enjoy.

Nutrition Information:
Calories per serving: 133.9; Protein: 3.2 g; Carbs: 14.3g; Fat: 7.1g

Asian Peanut Sauce Over Noodle Salad

Serves: 4, Cooking Time: 0 minutes
Ingredients:

- 1 cup shredded green cabbage
- 1 cup shredded red cabbage
- 1/4 cup chopped cilantro
- 1/4 cup chopped peanuts
- 1/4 cup chopped scallions
- 4 cups shiritake noodles (drained and rinsed)

Asian Peanut Sauce Ingredients:

- ¼ cup sugar-free peanut butter
- ¼ teaspoon cayenne pepper
- ½ cup filtered water
- ½ teaspoon kosher salt
- 1 tablespoon fish sauce (or coconut aminos for vegan)
- 1 tablespoon granulated erythritol sweetener
- 1 tablespoon lime juice
- 1 tablespoon toasted sesame oil
- 1 tablespoon wheat-free soy sauce
- 1 teaspoon minced garlic
- 2 tablespoons minced ginger

Directions for Cooking:

1) In a large salad bowl, combine all noodle salad ingredients and toss well to mix.
2) In a blender, mix all sauce ingredients and pulse until smooth and creamy.
3) Pour sauce over the salad and toss well to coat.
4) Evenly divide into four equal servings and enjoy.

Nutrition Information:
Calories per serving: 104; Protein: 7.0g; Carbs: 12.0g; Fat: 16.0g

Balela Salad from the Middle East

Serves: 6, Cooking Time: 0 minutes
Salad Ingredients:

- 1 jalapeno, finely chopped (optional)
- 1/2 green bell pepper, cored and chopped
- 2 1/2 cups grape tomatoes, slice in halves
- 1/2 cup sun-dried tomatoes
- 1/2 cup freshly chopped parsley leaves
- 1/2 cup freshly chopped mint or basil leaves
- 1/3 cup pitted Kalamata olives
- 1/4 cup pitted green olives
- 3 1/2 cups cooked chickpeas, drained and rinsed
- 3–5 green onions, both white and green parts, chopped

Dressing Ingredients:

- 1 garlic clove, minced

- 1 tsp ground sumac
- 1/2 tsp Aleppo pepper
- 1/4 cup Early Harvest Greek extra virgin olive oil
- 1/4 to 1/2 tsp crushed red pepper (optional)
- 2 tbsp lemon juice
- 2 tbsp white wine vinegar
- Salt and black pepper, a generous pinch to your taste

Directions for Cooking:

1) mix together the salad ingredients in a large salad bowl.
2) In a separate smaller bowl or jar, mix together the dressing ingredients.
3) Drizzle the dressing over the salad and gently toss to coat.
4) Set aside for 30 minutes to allow the flavors to mix.
5) Serve and enjoy.

Nutrition Information:
Calories per Serving: 257; Carbs: 30.5g; Protein: 8.4g; Fats: 12.6g

Asian Salad with pistachios

Serves: 6 , Cook Time: 0
Ingredients:
- ¼ cup chopped pistachios
- ¼ cup green onions, sliced
- 1 bunch watercress, trimmed
- 1 cup red bell pepper, diced
- 2 cups medium sized fennel bulb, thinly sliced
- 2 tbsp vegetable oil
- 3 cups Asian pears, cut into matchstick size
- 3 tbsp fresh lime juice

Directions for Cooking:

1) In a large salad bowl, mix pistachios, green onions, bell pepper, fennel, watercress and pears.
2) In a small bowl, mix vegetable oil and lime juice. Season with pepper and salt to taste.
3) Pour dressing to salad and gently mix before serving.

Nutrition Information:
Calories per Serving: 160; Protein: 3g; Fat: 1g; Carbs: 16g

Blue Cheese and Portobello Salad

Serves: 2, Cooking Time: 15 minutes
Ingredients:
- ½ cup croutons
- 1 tbsp merlot wine
- 1 tbsp water
- 1 tsp minced garlic
- 1 tsp olive oil
- 2 large Portobello mushrooms, stemmed, wiped clean and cut into bite sized pieces
- 2 pieces roasted red peppers (canned), sliced
- 2 tbsp balsamic vinegar
- 2 tbsp crumbled blue cheese
- 4 slices red onion
- 6 asparagus stalks cut into 1-inch sections
- 6 cups Bibb lettuce, chopped
- Ground pepper to taste

Directions for Cooking:
1) On medium fire, place a small pan and heat oil. Once hot, add onions and mushrooms. For 4 to 6 minutes, sauté until tender.

2) Add garlic and for a minute continue sautéing.
3) Pour in wine and cook for a minute.
4) Bring an inch of water to a boil in a pot with steamer basket. Once boiling, add asparagus, steam for two to three minutes or until crisp and tender, while covered. Once cooked, remove basket from pot and set aside.
5) In a small bowl whisk thoroughly black pepper, water, balsamic vinegar, and blue cheese.
6) To serve, place 3 cups of lettuce on each plate. Add 1 roasted pepper, ½ of asparagus, ½ of mushroom mixture, whisk blue cheese dressing before drizzling equally on to plates. Garnish with croutons, serve and enjoy.

Nutrition Information:
Calories per serving: 660.8; Protein: 38.5g; Carbs: 30.4g; Fat: 42.8g

Blue Cheese and Arugula Salad

Serves: 4, Cooking Time: 0 minutes

Ingredients:

- ¼ cup crumbled blue cheese
- 1 tsp Dijon mustard
- 1-pint fresh figs, quartered
- 2 bags arugula
- 3 tbsp Balsamic Vinegar
- 3 tbsp olive oil
- Pepper and salt to taste

Directions for Cooking:

1) Whisk thoroughly together pepper, salt, olive oil, Dijon mustard, and balsamic vinegar to make the dressing. Set aside in the ref for at least 30 minutes to marinate and allow the spices to combine.
2) On four serving plates, evenly arrange arugula and top with blue cheese and figs.
3) Drizzle each plate of salad with 1 ½ tbsp of prepared dressing.
4) Serve and enjoy.

Nutrition Information:

Calories per serving: 202; Protein: 2.5g; Carbs: 25.5g; Fat: 10g

Broccoli Salad Moroccan Style

Serves: 4, Cooking Time: 0 minutes

Ingredients:

- ¼ tsp sea salt
- ¼ tsp ground cinnamon
- ½ tsp ground turmeric
- ¾ tsp ground ginger
- ½ tbsp extra virgin olive oil
- ½ tbsp apple cider vinegar
- 2 tbsp chopped green onion
- 1/3 cup coconut cream
- ½ cup carrots, shredded
- 1 small head of broccoli, chopped

Directions for Cooking:

1) In a large salad bowl, mix well salt, cinnamon, turmeric, ginger, olive oil, and vinegar.
2) Add remaining ingredients, tossing well to coat.
3) Pop in the ref for at least 30 to 60 minutes before serving.

Nutrition Information:

Calories per serving: 90.5; Protein: 1.3g; Carbs: 4g; Fat: 7.7g

Charred Tomato and Broccoli Salad

Serves: 6, Cooking Time:0 minutes

Ingredients:

- ¼ cup lemon juice
- ½ tsp chili powder
- 1 ½ lbs. boneless chicken breast
- 1 ½ lbs. medium tomato
- 1 tsp freshly ground pepper
- 1 tsp salt
- 4 cups broccoli florets
- 5 tbsp extra virgin olive oil, divided to 2 and 3 tablespoons

Directions for Cooking:

1) Place the chicken in a skillet and add just enough water to cover the chicken. Bring to a simmer over high heat. Reduce the heat once the liquid boils and cook the chicken thoroughly for 12 minutes. Once cooked, shred the chicken into bite-sized pieces.
2) On a large pot, bring water to a boil and add the broccoli. Cook for 5 minutes until slightly tender. Drain and rinse the broccoli with cold water. Set aside.
3) Core the tomatoes and cut them crosswise. Discard the seeds and set the tomatoes cut side down on paper towels. Pat them dry.
4) In a heavy skillet, heat the pan over high heat until very hot. Brush the cut sides of the tomatoes with olive oil and place them on the pan. Cook the tomatoes until the sides are charred. Set aside.
5) In the same pan, heat the remaining 3 tablespoon olive oil over medium heat. Stir

the salt, chili powder and pepper and stir for 45 seconds. Pour over the lemon juice and remove the pan from the heat.

6) Plate the broccoli, shredded chicken and chili powder mixture dressing.

Nutrition Information:
Calories per serving: 210.8; Protein: 27.5g; Carbs: 6.3g; Fat: 8.4g

Chopped Chicken on Greek Salad

Serves: 4, Cooking Time: 0 minutes
Ingredients:

- ¼ tsp pepper
- ¼ tsp salt
- ½ cup crumbled feta cheese
- ½ cup finely chopped red onion
- ½ cup sliced ripe black olives
- 1 medium cucumber, peeled, seeded and chopped
- 1 tbsp chopped fresh dill
- 1 tsp garlic powder
- 1/3 cup red wine vinegar
- 2 ½ cups chopped cooked chicken
- 2 medium tomatoes, chopped
- 2 tbsp extra virgin olive oil
- 6 cups chopped romaine lettuce

Directions for Cooking:
1) In a large bowl, whisk well pepper, salt, garlic powder, dill, oil and vinegar.
2) Add feta, olives, onion, cucumber, tomatoes, chicken, and lettuce.
3) Toss well to combine.
4) Serve and enjoy.

Nutrition Information:
Calories per serving: 461.9; Protein: 19.4g; Carbs: 10.8g; Fat: 37.9g

Classic Greek Salad

Serves: 4, Cooking Time: 0 minutes
Ingredients:

- ¼ cup extra virgin olive oil, plus more for drizzling
- ¼ cup red wine vinegar
- 1 4-oz block Greek feta cheese packed in brine
- 1 cup Kalamata olives, halved and pitted
- 1 lemon, juiced and zested
- 1 small red onion, halved and thinly sliced
- 1 tsp dried oregano
- 1 tsp honey
- 14 small vine-ripened tomatoes, quartered
- 5 Persian cucumbers
- Fresh oregano leaves for topping, optional
- Pepper to taste
- Salt to taste

Directions for Cooking:
1) In a bowl of ice water, soak red onions with 2 tbsp salt.
2) In a large bowl, whisk well ¼ tsp pepper, ½ tsp salt, dried oregano, honey, lemon zest, lemon juice, and vinegar. Slowly pour olive oil in a steady stream as you briskly whisk mixture. Continue whisking until emulsified.
3) Add olives and tomatoes, toss to coat with dressing.
4) Alternatingly peel cucumber leaving strips of skin on. Trim ends slice lengthwise and chop in ½-inch thick cubes. Add into bowl of tomatoes.
5) Drain onions and add into bowl of tomatoes. Toss well to coat and mix.
6) Drain feta and slice into four equal rectangles.
7) Divide Greek salad into serving plates, top each with oregano and feta.
8) To serve, season with pepper and drizzle with oil and enjoy.

Nutrition Information:
Calories per serving: 365.5; Protein: 9.6g; Carbs: 26.2g; Fat: 24.7g

Cold Zucchini Noodle Bowl

Serves: 4, Cooking Time: 20 minutes
Ingredients:
- ¼ cup basil leaves, roughly chopped
- ¼ cup olive oil
- ¼ tsp sea salt
- ½ tsp salt1 tsp garlic powder
- 1 lb. peeled and uncooked shrimp
- 1 tsp lemon zest
- 1 tsp lime zest
- 2 tbsp almond oil
- 2 tbsp lemon juice
- 2 tbsp lime juice
- 3 clementine, peeled and separated
- 4 cups zucchini, spirals or noodles
- pinch of black pepper

Directions for Cooking:
1) Make zucchini noodles and set aside.
2) On medium fire, place a large nonstick saucepan and heat almond oil.
3) Meanwhile, pat dry shrimps and season with salt and garlic. Add into hot saucepan and sauté for 6 minutes or until opaque and cooked.
4) Remove from pan, transfer to a bowl and put aside.
5) Right away, add zucchini noodles to still hot pan and stir fry for a minute. Leave noodles on pan as you prepare the dressing.
6) Blend well salt, olive oil, juice and zest in a small bowl.
7) Then place noodles into salad bowl, top with shrimp, pour oil mixture, basil and clementine. Toss to mix well.
8) Refrigerate for an hour before serving.

Nutrition Information:
Calories per serving: 353.4; Carbs: 14.8g; Protein: 24.5g; Fat: 21.8g

Coleslaw Asian Style

Serves: 10 , Cook Time: 0 minutes
Ingredients:
- ½ cup chopped fresh cilantro
- 1 ½ tbsp minced garlic
- 2 carrots, julienned
- 2 cups shredded napa cabbage
- 2 cups thinly sliced red cabbage
- 2 red bell peppers, thinly sliced
- 2 tbsp minced fresh ginger root
- 3 tbsp brown sugar
- 3 tbsp soy sauce
- 5 cups thinly sliced green cabbage
- 5 tbsp creamy peanut butter
- 6 green onions, chopped
- 6 tbsp rice wine vinegar
- 6 tbsp vegetable oil

Directions for Cooking:
1) Mix thoroughly the following in a medium bowl: garlic, ginger, brown sugar, soy sauce, peanut butter, oil and rice vinegar.
2) In a separate bowl, blend well cilantro, green onions, carrots, bell pepper, Napa cabbage, red cabbage and green cabbage. Pour in the peanut sauce above and toss to mix well.
3) Serve and enjoy.

Nutrition Information:
Calories per Serving: 193.8; Protein: 4g; Fat: 12.6g; Carbs: 16.1g

Cucumber and Tomato Salad

Serves: 4, Cooking Time: 0 minutes
Ingredients:
- Ground pepper to taste
- Salt to taste
- 1 tbsp fresh lemon juice
- 1 onion, chopped
- 1 cucumber, peeled and diced
- 2 tomatoes, chopped
- 4 cups spinach

Directions for Cooking:
1) In a salad bowl, mix onions, cucumbers and tomatoes.

2) Season with pepper and salt to taste.
3) Add lemon juice and mix well.
4) Add spinach, toss to coat, serve and enjoy.

Nutrition Information:
Calories per Serving: 70.3; Fat: 0.3g; Protein: 1.3g; Carbohydrates: 7.1g

Cucumber Salad Japanese Style

Serves: 5 servings , Cook Time: 0 minutes
Ingredients:
- 1 ½ tsp minced fresh ginger root
- 1 tsp salt
- 1/3 cup rice vinegar
- 2 large cucumbers, ribbon cut
- 4 tsp sugar

Directions for Cooking:

1) Mix well ginger, salt, sugar and vinegar in a small bowl.
2) Add ribbon cut cucumbers and mix well.
3) Let stand for at least one hour in the ref before serving.

Nutrition Information
Calories per Serving: 29; Fat: .2g; Protein: .7g; Carbs: 6.1g

Easy Garden Salad with Arugula

Serves: 2 , Cook Time: 0
Ingredients:
- ¼ cup grated parmesan cheese
- ¼ cup pine nuts
- 1 cup cherry tomatoes, halved
- 1 large avocado, sliced into ½ inch cubes
- 1 tbsp rice vinegar
- 2 tbsp olive oil or grapeseed oil
- 4 cups young arugula leaves, rinsed and dried
- Black pepper, freshly ground
- Salt to taste

Directions For Cooking:

1) Get a bowl with cover, big enough to hold the salad and mix together the parmesan cheese, vinegar, oil, pine nuts, cherry tomatoes and arugula.
2) Season with pepper and salt according to how you like it. Place the lid and jiggle the covered bowl to combine the salad.
3) Serve the salad topped with sliced avocadoes.

Nutrition Information:
Calories per Serving: 490.8; Fat: 43.6g; Protein: 9.1g; Carbs: 15.5g

Easy Quinoa & Pear Salad

Serves: 6, Cooking Time: 0 minutes
Ingredients:
- ¼ cup chopped parsley
- ¼ cup chopped scallions
- ¼ cup lime juice
- ¼ cup red onion, diced
- ½ cup diced carrots
- ½ cup diced celery
- ½ cup diced cucumber
- ½ cup diced red pepper
- ½ cup dried wild blueberries
- ½ cup olive oil
- ½ cup spicy pecans, chopped
- 1 tbsp chopped parsley
- 1 tsp honey
- 1 tsp sea salt
- 2 fresh pears, cut into chunks
- 3 cups cooked quinoa

Directions for Cooking:
1) In a small bowl mix well olive oil, salt, lime juice, honey, and parsley. Set aside.
2) In large salad bowl, add remaining ingredients and toss to mix well.
3) Pour dressing and toss well to coat.
4) Serve and enjoy.

Nutrition Information:
Calories per serving: 382; Protein: 5.6g; Carbs: 31.4g; Fat: 26g

Easy-Peasy Club Salad

Serves: 3, Cooking Time: 0 minutes
Ingredients:
- ½ cup cherry tomatoes, halved
- ½ teaspoon garlic powder
- ½ teaspoon onion powder
- 1 cup diced cucumber
- 1 tablespoon Dijon mustard
- 1 tablespoon milk
- 1 teaspoon dried parsley
- 2 tablespoons mayonnaise
- 2 tablespoons sour cream
- 3 cups romaine lettuce, torn into pieces
- 3 large hard-boiled eggs, sliced
- 4 ounces cheddar cheese, cubed

Directions for Cooking:

1) Make the dressing by mixing garlic powder, onion powder, dried parsley, mayonnaise, and sour cream in a small bowl. Add a tablespoon of milk and mix well. If you want the dressing thinner, you can add more milk.
2) In a salad platter, layer salad ingredients with Dijon mustard in the middle.
3) Evenly drizzle with dressing and toss well to coat.
4) Serve and enjoy.

Nutrition Information:
Calories per serving: 335.5; Protein: 16.8g; Carbs: 7.9g; Fat: 26.3g

Fennel and Seared Scallops Salad

Serves: 4, Cooking Time: 10 minutes
Ingredients:
- ¼ tsp salt
- ½ large fennel bulb, halved, cored and very thinly sliced
- ½ tsp whole fennel seeds, freshly ground
- 1 large pink grapefruit
- 1 lb. fresh sea scallops, muscle removed, room temperature
- 1 tbsp olive oil, divided
- 1 tsp raw honey
- 12 whole almonds chopped coarsely and lightly toasted
- 4 cups red leaf lettuce, cored and torn into bite sized pieces
- A pinch of ground pepper

Directions for Cooking:
1) To catch the juices, work over a bowl. Peel and segment grapefruit. Strain the juice in a cup.
2) For the dressing, whisk together in a small bowl black pepper, 1/8 tsp salt, 1/8 tsp ground fennel, honey, 2 tsp water, 2 tsp oil and 3 tbsp of pomegranate juice. Set aside 1 tbsp of the dressing.
3) Pat scallops dry with a paper towel and season with remaining salt and ½ tsp ground fennel.
4) On medium fire, place a nonstick skillet and brush with 1 tsp oil. Once heated, add ½ of scallops and cook until lightly browned or for 5 minutes each side. Transfer to a plate and keep warm as you cook the second batch using the same process.
5) Mix together dressing, lettuce and fennel in a large salad bowl. Divide evenly onto 4 salad plates.
6) Evenly top each salad with scallops, grapefruit segments and almonds. Drizzle with reserved dressing, serve and enjoy.

Nutrition Information:
Calories per serving: 231.9; Protein: 25.3g; Carbs: 18.5g; Fat: 6.3g

Fruity Asparagus-Quinoa Salad

Serves: 8, Cooking Time: 25 minutes
Salad Ingredients:
- ¼ cup chopped pecans, toasted
- ½ cup finely chopped white onion
- ½ jalapeno pepper, diced
- ½ lb. asparagus, sliced to 2-inch lengths, steamed and chilled
- ½ tsp kosher salt

- 1 cup fresh orange sections
- 1 cup uncooked quinoa
- 1 tsp olive oil
- 2 cups water
- 2 tbsp minced red onion
- 5 dates, pitted and chopped

Dressing Ingredients:
- ¼ tsp ground black pepper
- ¼ tsp kosher salt
- 1 garlic clove, minced
- 1 tbsp olive oil
- 2 tbsp chopped fresh mint
- 2 tbsp fresh lemon juice
- Mint sprigs – optional

Directions for Cooking:
1) Wash and rub with your hands the quinoa in a bowl at least three times, discarding water each and every time.

2) On medium-high fire, place a large nonstick fry pan and heat 1 tsp olive oil. For two minutes, sauté onions before adding quinoa and sautéing for another five minutes.
3) Add ½ tsp salt and 2 cups water and bring to a boil. Lower fire to a simmer, cover and cook for 15 minutes. Turn off fire and let stand until water is absorbed.
4) Add pepper, asparagus, dates, pecans and orange sections into a salad bowl. Add cooked quinoa, toss to mix well.
5) In a small bowl, whisk mint, garlic, black pepper, salt, olive oil and lemon juice to create the dressing.
6) Pour dressing over salad, serve and enjoy.

Nutrition Information:
Calories per Serving: 173; Fat: 6.3g; Protein: 4.3g; Carbohydrates: 24.7g

Garden Salad with Balsamic Vinegar

Serves: 1, Cooking Time: 0 minutes
Ingredients:
- 1 cup baby arugula
- 1 cup spinach
- 1 tbsp craisins
- 1 tbsp almonds, shaved or chopped
- 1 tbsp balsamic vinegar
- ½ tbsp extra virgin olive oil

Directions for Cooking:

1) In a plate, mix arugula and spinach.
2) Top with craisins and almonds.
3) Drizzle olive oil and balsamic vinegar.
4) Serve and enjoy.

Nutrition Information:
Calories per serving: 206; Fat: 15 g; Protein: 5g; Carbohydrates: 14g

Garden Salad with Grapes

Serves: 6, Cooking Time: 0 minutes
Ingredients:
- ¼ tsp black pepper
- ¼ tsp salt
- ½ tsp stone-ground mustard
- 1 tsp chopped fresh thyme
- 1 tsp honey
- 1 tsp maple syrup
- 2 cups red grapes, halved
- 2 tbsp toasted sunflower seed kernels
- 2 tsp grapeseed oil
- 3 tbsp red wine vinegar
- 7 cups loosely packed baby arugula

Directions for Cooking:
1) In a small bowl whisk together mustard, syrup, honey and vinegar. Whisking continuously, slowly add oil.
2) In a large salad bowl, mix thyme, seeds, grapes and arugula.
3) Drizzle with the oil dressing, season with pepper and salt.
4) Gently toss to coat salad with the dressing.

Nutrition Information:
Calories per serving: 85.7; Protein: 1.6g; Carbs: 12.4g; Fat: 3.3g

Garden Salad with Oranges and Olives

Serves: 4 , Cooking Time: 15 minutes

Ingredients:

- ½ cup red wine vinegar
- 1 tbsp extra virgin olive oil
- 1 tbsp finely chopped celery
- 1 tbsp finely chopped red onion
- 16 large ripe black olives
- 2 garlic cloves
- 2 navel oranges, peeled and segmented
- 4 boneless, skinless chicken breasts, 4-oz each
- 4 garlic cloves, minced
- 8 cups leaf lettuce, washed and dried
- Cracked black pepper to taste

Directions for Cooking:

1) Prepare the dressing by mixing pepper, celery, onion, olive oil, garlic and vinegar in a small bowl. Whisk well to combine.
2) Lightly grease grate and preheat grill to high.
3) Rub chicken with the garlic cloves and discard garlic.
4) Grill chicken for 5 minutes per side or until cooked through.
5) Remove from grill and let it stand for 5 minutes before cutting into ½-inch strips.
6) In 4 serving plates, evenly arrange two cups lettuce, ¼ of the sliced oranges and 4 olives per plate.
7) Top each plate with ¼ serving of grilled chicken, evenly drizzle with dressing, serve and enjoy.

Nutrition Information:
Calories per serving: 259.8; Protein: 48.9g; Carbs: 12.9g; Fat: 1.4g

Ginger Yogurt Dressed Citrus Salad

Serves: 6, Cooking Time: minutes

Ingredients:

- 2/3 cup minced crystallized ginger
- 1 16-oz Greek yogurt
- ¼ tsp ground cinnamon
- 2 tbsp honey
- ½ cup dried cranberries
- 3 navel oranges
- 2 large tangerines, peeled
- 1 pink grapefruit, peeled

Directions for Cooking:

1) Into sections, break tangerines and grapefruit.
2) Cut tangerine sections into half.
3) Into thirds, slice grapefruit sections.
4) Cut orange pith and peel in half and slice oranges into ¼ inch thick rounds, then quartered.
5) In a medium bowl, mix oranges, grapefruit, tangerines and its juices.
6) Add cinnamon, honey and ½ cup of cranberries.
7) Cover and place in the ref for an hour.
8) In a small bowl, mix ginger and yogurt.
9) To serve, add a dollop of yogurt dressing onto a serving of fruit and sprinkle with cranberries.

Nutrition Information:
Calories per serving: 190; Protein: 2.9g; Carbs: 16.7g; Fat: 12.4g

Goat Cheese and Oregano Dressing Salad

Serves: 4, Cooking Time: 0 minutes

Ingredients:

- ¾ cup crumbled soft fresh goat cheese
- 1 ½ cups diced celery
- 1 ½ large red bell peppers, diced
- 1 tbsp chopped fresh oregano
- 1/3 cup chopped red onion
- 2 tbsp extra virgin olive oil
- 2 tbsp fresh lemon juice
- 4 cups baby spinach leaves, coarsely chopped

Directions for Cooking:

1) In a large salad bowl, mix oregano, lemon juice and oil.
2) Add pepper and salt to taste.

3) Mix in red onion, goat cheese, celery, bell peppers and spinach.
4) Toss to coat well, serve and enjoy.

Nutrition Information:
Calories per serving: 110.9; Protein: 6.9g; Carbs: 10.7g; Fat: 4.5g

Grape and Walnut Garden Salad

Serves: 2, Cooking Time: 0 minutes
Ingredients:
- ½ cup chopped walnuts, toasted
- 1 ripe persimmon
- ½ cup red grapes, halved lengthwise
- 1 shallot, minced
- 1 tsp minced garlic
- 1 tsp whole grain mustard
- 2 tbsp fresh lemon juice
- 3 tbsp extra virgin olive oil
- 6 cups baby spinach

Directions for Cooking:
1) Cut persimmon and red pear into ½-inch cubes. Discard seeds.
2) In a medium bowl, whisk garlic, shallot, olive oil, lemon juice and mustard to make the dressing.
3) In a medium salad bowl, toss to mix spinach, pear and persimmon.
4) Pour in dressing and toss to coat well.
5) Garnish with pecans.
6) Serve and enjoy.

Nutrition Information:
Calories per serving: 440; Protein: 6.1g; Carbs: 39.1g; Fat: 28.8g

Greek Antipasto Salad

Serves: 4, Cooking Time: 0 minutes
Ingredients:
- ½ cup artichoke hearts, chipped
- ½ cup olives, sliced
- ½ cup sweet peppers, roasted
- 1 large head romaine lettuce, chopped
- 4 ounces cooked prosciutto, cut into thin strips
- 4 ounces cooked salami, cubed
- Italian dressing to taste

Directions for Cooking:
1) In a large mixing bowl, add all the ingredients except the Italian dressing. Mix everything until the vegetables are evenly distributed.
2) Add the Italian dressing and toss to combine.
3) Serve chilled.

Nutrition Information:
Calories per Serving: 425.8; Fat: 38.9 g; Protein: 39.2 g; Carbs: 12.6 g

Grilled Halloumi Cheese Salad

Serves: 1, Cooking Time: 10 minutes
Ingredients:
- 0.5 oz chopped walnuts
- 1 handful baby arugula
- 1 Persian cucumber, sliced into circles about ½-inch thick
- 3 oz halloumi cheese
- 5 grape tomatoes, sliced in half
- balsamic vinegar
- olive oil
- salt

Directions for Cooking:
1) Into 1/3 slices, cut the cheese. For 3 to 5 minutes each side, grill the kinds of cheese until you can see grill marks.
2) In a salad bowl, add arugula, cucumber, and tomatoes. Drizzle with olive oil and balsamic vinegar. Season with salt and toss well coat.
3) Sprinkle walnuts and add grilled halloumi.
4) Serve and enjoy.

Nutrition Information:
Calories per serving: 543; Protein: 21.0g; Carbs: 9.0g; Fat: 47.0g

Grilled Eggplant Salad

Serves: 4, Cooking Time: 18 minutes

Ingredients:

- 1 avocado, halved, pitted, peeled and cubed
- 1 Italian eggplant, cut into 1-inch thick slices
- 1 large red onion, cut into rounds
- 1 lemon, zested
- 1 tbsp coarsely chopped oregano leaves
- 1 tbsp red wine vinegar
- 1 tsp Dijon mustard
- Canola oil
- Freshly ground black pepper
- Honey
- Olive oil
- Parsley sprigs for garnish
- Salt

Directions for Cooking:

1) With canola oil, brush onions and eggplant and place on grill.
2) Grill on high until onions are slightly charred and eggplants are soft around 5 minutes for onions and 8 to 12 minutes for eggplant.
3) Remove from grill and let cool for 5 minutes.
4) Roughly chop eggplants and onions and place in salad bowl.
5) Add avocado and toss to mix.
6) Whisk oregano, mustard and red wine vinegar in a small bowl.
7) Whisk in olive oil and honey to taste. Season with pepper and salt to taste.
8) Pour dressing to eggplant mixture, toss to mix well.
9) Garnish with parsley sprigs and lemon zest before serving.

Nutrition Information:
Calories per serving: 190; Protein: 2.9g; Carbs: 16.7g; Fat: 12.4g

Grilled Vegetable Salad

Serves: 3 , Cook Time: 7 minutes

Ingredients:

- ¼ cup extra virgin olive oil, for brushing
- ¼ cup fresh basil leaves
- ¼ lb. feta cheese
- ½ bunch asparagus, trimmed and cut into bite-size pieces
- 1 medium onion, cut into ½ inch rings
- 1-pint cherry tomatoes
- 1 red bell pepper, quartered, seeds and ribs removed
- 1 yellow bell pepper, quartered, seeds and ribs removed
- Pepper and salt to taste

Directions for Cooking:

1) Toss olive oil and vegetables in a big bowl. Season with salt and pepper.
2) Frill vegetables in a preheated griller for 5-7 minutes or until charred and tender.
3) Transfer veggies to a platter, add feta and basil.
4) In a separate small bowl, mix olive oil, balsamic vinegar, garlic seasoned with pepper and salt.
5) Drizzle dressing over vegetables and serve.

Nutritional Information:
Calories per Serving: 147.6; Protein: 3.8g; Fat: 19.2g; Carbs: 13.9 g

Healthy Detox Salad

Serves: 4, Cooking Time: 0 minutes

Ingredients:

- 4 cups mixed greens
- 2 tbsp lemon juice
- 2 tbsp pumpkin seed oil
- 1 tbsp chia seeds
- 2 tbsp almonds, chopped
- 1 large apple, diced
- 1 large carrot, coarsely grated
- 1 large beet, coarsely grated

Directions for Cooking:

1) In a medium salad bowl, except for mixed greens, combine all ingredients thoroughly.

2) Into 4 salad plates, divide the mixed greens.
3) Evenly top mixed greens with the salad bowl mixture.
4) Serve and enjoy.

Nutrition Information:
Calories per serving: 141; Protein: 2.1g; Carbs: 14.7g; Fat: 8.2g

Herbed Calamari Salad

Serves: 6, Cooking Time: 25 minutes
Ingredients:
- ¼ cup finely chopped cilantro leaves
- ¼ cup finely chopped mint leaves
- ¼ tsp freshly ground black pepper
- ½ cup finely chopped flat leaf parsley leaves
- ¾ tsp kosher salt
- 2 ½ lbs. cleaned and trimmed uncooked calamari rings and tentacles, defrosted
- 3 medium garlic cloves, smashed and minced
- 3 tbsp extra virgin olive oil
- A pinch of crushed red pepper flakes
- Juice of 1 large lemon
- Peel of 1 lemon, thinly sliced into strips

Directions for Cooking:
1) On a nonstick large fry pan, heat 1 ½ tbsp olive oil. Once hot, sauté garlic until fragrant around a minute.
2) Add calamari, making sure that they are in one layer, if pan is too small then cook in batches.
3) Season with pepper and salt, after 2 to 4 minutes of searing, remove calamari from pan with a slotted spoon and transfer to a large bowl. Continue cooking remainder of calamari.
4) Season cooked calamari with herbs, lemon rind, lemon juice, red pepper flakes, pepper, salt, and remaining olive oil.
5) Toss well to coat, serve and enjoy.

Nutrition Information:
Calories per serving: 551.7; Protein: 7.3g; Carbs: 121.4g; Fat: 4.1g

Herbed Chicken Salad Greek Style

Serves: 6 , Cook Time: 0 minutes
Ingredients:
- ¼ cup or 1 oz crumbled feta cheese
- ½ tsp garlic powder
- ½ tsp salt
- ¾ tsp black pepper, divided
- 1 cup grape tomatoes, halved
- 1 cup peeled and chopped English cucumbers
- 1 cup plain fat-free yogurt
- 1 pound skinless, boneless chicken breast, cut into 1-inch cubes
- 1 tsp bottled minced garlic
- 1 tsp ground oregano
- 2 tsp sesame seed paste or tahini
- 5 tsp fresh lemon juice, divided
- 6 pitted kalamata olives, halved
- 8 cups chopped romaine lettuce
- Cooking spray

Directions for Cooking:
1) In a bowl, mix together ¼ tsp salt, ½ tsp pepper, garlic powder and oregano. Then on medium-high heat place a skillet and coat with cooking spray and sauté together the spice mixture and chicken until chicken is cooked. Before transferring to bowl, drizzle with juice.
2) In a small bowl, mix thoroughly the following: garlic, tahini, yogurt, ¼ tsp pepper, ¼ tsp salt, and 2 tsp juice.
3) In another bowl, mix together olives, tomatoes, cucumber and lettuce.
4) To Serve salad, place 2 ½ cups of lettuce mixture on plate, topped with ½ cup chicken mixture, 3 tbsp yogurt mixture and 1 tbsp of cheese.

Nutrition Information:
Calories per Serving: 170.1; Fat: 3.7g; Protein: 20.7g; Carbs: 13.5g

Kale Salad Recipe

Serves: 4, Cooking Time: 7 minutes
Ingredients:
- ¼ cup Kalamata olives
- ½ of a lemon
- 1 ½ tbsp flaxseeds
- 1 garlic clove, minced
- 1 small cucumber, sliced thinly
- 1 tbsp extra virgin olive oil
- 2 tbsp green onion, chopped
- 2 tbsp red onion, minced
- 6 cups dinosaur kale, chopped
- a pinch of dried basil
- a pinch of salt

Directions for Cooking:

1) Bring a medium pot, half-filled with water to a boil.
2) Rinse kale and cut into small strips. Place in a steamer and put on top of boiling water and steam for 5 – 7 minutes.
3) Transfer steamed kale to a salad bowl.
4) Season kale with oil, salt, basil and lemon. Toss to coat well.
5) Add remaining ingredients into salad bowl, toss to mix.
6) Serve and enjoy.

Nutrition Information:
Calories per serving: 92.7; Protein: 2.4g; Carbs: 6.6g; Fat: 6.3g

Lemony Lentil Salad with Salmon

Serves: 6, Cooking Time: 0 minutes
Ingredients:
- ¼ tsp salt
- ½ cup chopped red onion
- 1 cup diced seedless cucumber
- 1 medium red bell pepper, diced
- 1/3 cup extra virgin olive oil
- 1/3 cup fresh dill, chopped
- 1/3 cup lemon juice
- 2 15oz cans of lentils
- 2 7oz cans of salmon, drained and flaked
- 2 tsp Dijon mustard

- Pepper to taste

Directions for Cooking:
1) In a bowl, mix together, lemon juice, mustard, dill, salt and pepper.
2) Gradually add the oil, bell pepper, onion, cucumber, salmon flakes and lentils.
3) Toss to coat evenly.

Nutrition Information:
Calories per serving: 349.1; Protein: 27.1g; Carbs: 35.2g; Fat: 11.1g

Mouthwatering Steakhouse Salad

Serves: 4, Cooking Time: 30 minutes
Ingredients:
- ½ tsp pepper
- ½ tsp salt
- 1 lb. green beans, trimmed
- 10oz timed filet mignon
- 2 garlic cloves
- 2 tsp extra virgin olive oil
- 3 tbsp balsamic vinegar
- 4 medium red bell peppers, seeded and halved
- 6 medium tomatoes cut into ¼ wedges
- 8 cups mesclun

Directions for Cooking:

1) Preheat the grill or the broiler. Put the red peppers on the grill and cook until the skin blisters and chars. Peel away blackened skins and cut into chunks.
2) Meanwhile, lay the filet mignon on a cutting board and slit it lengthwise until it opens like a book when pressed flat. Sprinkle with ¼ teaspoon salt and ¼ teaspoon pepper. Cut 1 garlic clove and rub the cut sides all over the steak. Grill the beef until done. Slice it thinly and set aside.

3) In a saucepan, cook the beans in the boiling water until tender. Drain and rinse with cold water. Set aside.
4) Mince the remaining garlic and add to vinegar, oil and shallot. Season with salt and pepper.

5) In a plate, prepare a mesclun bead and arrange the steak, beans, tomatoes and red peppers on top. Drizzle with the dressing. Serve warm.

Nutrition Information:
Calories per serving: 220.3; Protein: 21.6g; Carbs: 21.1g; Fat: 5.5g

Mozzarella and Fig Salad

Serves: 4 , Cook Time: 3 minutes
Ingredients:
- 0.10 lbs of toasted and chopped hazelnut
- 0.45 lb of trimmed green beans
- ¼ lb mozzarella, ripped into chunks
- 1 shallot, sliced thinly
- 1 tbsp fig jam or relish
- 3 tbsp balsamic vinegar
- 3 tbsp extra virgin olive oil
- 6 small figs, quartered
- Small handful of basil leaves, torn

Directions for Cooking:
1) For two to three minutes, blanch beans in salted water. Then remove the water, wash with cold tap water, drain and let dry on top of kitchen towel.
2) Once the beans are dried, place on a food platter and add basil, hazelnuts, mozzarella, shallots and figs.
3) To create dressing, use a medium lidded jar and add your choice of seasoning, olive oil, fig jam and vinegar. Cover the jar and shake vigorously before pouring over the salad.

Nutrition Information:
Calories per Serving: 294.8; Fat: 17.6g; Protein: 12.7g; Carbs: 21.4g

Mustard Potato Salad

Serves: 6, Cooking Time: 6 minutes
Ingredients:
- 1 1/2 lb. baby potatoes (gold or red potatoes), unpeeled
- Water
- 2 tsp salt
- 1/4 cup chopped red onions
- 1/4 cup fresh chopped parsley
- 1/4 cup chopped dill
- 2 tbsp capers

Dijon Vinaigrette Ingredients:
- 1/3 cup extra virgin olive oil
- 2 tbsp white wine vinegar
- 2 tsp Dijon mustard
- 1/2 tsp ground sumac
- 1/2 tsp black pepper
- 1/4 tsp ground coriander

Directions for Cooking:
1) Wash and dry potatoes.
2) Slice potatoes thinly with a mandolin.

3) In a pot, place potatoes. Add 3 cups water and bring to a boil. Once simmering, add salt and simmer for 6 minutes.
4) In the meantime, add vinaigrette ingredients to a small bowl and whisk until well-combined
5) Once potatoes are cooked, drain. Place potatoes on a tray and immediately add the vinaigrette (while potatoes are warm), toss to coat.
6) Let potatoes sit for 10 minutes until flavors meld.
7) Add onions, fresh herbs, and capers. Toss gently to combine.
8) Evenly divide potatoes into bowls, serve, and enjoy.

Nutrition Information:
Calories per Serving: 199; Carbs: 20.3g; Protein: 2.7g; Fats: 12.7g

Nutty, Curry-Citrus Garden Salad

Serves: 2, Cooking Time: 0 minutes
Ingredients:

- ¼ tsp curry powder
- 1 medium carrot, shredded
- 1 tsp Balsamic vinegar
- 2 cups spring mix salad greens
- 2 tbsp orange juice
- 2 tsp extra virgin olive oil
- 8 pecan halves, chopped
- Pepper and salt to taste

Directions for Cooking:

1) In a small bowl, whisk well curry powder, balsamic vinegar, olive oil, and orange juice.
2) Season with pepper and salt to taste. Mix well.
3) In a salad bowl, mix shredded carrot and salad greens.
4) Pour in dressing, toss well to coat.
5) To serve, top with chopped pecans and enjoy.

Nutrition Information:
Calories per serving: 117; Protein: 2.39g; Carbs: 10.2g; Fat: 7.4g

Pecans and Spinach Salad

Serves: 2, Cooking Time: 15 minutes
Ingredients:

- ½ avocado
- ½ cup cherry tomatoes
- ½ ripe nectarine
- 1/3 cup raw pecans
- 2 cups baby spinach leaves
- 2 tsp avocado oil
- 6 oz. wild caught salmon fillet with skin

Vinaigrette Ingredients:

- ¼ tsp Paleo Dijon style mustard
- 2 tsp fresh lemon juice
- 3 tsp walnut oil
- Freshly ground black pepper to taste

Directions for Cooking:

1) Place a cast iron pan on medium-high fire and melt avocado oil. Preheat oven to 400 degrees F.
2) Once oil is hat sear salmon on both sides for 2 minutes per side. Pop in oven and bake for 10 minutes.
3) In a small bowl whisk all vinaigrette ingredients until emulsified. Season with pepper to taste and set aside.
4) Chop pecans into small pieces. Chop avocado, tomatoes, and nectarines into bite-sized pieces and place in a large salad bowl.
5) Add spinach and chopped pecans in bowl. Pour dressing and toss to coat well.
6) Serve salad with roasted salmon on top.

Nutrition Information:
Calories per serving: 388.4; Protein: 4.1g; Carbs: 23.7g; Fat: 30.8g

Riced Cauliflower & Snap Peas

Serves: 4, Cooking Time: 10 minutes
Ingredients:

- 1 clove garlic crushed
- 8 ounces cauliflower riced
- 1/2 cup sliced almonds
- 1/2 cup sugar snap peas end removed, and each pod cut into three pieces
- 1/2 teaspoon coarse grain Dijon mustard
- 1/2 teaspoon sea salt
- 1/4 cup chives
- 1/4 cup lemon juice
- 1/4 cup olive oil
- 1/4 cup red onions minced
- 1/4 teaspoon pepper

Directions for Cooking:

1) Place riced cauliflower in a large microwave safe bowl and microwave on high for 3 minutes. Stir and microwave again for another 2 minutes. Stir and let it cool in the fridge.

2) Meanwhile, make the dressing by adding olive oil in a medium bowl. With a wire whisk, continuously whisk as you slowly add lemon juice. Whisk in salt, pepper, mustard, and garlic.
3) Take out the cooled the bowl of cooked riced cauliflower. Add red onion, almonds, chives, and peas. Mix well. Add dressing and toss well to coat.

4) Transfer mixture into a container with an airtight lid and let it sit covered in the fridge for at least 4 hours to allow the flavors to settle.
5) Serve and enjoy cold.

Nutrition Information:
Calories per serving: 220; Protein: 4.0g; Carbs: 6.0g; Fat: 20.0g

Raw Winter Persimmon Salad

Serves: 2 , Cook Time: 0 minutes
Ingredients:

- ½ cup coarsely chopped pistachio
- ½ cup sweet potato, spiralized
- 1 red bell pepper, diced
- 1 red bell pepper, julienned
- 1 ripe fuyu persimmon, diced
- 1 tbsp chili powder
- 2 fuyu persimmon, sliced
- 3 tbsp lime juice
- 4 cups mixed greens
- a pinch of chipotle powder
- salt to taste

Directions for Cooking:
1) In a salad bowl, mix and arrange persimmons, bell pepper and sweet potatoes. Set aside.
2) In a food processor, puree salt, lime juice, chipotle powder, chili powder, diced persimmon and diced bell pepper until smooth and creamy.
3) Pour over salad, toss to mix.
4) Serve and enjoy.

Nutrition Information:
Calories per Serving: 467.4; Fat: 15.4g; Protein: 11.3g; Carbs: 70.9g

Sunflower Seeds and Arugula Garden Salad

Serves: 6, Cooking Time: 0 minutes
Ingredients:

- ¼ tsp black pepper
- ¼ tsp salt
- 1 tsp fresh thyme, chopped
- 2 tbsp sunflower seeds, toasted
- 2 cups red grapes, halved
- 7 cups baby arugula, loosely packed
- 1 tbsp olive oil
- 2 tsp honey
- 3 tbsp red wine vinegar
- ½ tsp stone-ground mustard

Directions for Cooking:
1) In a small bowl, whisk together mustard, honey and vinegar. Slowly pour oil as you whisk.
2) In a large salad bowl, mix thyme, seeds, grapes and arugula.
3) Drizzle with dressing and serve.

Nutrition Information:
Calories per serving: 86.7; Protein: 1.6g; Carbs: 13.1g; Fat: 3.1g

Red Wine Dressed Arugula Salad

Serves: 2, Cooking Time: 12 minutes
Ingredients:

- ¼ cup red onion, sliced thinly
- 1 ½ tbsp fresh lemon juice
- 1 ½ tbsp olive oil
- 1 tbsp extra-virgin olive oil

- 1 tbsp red-wine vinegar
- 2 center cut salmon fillets (6-oz each)
- 2/3 cup cherry tomatoes, halved
- 3 cups baby arugula leaves

- Pepper and salt to taste

Directions for Cooking:
1) In a shallow bowl, mix pepper, salt, 1 ½ tbsp olive oil and lemon juice. Toss in salmon fillets and rub with the marinade. Allow to marinate for at least 15 minutes.
2) Grease a baking sheet and preheat oven to 350 degrees F.

3) Bake marinated salmon fillet for 10 to 12 minutes or until flaky with skin side touching the baking sheet.
4) Meanwhile, in a salad bowl mix onion, tomatoes and arugula.
5) Season with pepper and salt. Drizzle with vinegar and oil. Toss to combine and serve right away with baked salmon on the side.

Nutrition Information:
Calories per serving: 400; Protein: 36.6g; Carbs: 5.8g; Fat: 25.6g

Salad Greens with Pear and Persimmon

Serves: 2, Cooking Time: 0 minutes

Ingredients:
- ½ cup chopped pecans, toasted
- 1 ripe persimmon, sliced
- 1 ripe red pear, sliced
- 1 shallot, minced
- 1 tsp minced garlic
- 1 tsp whole grain mustard
- 2 tbsp fresh lemon juice
- 3 tbsp extra virgin olive oil
- 6 cups baby spinach

Directions for Cooking:

1) In a big mixing bowl, mix garlic, olive oil, lemon juice and mustard.
2) Once thoroughly mixed, add remaining ingredients.
3) Toss to coat.
4) Equally divide into two bowls, serve and enjoy.

Nutrition Information:
Calories per serving: 429.1; Protein: 6.2g; Carbs: 39.2g; Fat: 27.5g

Salmon & Arugula Salad

Serves: 2, Cooking Time: 12 minutes

Ingredients:
- ¼ cup red onion, sliced thinly
- 1 ½ tbsp fresh lemon juice
- 1 ½ tbsp olive oil
- 1 tbsp extra-virgin olive oil
- 1 tbsp red-wine vinegar
- 2 center cut salmon fillets (6-oz each)
- 2/3 cup cherry tomatoes, halved
- 3 cups baby arugula leaves
- Pepper and salt to taste

Directions for Cooking:
1) In a shallow bowl, mix pepper, salt, 1 ½ tbsp olive oil and lemon juice. Toss in salmon fillets and rub with the marinade. Allow to marinate for at least 15 minutes.

2) Grease a baking sheet and preheat oven to 350 degrees F.
3) Bake marinated salmon fillet for 10 to 12 minutes or until flaky with skin side touching the baking sheet.
4) Meanwhile, in a salad bowl mix onion, tomatoes and arugula.
5) Season with pepper and salt. Drizzle with vinegar and oil. Toss to combine and serve right away with baked salmon on the side.

Nutrition Information:
Calories per serving: 400; Protein: 36.6g; Carbs: 5.8g; Fat: 25.6g

Spinach and Cranberry Salad

Serves: 4 , Cook Time: 5 minutes

Ingredients:

- ¼ cup cider vinegar
- ¼ cup honey
- ¼ cup white wine vinegar
- ¼ tsp paprika
- ½ cup olive oil
- ½ cup pumpkin seeds
- 1 cup dried cranberries
- 1 lb spinach, rinsed and torn into bite sized pieces
- 2 tsp minced onion

Directions for Cooking:

1) Toast pumpkin seeds by placing in a nonstick saucepan on medium fire. Stir frequently and toast for at least 3 to 5 minutes. Remove from fire and set aside.
2) In a medium bowl, mix well olive oil, cider vinegar, white wine vinegar, paprika, onion, and honey. Whisk well until mixture is uniform.
3) In a large salad bowl, add torn spinach.
4) Drizzle with dressing and toss well to coat.
5) Garnish with cooled and toasted pumpkin seeds and dried cranberries.
6) Serve and enjoy.

Nutrition Information:
Calories per Serving: 531.3; Fat: 34.9g; Protein: 9.1g; Carbs: 45.2g

Supreme Caesar Salad

Serves: 4, Cook Time: 10 minutes

Ingredients:

- ¼ cup olive oil
- ¾ cup mayonnaise
- 1 head romaine lettuce, torn into bite sized pieces
- 1 tbsp lemon juice
- 1 tsp Dijon mustard
- 1 tsp Worcestershire sauce
- 3 cloves garlic, peeled and minced
- 3 cloves garlic, peeled and quartered
- 4 cups day old bread, cubed
- 5 anchovy filets, minced
- 6 tbsp grated Parmesan cheese, divided
- Ground black pepper to taste
- Salt to taste

Directions for Cooking:

1) In a small bowl, whisk well lemon juice, mustard, Worcestershire sauce, 2 tbsp Parmesan cheese, anchovies, mayonnaise, and minced garlic. Season with pepper and salt to taste. Set aside in the ref.
2) On medium fire, place a large nonstick saucepan and heat oil.
3) Sauté quartered garlic until browned around a minute or two. Remove and discard.
4) Add bread cubes in same pan, sauté until lightly browned. Season with pepper and salt. Transfer to a plate.
5) In large bowl, place lettuce and pour in dressing. Toss well to coat. Top with remaining Parmesan cheese.
6) Garnish with bread cubes, serve, and enjoy.

Nutrition Information:
Calories per Serving: 443.3; Fat: 32.1g; Protein: 11.6g; Carbs: 27g

Summer Jicama & Cabbage Slaw

Serves: 4, Cooking Time: 0 minutes

Ingredients:

- ½ head green cabbage, shredded
- ½ head purple cabbage, shredded
- ½ lb. jicama, peeled, and sliced
- ½ red onion, sliced thinly
- 1 handful parsley, finely chopped
- Salt to taste

Dressing Ingredients:

- ¼ tsp salt
- ½ cup coconut concentrate warmed in a bowl of hot water

- ½ cup warm filtered water
- ½ lemon, juiced
- 1/3 cup extra virgin olive oil
- 2 tbsp apple cider vinegar

Directions for Cooking:
1) In blender, add all dressing ingredients except for warm water. Puree until smooth and creamy. Add warm water by teaspoonful to reach desired consistency.

2) In a large salad bowl, add shredded cabbages and add salt. Massage for a minute or two to soften some tough fibers.
3) Add parsley, jicama, and red onion into bowl. Pour dressing and toss well to combine.
4) Serve and enjoy.

Nutrition Information:
Calories per serving: 156.1; Protein: 3g; Carbs: 17.8g; Fat: 8.1g

Sunflower Seed, Grape, and Arugula Salad

Serves: 2 , Cook Time: 0
Ingredients:
- ¼ tsp ground black pepper
- ¼ tsp salt
- ½ tsp stone-ground mustard
- 1 tsp chopped fresh thyme
- 1 tsp honey
- 1 tsp maple syrup
- 2 cups red grapes, halved
- 2 tbsp toasted sunflower seed kernels
- 2 tsp grapeseed oil
- 3 tbsp red wine vinegar
- 7 cups loosely packed baby arugula

Directions for Cooking:
1) In a small bowl, whisk well mustard, syrup, honey, and vinegar. Slowly add oil while whisking continuously.
2) I large salad bowl, mix thyme, seeds, grapes, and arugula.
3) Pour mustard mixture into bowl of salad and toss well to coat evenly with dressing.

Nutrition Information:
Calories per Serving: 531.3; Fat: 10.3g; Protein: 5.1g; Carbs: 37.8g

Tabbouleh- Arabian Salad

Serves: 6 , Cook Time: 0 minutes
Ingredients:
- ¼ cup chopped fresh mint
- 1 2/3 cups boiling water
- 1 cucumber, peeled, seeded and chopped
- 1 cup bulgur
- 1 cup chopped fresh parsley
- 1 cup chopped green onions
- 1 tsp salt
- 1/3 cup lemon juice
- 1/3 cup olive oil
- 3 tomatoes, chopped
- Ground black pepper to taste

Directions for Cooking:
1) In a large bowl, mix together boiling water and bulgur. Let soak and set aside for an hour while covered.
2) After one hour, toss in cucumber, tomatoes, mint, parsley, onions, lemon juice and oil. Then season with black pepper and salt to taste. Toss well and refrigerate for another hour while covered before serving.

Nutrition Information:
Calories per serving: 185.5; Fat: 13.1g; Protein: 4.1g; Carbs: 12.8g

Tangy Citrus Salad with Grilled Cod

Serves: 2, Cooking Time: 10 minutes
Ingredients:
- ½ cup orange segments
- ¾ cup chopped red bell pepper
- 1 ½ cups shredded carrot

- 1 ½ cups shredded kohlrabi
- 1 ½ cups shredded spinach
- 1 ½ tbsp olive oil

- 1 cup grapefruit segments
- 1 cup shredded celery
- 1 tbsp minced garlic
- 1 tbsp shredded fresh basil
- 1 tsp black pepper
- 6-oz baked or broiled cod
- Zest and juice of 1 lemon
- Zest and juice of 1 lime
- Zest and juice of 1 orange

Directions for Cooking:
1) Grease grill grate with cooking spray and preheat to medium-high fire. Once grate is hot,

grill cod until flaky, around 5 minutes per side.
2) Meanwhile, mix remaining ingredients, except for citrus pieces, in a large salad bowl and toss well to combine.
3) To serve, evenly divide salad into two plates, top with ½ of grilled cod and garnish with citrus pieces.

Nutrition Information:
Calories per serving: 381.9; Protein: 22g; Carbs: 47.6g; Fat: 11.5g

Thai Salad with Cilantro Lime Dressing

Serves: 2, Cooking Time: 20 minutes
Ingredients:
- ¼ cup cashews
- ¼ cup fresh mint leaves
- ¼ cup fresh Thai basil leaves
- ¼ teaspoon fish sauce
- ½ cup green papaya, julienned
- ½ teaspoon honey
- 1 head green leaf lettuce, chopped
- 1 loose handful fresh cilantro
- 1 tablespoon lime juice
- 1 teaspoon coconut aminos
- 3 tablespoon olive oil
- 3 tangerines, peeled and segmented

Directions for Cooking:
1) Prepare the lime cilantro dressing by mixing honey, fresh cilantro, fish sauce, coconut aminos, lime juice and oil in a mixing bowl. Mix then set aside.
2) Prepare the salad by mixing the remaining six ingredients. Toss everything to distribute the ingredients.
3) Toss the salad dressing into the vegetables.
4) Serve chilled.

Nutrition Information:
Calories per Serving: 649.8; Fat: 57.4 g; Protein: 7.5 g; Carbs: 25.8 g;

Truffle Oil, Mushrooms and Cauliflower Salad

Serves: 4, Cooking Time: 25 minutes
Ingredients:
- ¼ tsp fresh ground black pepper
- ¼ tsp salt
- 1 ½ oz grate Pecorino-Romano cheese, divided
- 1 15-oz BPA free can unsalted cannellini beans, drained and rinsed (try Eden organic cannellini beans)
- 1 cup low-sodium chicken broth
- 1 large head cauliflower, chopped into florets
- 1 yellow onion, chopped
- 1/3 cup chopped fresh flat leaf parsley leaves
- 2 tbsp fresh lemon juice
- 3 cloves garlic, minced
- 4 tsp truffle oil
- 8 oz cremini mushrooms, sliced

- Olive oil cooking spray

Directions for Cooking:
1) Divide cauliflower in 3 batches and process in a food processor until the size of a rice grain. Repeat until all batches are done.
2) Next blend together broth and beans for a minute or until smooth.
3) On medium low fire, place a large pan and grease with cooking spray.
4) Add onions and mushrooms; stir fry until liquid is almost gone around 5-7 minutes.
5) Add pepper, salt and garlic. Cook for a minute more.
6) Increase fire to medium high and add lemon juice. Cook and stir for a minute or until liquid has evaporated.

7) Add pureed beans and bring to a simmer. Once simmering, add cauliflower and mix well. Cover, reduce fire to medium, and stir occasionally as you cook cauliflower until tender, around 8-10 minutes.
8) Once cauliflower is tender, turn off heat.

9) Add truffle oil, parsley and ¾ oz cheese. Mix well.
10) Evenly divide on to bowls, top with remaining cheese and serve.

Nutrition Information:
Calories per serving: 506.1; Protein: 19.3g; Carbs: 76.4g; Fat: 13.7g

Tuna Avocado Salad

Serves: 4, Cooking Time: 0 minutes
Ingredients:
- 1 avocado, pit removed and sliced
- 1 lemon, juiced
- 1 tablespoon chopped onion
- 5 ounces cooked or canned tuna
- Salt and pepper to taste

Directions for Cooking:

1) In a mixing bowl, combine the avocado and lime juice. Mash the avocado and add the tuna.
2) Season with salt and pepper to taste.
3) Serve chilled.

Nutrition Information:
Calories per Serving: 695.5; Fat: 50.7 g; Protein: 41.5 g; Carbs: 18.3 g

Tuna-Mediterranean Salad

Serves: 6 , Cook Time: 0 minutes
Ingredients:
- ¼ cup chopped pitted ripe olives
- ¼ cup drained and chopped roasted red peppers
- ¼ cup Mayonnaise dressing with olive oil
- 1 tbsp small capers, rinsed and drained
- 2 green onions, sliced
- 2 pcs of 6 oz cans of tuna, drained and flaked
- 6 slices whole wheat bread optional

- Salad greens like lettuce optional

Directions for Cooking:
1) With the exception of salad greens or bread, mix together all of the ingredients in a bowl. If desired, you can arrange it on top of salad greens or serve with bread

Nutrition Information:
Calories per Serving: 197.1; Protein: 6.9g; Fat: 5.7g; Carbs: 16.3g

Tuna, Ripe Olive and Artichoke Salad

Serves: 5, Cooking Time: 0 minutes
Ingredients:
- ½ cup chopped olives
- 1 1/ 2 tsp chopped fresh oregano
- 1 12-oz can chunk light tuna, drained and flaked
- 1 cup chopped canned artichoke hearts
- 1/3 cup reduced fat mayonnaise
- 2 tsp lemon juice

Directions for Cooking:
1) In a medium salad bowl, mix well oregano, lemon juice, mayonnaise, olives, artichokes, and tuna.
2) Serve and enjoy.

Nutrition Information:
Calories per serving: 154.8; Protein: 14.5g; Carbs: 5.3g; Fat: 8.4g

Tuna-Dijon Salad

Serves: 6, Cooking Time: minutes

Tuna Salad Ingredients:

- 5 whole small radishes, stems removed and chopped
- 3 stalks green onions, chopped
- 1 cup chopped parsley leaves
- ½ cup chopped fresh mint leaves, stems removed
- Six slices heirloom tomatoes for serving
- Pita chips or pita pockets for serving
- 2 1/2 celery stalks, chopped
- 1/2 English cucumber, chopped
- 1/2 medium-sized red onion, finely chopped
- 1/2 cup pitted Kalamata olives, halved
- 3 5-ounce cans Genova tuna in olive oil

Dijon vinaigrette Ingredients:

- 1 1/2 limes, juice of
- 1/2 tsp crushed red pepper flakes, optional
- 1/2 tsp sumac
- 1/3 cup Early Harvest extra virgin olive oil
- 2 1/2 tsp good quality Dijon mustard
- Pinch of salt and pepper
- Zest of 1 lime

Directions for Cooking:

1) Make the dressing by mixing all ingredients in a small bowl until thoroughly blended. Set aside to allow flavors to mix.
2) In a large salad bowl, make the salad.
3) Mix well mint leaves, parsley. Olives, chopped veggies, and tuna.
4) Drizzle with vinaigrette and toss well to coat.
5) Put in the fridge for at least half an hour to allow flavors to mix.
6) Toss again. Top with tomatoes.
7) Serve with pita chips on the side and enjoy.

Nutrition Information:
Calories per Serving: 299; Carbs: 6.6g; Protein: 25.7g; Fats: 19.2g

Warm Arugula Salad with Bread

Serves: 4, Cooking Time: 15 minutes

Ingredients:

- ½ cup grated Parmesan cheese
- 1 cup cherry tomatoes, halved
- 1 tbsp minced garlic
- 1/8 tsp pepper
- 1/8 tsp salt
- 2 slices crusty whole-wheat bread, cut into 1-inch cubes
- 2 tbsp balsamic vinegar
- 3 tbsp extra virgin olive oil, divided
- 8 cups arugula

Directions for Cooking:

1) On medium-high fire, place a large nonstick saucepan and heat 2 tbsp oil.
2) Add bread and stir fry for 5 to 6 minutes or until browned.
3) Stir in arugula and tomatoes, cook for a minute or until arugula is lightly wilted.
4) Push mixture to one side of pan and add remaining oil to empty side of pan.
5) Add garlic and sauté for 30 seconds or until sizzling and fragrant.
6) Mix bread mixture with garlic and turn off fire.
7) While pan is still hot, season with balsamic vinegar, pepper and salt.
8) Toss well to coat and combine.
9) Transfer to a serving platter, op with Parmesan cheese, and enjoy.

Nutrition Information:
Calories per serving: 156.8; Protein: 6.8g; Carbs: 12.6g; Fat: 8.8g

Warm Brussels Sprouts Salad with Nuts

Serves: 6, Cooking Time: 15 minutes

Ingredients:
- ¼ tsp salt
- ½ oz shaved Asiago cheese
- ¾ lb. Brussels sprouts, trimmed and halved
- 1 ½ tbsp finely chopped walnuts, toasted
- 1 ½ tsp extra virgin olive oil, divided
- 1 garlic clove, minced
- 1/3 cup fresh breadcrumbs
- 1/8 tsp ground black pepper

Directions for Cooking:
1) On medium fire, place a large nonstick pan and heat 1 tsp oil.
2) Add garlic and sauté until golden brown, around a minute.
3) Add breadcrumbs and cook until lightly browned, around a minute. Transfer to a large salad bowl.
4) Separate the Brussels sprouts leaves and quarter the cores.
5) In same pan on medium fire, heat remaining oil. Add the Brussels sprouts cores and leaves. Stir fry for 8 minutes or until leaves are wilted and cores are tender yet crisp.
6) Turn off fire, transfer Brussels sprouts to bowl of crumbs and toss to mix well.
7) Add pepper and salt, mix again.
8) To serve, top with cheese and walnuts.

Nutrition Information:
Calories per serving: 62.9; Protein: 3.3g; Carbs: 6.8g; Fat: 2.5g

Warm Brussels Sprouts with Slivered Almonds

Serves: 6, Cooking Time: 10 minutes

Ingredients:
- ¼ tsp salt
- ½ oz Parmesan cheese, shaved
- ¾ lb. Brussels sprouts
- 1 ½ tbsp slivered walnuts
- 1 ½ tsp avocado oil, divided
- 1 garlic clove, minced
- 1/3 cup fresh breadcrumbs
- 1/8 tsp black pepper

Directions for Cooking:
1) Slice Brussels sprouts in half then separate the leaves from the cores. Cut the cores in quarters and set aside.
2) On medium fire, place a large nonstick saucepan and heat 1 tsp oil. Sauté garlic for a minute.
3) Add breadcrumbs and sauté for another minute or until lightly browned. Transfer to a bowl.
4) In same pan, add remaining oil and cook Brussels sprouts until crisp tender around 8 minutes.
5) Transfer to serving bowl, pour in breadcrumb mixture and toss to mix.
6) Garnish with cheese and nuts before serving.

Nutrition Information:
Calories per serving: 77.5; Protein: 3.5g; Carbs: 8.9g; Fat: 3.1g

Warm Cauliflower Salad

Serves: 2 , Cook Time: 0 minutes

Ingredients:

- ½ cup raisins
- ½ cup toasted pine nuts
- ½ tsp ground cinnamon
- 1 tbsp olive oil
- 1 tsp fennel seeds
- 1 tsp ground turmeric
- 2 tsp ground cumin
- 50g baby spinach
- 600 g cauliflower, trimmed, cut into florets
- Lemon wedges, to serve

Directions for Cooking:

1) In a boiling pot of water, blanch cauliflower for 3 minutes, and drain. Set aside.
2) On medium-high fire, place a large saucepan and heat olive oil for 30 seconds.
3) Add turmeric and cumin. Sauté until fragrant, around a minute.
4) Add drained cauliflower and cook until golden, around 5 minutes.
5) Stir in spinach, raisins, and pine nuts.
6) Season with pepper and salt to taste.
7) Turn off fire, transfer to a serving plate, garnish with lemon wedges, serve and enjoy.

Nutrition Information:

Calories per Serving: 422.3; Fat: 31.1g; Protein: 11.5g; Carbs: 24.1g

Warm Brussels Sprouts Salad with Nuts

Serves: 6, Cooking Time: 10 minutes

Ingredients:

- ¼ tsp salt
- ½ oz. Asiago cheese, shaved
- ¾ lb. Brussels sprouts
- 1 ½ tbsp toasted walnuts, finely chopped
- 1 ½ tsp olive oil, divided
- 1 garlic clove, minced
- 1/3 cup fresh breadcrumbs
- 1/8 tsp black pepper

Directions for Cooking:

1) Slice Brussels sprouts in half then separate the leaves from the cores. Cut the cores in quarters and set aside.
2) On medium fire, place a large nonstick saucepan and heat 1 tsp oil. Sauté garlic for a minute.
3) Add breadcrumbs and sauté for another minute or until lightly browned. Transfer to a bowl.
4) In same pan, add remaining oil and cook Brussels sprouts until crisp tender around 8 minutes.
5) Transfer to serving bowl, pour in breadcrumb mixture and toss to mix.
6) Garnish with cheese and nuts before serving.

Nutrition Information:

Calories per Serving: 77.5; Fat: 3.1g; Protein: 3.5g; Carbohydrates: 8.9g

Chapter 8 Beans Recipes

Black Eyed Peas Stew

Serves: 4, Cooking Time: 20 minutes

Ingredients:
- ½ cup extra virgin olive oil, divided
- 1 cup fresh dill, stems removed, chopped
- 1 cup fresh parsley, stems removed, chopped
- 1 cup water
- 2 bay leaves
- 2 carrots, peeled and sliced
- 2 cups black eyed beans, drained and rinsed
- 2 slices orange with peel and flesh
- 2 Tablespoons tomato paste
- 4 green onions, thinly sliced
- Salt and pepper, to taste

Directions for Cooking:
1) Place a pot on medium-high fire and heat. Add ¼ cup oil and heat for 3 minutes.
2) Stir in bay leaves and tomato paste. Sauté for 2 minutes.
3) Stir in carrots and a up of water. Cover and simmer for 5 minutes.
4) Stir in dill, parsley, beans, and orange. Cover and cook for 3 minutes or until heated through.
5) Season with pepper and salt to taste.
6) Stir in remaining oil and green onions cook for 2 minutes.
7) Serve and enjoy.

Nutrition Information:
Calories per serving: 376; Protein: 8.8g; Carbs: 25.6g; Fat: 27.8g

Brussels Sprouts 'n White Bean Medley

Serves: 4, Cooking Time: 15 minutes

Ingredients:
- 1 tsp salt
- 2 tbsp olive oil
- 3 cans white beans, drained and rinsed
- 3 medium onions, peeled and sliced
- 3tbsp lemon juice
- 4 ½ cups Brussels sprouts, cleaned and sliced in half
- 6 garlic cloves, smashed, peeled, and minced
- Pepper to taste

Directions for Cooking:
1) Place a saucepan on medium-high fire and heat for 2 minutes.
2) Add oil and heat for a minute.
3) Sauté garlic and onions for 3 minutes.
4) Stir in Brussels Sprouts and sauté for 5 minutes.
5) Stir in white beans and sauté for 5 minutes.
6) Season with pepper and salt.

Nutrition Information:
Calories per serving: 371; Protein: 21.4g; Carbs: 57.8g; Fat: 8.1g

Bean and Toasted Pita Salad

Serves: 4, Cooking Time: 10 minutes

Ingredients:
- 3 tbsp chopped fresh mint
- 3 tbsp chopped fresh parsley
- 1 cup crumbled feta cheese
- 1 cup sliced romaine lettuce
- ½ cucumber, peeled and sliced
- 1 cup diced plum tomatoes
- 2 cups cooked pinto beans, well drained and slightly warmed
- Pepper to taste
- 3 tbsp extra virgin olive oil
- 2 tbsp ground toasted cumin seeds
- 2 tbsp fresh lemon juice
- 1/8 tsp salt
- 2 cloves garlic, peeled
- 2 6-inch whole wheat pita bread, cut or torn into bite-sized pieces

Directions for Cooking:

1) In large baking sheet, spread torn pita bread and bake in a preheated 400 degrees F oven for 6 minutes.
2) With the back of a knife, mash garlic and salt until paste like. Add into a medium bowl.
3) Whisk in ground cumin and lemon juice. In a steady and slow stream, pour oil as you whisk continuously. Season with pepper.
4) In a large salad bowl, mix cucumber, tomatoes and beans. Pour in dressing, toss to coat well.
5) Add mint, parsley, feta, lettuce and toasted pita, toss to mix once again and serve.

Nutrition Information:
Calories per serving: 427; Protein: 17.7g; Carbs: 47.3g; Fat: 20.4g

Beans and Spinach Mediterranean Salad

Serves: 4, Cooking Time: 30 minutes
Ingredients:

- 1 can (14 ounces) water-packed artichoke hearts, rinsed, drained and quartered
- 1 can (14-1/2 ounces) no-salt-added diced tomatoes, undrained
- 1 can (15 ounces) cannellini beans, rinsed and drained
- 1 small onion, chopped
- 1 tablespoon olive oil
- 1/4 teaspoon pepper
- 1/4 teaspoon salt
- 1/8 teaspoon crushed red pepper flakes
- 2 garlic cloves, minced
- 2 tablespoons Worcestershire sauce
- 6 ounces fresh baby spinach (about 8 cups)
- Additional olive oil, optional

Directions for Cooking:

1) Place a saucepan on medium-high fire and heat for a minute.
2) Add oil and heat for 2 minutes. Stir in onion and sauté for 4 minutes. Add garlic and sauté for another minute.
3) Stir in seasonings, Worcestershire sauce, and tomatoes. Cook for 5 minutes while stirring continuously until sauce is reduced.
4) Stir in spinach, artichoke hearts, and beans. Sauté for 3 minutes until spinach is wilted and other ingredients are heated through.
5) Serve and enjoy.

Nutrition Information:
Calories per serving: 187; Protein: 8.0g; Carbs: 30.0g; Fat: 4.0g

Black Bean Hummus

Serves: 8, Cooking Time: 0 minutes
Ingredients:

- 10 Greek olives
- ¼ tsp paprika
- ¼ tsp cayenne pepper
- ½ tsp salt
- ¾ tsp ground cumin
- 1 ½ tbsp tahini
- 2 tbsp lemon juice
- 1 15-oz can black beans, drain and reserve liquid
- 1 clove garlic

Directions for Cooking:

1) In food processor, mince garlic.
2) Add cayenne pepper, salt, cumin, tahini, lemon juice, 2 tbsp reserved black beans liquid, and black beans.
3) Process until smooth and creamy. Scrape the side of processor as needed and continue pureeing.
4) To serve, garnish with Greek olives and paprika.
5) Best eaten as a dip for pita bread or chips.

Nutrition Information:
Calories per serving: 205; Protein: 12.1g; Carbs: 34.4g; Fat: 2.9g

Chicken and White Bean

Serves: 8, Cooking Time: 70 minutes

Ingredients:

- 2 tbsp fresh cilantro, chopped
- 2 cups grated Monterey Jack cheese
- 3 cups water
- 1/8 tsp cayenne pepper
- 2 tsp pure chile powder
- 2 tsp ground cumin
- 1 4-oz can chopped green chiles
- 1 cup corn kernels
- 2 15-oz cans shite beans, drained and rinsed
- 2 garlic cloves
- 1 medium onion, diced
- 2 tbsp extra virgin olive oil
- 1 lb. chicken breasts, boneless and skinless

Directions for Cooking:

1) Slice chicken breasts into ½-inch cubes and with pepper and salt, season it.
2) On high fire, place a large nonstick fry pan and heat oil.
3) Sauté chicken pieces for three to four minutes or until lightly browned.
4) Reduce fire to medium and add garlic and onion.
5) Cook for 5 to 6 minutes or until onions are translucent.
6) Add water, spices, chilies, corn and beans. Bring to a boil.
7) Once boiling, slow fire to a simmer and continue simmering for an hour, uncovered.
8) To serve, garnish with a sprinkling of cilantro and a tablespoon of cheese.

Nutrition Information:

Calories per serving: 433; Protein: 30.6g; Carbs: 29.5g; Fat: 21.8g

Chickpea Alfredo Sauce

Serves: 4, Cooking Time: 0 minutes

Ingredients:

- ¼ teaspoon ground nutmeg
- ¼ teaspoon sea salt or to taste
- 1 clove garlic minced
- 2 cups chickpeas, rinsed and drained
- 1 tablespoon white miso paste
- 1-½ cups water
- 2 tablespoons lemon juice
- 3 tablespoons nutritional yeast

Directions for Cooking:

1) Add all ingredients in a blender.
2) Puree until smooth and creamy.

Nutrition Information:

Calories per serving: 123; Protein: 6.2g; Carbs: 20.2g; Fat: 2.4g

Chickpea Fried Eggplant Salad

Serves: 4, Cooking Time: 10 minutes

Ingredients:

- 1 cup chopped dill
- 1 cup chopped parsley
- 1 cup cooked or canned chickpeas, drained
- 1 large eggplant, thinly sliced (no more than 1/4 inch in thickness)
- 1 small red onion, sliced in 1/2 moons
- 1/2 English cucumber, diced
- 3 Roma tomatoes, diced
- 3 tbsp Za'atar spice, divided
- oil for frying, preferably extra virgin olive oil
- Salt

Garlic Vinaigrette Ingredients:

- 1 large lime, juice of
- 1/3 cup extra virgin olive oil
- 1–2 garlic cloves, minced
- Salt & Pepper to taste

Directions for Cooking:

1) On a baking sheet, spread out sliced eggplant and season with salt generously. Let it sit for 30 minutes. Then pat dry with paper towel.
2) Place a small pot on medium-high fire and fill halfway with oil. Heat oil for 5 minutes. Fry eggplant in batches until golden brown, around 3 minutes per side. Place cooked eggplants on a paper towel lined plate.

3) Once eggplants have cooled, assemble the eggplant on a serving dish. Sprinkle with 1 tbsp of Za'atar.
4) Mix dill, parsley, red onions, chickpeas, cucumbers, and tomatoes in a large salad bowl. Sprinkle remaining Za'atar and gently toss to mix.
5) Whisk well the vinaigrette ingredients in a small bowl. Drizzle 2 tbsp of the dressing over the fried eggplant. Add remaining dressing over the chickpea salad and mix.
6) Add the chickpea salad to the serving dish with the fried eggplant.
7) Serve and enjoy.

Nutrition Information:
Calories per serving: 642; Protein: 16.6g; Carbs: 25.9g; Fat: 44.0g

Chickpea Salad Moroccan Style

Serves: 6, Cooking Time: 0 minutes
Ingredients:
- 1/3 cup crumbled low-fat feta cheese
- ¼ cup fresh mint, chopped
- ¼ cup fresh cilantro, chopped
- 1 red bell pepper, diced
- 2 plum tomatoes, diced
- 3 green onions, sliced thinly
- 1 large carrot, peeled and julienned
- 3 cups BPA free canned chickpeas or garbanzo beans
- Pinch of cayenne pepper
- ¼ tsp salt
- ¼ tsp pepper
- 2 tsp ground cumin
- 3 tbsp fresh lemon juice
- 3 tbsp olive oil

Directions for Cooking:
1) Make the dressing by whisking cayenne, black pepper, salt, cumin, lemon juice and oil in a small bowl and set aside.
2) Mix together feta, mint, cilantro, red pepper, tomatoes, onions, carrots and chickpeas in a large salad bowl.
3) Pour dressing over salad and toss to coat well.
4) Serve and enjoy.

Nutrition Information:
Calories per serving: 300; Protein: 13.2g; Carbs: 35.4g; Fat: 12.8g

Chickpea-Crouton Kale Caesar Salad

Serves: 4, Cooking Time: 35 minutes
Salad Ingredients:
- 1 large bunch Tuscan kale, stem removed & thinly sliced
- ½ cup toasted pepitas

Chickpeas Crouton Ingredients:
- 1 cup chickpeas, rinsed and drained
- 1 tbsp Dijon mustard
- 1 tbsp nutritional yeast
- 2 tbsp olive oil
- salt and pepper, to taste

Dressing Ingredients:
- ½ cup silken tofu
- 2 tablespoons olive oil
- 1 lemon, zested and juiced
- 1 clove garlic
- 2 teaspoons capers, drained
- 2 tablespoons nutritional yeast
- 1 teaspoon Dijon mustard
- salt and pepper, to taste

Directions for Cooking:
1) Heat oven to 350 degrees F. Toss the chickpeas in the garlic, Dijon, nutritional yeast, olive oil, and salt and pepper. Roast for 30-35 minutes, until browned and crispy.
2) In a blender, add all dressing ingredients. Puree until smooth and creamy.
3) In a large salad bowl, toss the kale with dressing to taste, massaging lightly to tenderize the kale.
4) Top with the chickpea croutons, pepitas, and enjoy!

Nutrition Information:
Calories per serving: 327; Protein: 11.9g; Carbs: 20.3g; Fat: 23.8g

Chickpea-Curry Salad

Serves: 4, Cooking Time: 0 minutes
Ingredients:

- 2 Tablespoons extra-virgin olive oil
- 2 teaspoons apple cider vinegar
- 2 teaspoons curry powder
- 2 teaspoons pure maple syrup
- 2 (15 oz) cans chickpeas, rinsed and drained
- 1 cup chopped red bell pepper
- 2 celery hearts, chopped
- 2 Tablespoons finely chopped red onion
- chopped cashews (optional)
- spinach or spring mix for serving
- juice from 1/2 a lime
- 1/2 teaspoon sea salt
- 1/2 teaspoon turmeric
- 4 Medjool dates, pitted and chopped (or 1/2 cup raisins)
- 1/3 cup fresh cilantro, chopped
- 1/4 teaspoon garam masala

Directions for Cooking:

1) In a small bowl, whisk well garam masala, turmeric, salt, maple syrup, curry powder, cider vinegar, lime juice, and oil.
2) In a large salad bowl, toss well to mix the cilantro, red onion, dates, red pepper, celery, and chickpeas.
3) Drizzle with dressing and toss well to coat.
4) Add the salad greens and cashers, toss well to mix.
5) Serve and enjoy.

Nutrition Information:
Calories per serving: 352; Protein: 12.0g; Carbs: 61.0g; Fat: 12.0g

Chorizo-Kidney Beans Quinoa Pilaf

Serves: 4, Cooking Time: 35 minutes
Ingredients:

- ¼ pound dried Spanish chorizo diced (about 2/3 cup)
- ¼ teaspoon red pepper flakes
- ¼ teaspoon smoked paprika
- ½ teaspoon cumin
- ½ teaspoon sea salt
- 1 3/4 cups water
- 1 cup quinoa
- 1 large clove garlic minced
- 1 small red bell pepper finely diced
- 1 small red onion finely diced
- 1 tablespoon tomato paste
- 1 15-ounce can kidney beans rinsed and drained

Directions for Cooking:

1) Place a nonstick pot on medium-high fire and heat for 2 minutes. Add chorizo and sauté for 5 minutes until lightly browned.
2) Stir in peppers and onion. Sauté for 5 minutes.
3) Add tomato paste, red pepper flakes, salt, paprika, cumin, and garlic. Sauté for 2 minutes.
4) Stir in quinoa and mix well. Sauté for 2 minutes.
5) Add water and beans. Mix well. Cover and simmer for 20 minutes or until liquid is fully absorbed.
6) Turn off fire and fluff quinoa. Let it sit for 5 minutes more while uncovered.
7) Serve and enjoy.

Nutrition Information:
Calories per serving: 260; Protein: 9.6g; Carbs: 40.9g; Fat: 6.8g

Cilantro-Dijon Vinaigrette on Kidney Bean Salad

Serves: 4, Cooking Time: 0 minutes
Salad Ingredients:

- 1 15-oz. can kidney beans, drained and rinsed
- 1/2 English cucumbers, chopped
- 1 Medium-sized heirloom tomato, chopped
- 1 bunch fresh cilantro, stems removed, chopped (about 1 1/4 cup)
- 1 red onion, chopped (about 1 cup)

Cilantro-Dijon Vinaigrette Ingredients:
- 1 large lime or lemon, juice of
- 3 tbsp Private Reserve or Early Harvest Greek extra virgin olive oil
- 1 tsp Dijon mustard
- ½ tsp fresh garlic paste, or finely chopped garlic
- 1 tsp sumac
- Salt and pepper, to taste

Directions for Cooking:

1) In a small bowl, whisk well all vinaigrette ingredients.
2) In a salad bowl, combine cilantro chopped veggies, and kidney beans.
3) Add vinaigrette to salad and toss well to mix.
4) For 30 minutes allow for flavors to mix and set in the fridge.
5) Mix and adjust seasoning if needed before serving.

Nutrition Information:
Calories per serving: 154; Protein: 5.5g; Carbs: 18.3g; Fat: 7.4g

Extraordinary Green Hummus

Serves: 8, Cooking Time: 0 minutes
Ingredients:
- ¼ cup fresh lemon juice (about 1 large lemon's worth)
- ¼ cup roughly chopped, loosely packed fresh tarragon or basil
- ¼ cup tahini
- ½ cup roughly chopped, loosely packed fresh parsley
- ½ teaspoon salt, more to taste
- 1 large garlic clove, roughly chopped
- 1 to 2 tablespoons water, optional
- 2 tablespoons olive oil, plus more for serving
- 2 to 3 tablespoons roughly chopped fresh chives or green onion
- Garnish with extra olive oil and a sprinkling of chopped fresh herbs
- One (15-ounce) can of chickpeas, also called garbanzo beans, drained and rinsed

Directions for Cooking:
1) Place all ingredients in a blender and puree until smooth and creamy.
2) Transfer to a bowl and adjust seasoning if needed.
3) Serve with pita chips.

Nutrition Information:
Calories per serving: 8; Protein: 3.8g; Carbs: 10.0g; Fat: 8.3g

Curried Chicken, Chickpeas and Raita Salad

Serves: 8, Cooking Time: 15 minutes
Curried Chicken Ingredients:
- 1 cup red grapes, halved
- 3-4 cups rotisserie chicken, meat coarsely shredded
- 2 tbsp cilantro
- 1 cup plain yogurt
- 2 medium tomatoes, chopped
- 1 tsp ground cumin
- 1 tbsp curry powder
- 2 tbsp olive oil
- 1 tbsp minced peeled ginger
- 1 tbsp minced garlic
- 1 medium onion, chopped

Chickpeas Ingredients:
- ¼ tsp cayenne
- ½ tsp turmeric
- 1 tsp ground cumin
- 1 19-oz can chickpeas, rinsed, drained and patted dry
- 1 tbsp olive oil

Topping and Raita Ingredients:
- ½ cup sliced and toasted almonds
- 2 tbsp chopped mint
- 2 cups cucumber, peeled, cored and chopped
- 1 cup plain yogurt

Directions for Cooking:
1) To make the chicken salad, on medium low fire, place a medium nonstick saucepan and heat oil.
2) Sauté ginger, garlic and onion for 5 minutes or until softened while stirring occasionally.

3) Add 1 ½ tsp salt, cumin and curry. Sauté for two minutes.
4) Increase fire to medium high and add tomatoes. Stirring frequently, cook for 5 minutes.
5) Pour sauce into a bowl, mix in chicken, cilantro and yogurt. Stir to combine and let it stand to cool to room temperature.
6) To make the chickpeas, on a nonstick fry pan, heat oil for 3 minutes.
7) Add chickpeas and cook for a minute while stirring frequently.
8) Add ¼ tsp salt, cayenne, turmeric and cumin. Stir to mix well and cook for two minutes or until sauce is dried.
9) Transfer to a bowl and let it cool to room temperature.
10) To make the raita, mix ½ tsp salt, mint, cucumber and yogurt. Stir thoroughly to combine and dissolve salt.
11) To assemble, in four 16-oz lidded jars or bowls layer the following: curried chicken, raita, chickpeas and garnish with almonds.
12) You can make this recipe one day ahead and refrigerate for 6 hours before serving.

Nutrition Information:
Calories per serving: 381; Protein: 36.1g; Carbs: 27.4g; Fat: 15.5g

Exotic Chickpea Tagine

Serves: 4, Cooking Time: 45 minutes

Ingredients:
- 4 tsp sliced toasted almonds
- 1 cup whole wheat couscous, cooked according to manufacturer's instructions
- Freshly squeezed juice of ½ lemon, plus additional to taste
- 1 19-oz can chickpeas, drained and rinsed
- ½ cup water
- ¼ cup packed dried apricots, sliced
- 1 medium zucchini, quartered and cut into ½-inch chunks
- 4 plum tomatoes, cored and chopped
- ¼ tsp turmeric
- 1 whole cinnamon stick
- 1 tsp ground cumin
- 2 tsp honey, plus additional to taste
- ½ tsp harissa paste plus additional to taste
- 3 quarter-sized pieces of peeled fresh ginger
- 2 garlic cloves, roughly chopped
- 2 small carrots, sliced lengthwise, then cut into ½-inch thick slices
- 1 ½ cups cubed, peeled butternut squash
- ½ tsp salt plus additional to taste
- 1 red onion, quartered and thickly sliced
- 1 ½ tbsp extra virgin olive oil

Directions for Cooking:
1) On medium low fire, place a heavy and large pot. Heat oil and sauté onions and salt until onions are soft and translucent.
2) Add carrots and sauté for another 5 minutes. Add ginger, garlic and butternut squash. Sauté for 5 minutes and lower fire to medium.
3) Add turmeric, cinnamon stick, cumin, honey and harissa. Sauté for a minute or until fragrant. Stir in apricots, zucchini and tomatoes. Add water and bring to a boil. Once boiling, lower fire to a simmer, cover and cook for 20 minutes or until vegetables are tender.
4) Stir in lemon juice and chickpeas. Increase fire to medium and continue cooking dish uncovered for 5 to 10 minutes or until sauce has thickened.
5) Season dish to taste. Adjust seasoning like lemon, honey and harissa if needed.
6) Serve tagine over couscous and garnished with sliced almonds.

Nutrition Information:
Calories per serving: 345; Protein: 13.2g; Carbs: 54.1g; Fat: 10.0g

Fasolakia – Potatoes & Green Beans in Olive Oil

Serves: 4, Cooking Time: 25 minutes

Ingredients:

- 1 1/2 onion, sliced thin
- 1 bunch of dill, chopped
- 1 cup water
- 1 large zucchini, quartered
- 1 lb. green beans frozen
- 1 tsp dried oregano
- 1/2 bunch parsley, chopped
- 1/2 cup extra virgin olive oil
- 15 oz can diced tomatoes
- 2 potatoes, quartered
- salt and pepper, to taste

Directions for Cooking:

1) Place a pot on medium-high fire and heat pot for 2 minutes.

2) Add oil and heat for 3 minutes.

3) Stir in onions and sauté for 2 minutes. Stir in dill, oregano, and potatoes. Cook for 3 minutes. Season with pepper and salt.

4) Add dice tomatoes and water. Cover and simmer for 10 minutes.

5) Stir in zucchini and green beans. Cook for 5 minutes.

6) Adjust seasoning to taste, turn off fire, and stir in parsley.

7) Serve and enjoy.

Nutrition Information:

Calories per serving: 384; Protein: 5.9g; Carbs: 30.6g; Fat: 27.9g

Feta on Tomato-Black Bean

Serves: 8, Cooking Time: 0 minutes

Ingredients:

- 1/2 red onion, sliced
- 1/4 cup crumbled feta cheese
- 1/4 cup fresh dill, chopped
- 2 14.5-ounce cans black beans, drained and rinsed
- 2 tablespoons extra-virgin olive oil
- 4 Roma or plum tomatoes, diced
- Juice of 1 lemon
- Salt to taste

Directions for Cooking:

1) Except for feta, mix well all ingredients in a salad bowl.

2) Sprinkle with feta.

3) Serve and enjoy.

Nutrition Information:

Calories per serving: 121; Protein: 6.0g; Carbs: 15.0g; Fat: 5.0g

Garbanzo and Kidney Bean Salad

Serves: 4, Cooking Time: 0 minutes

Ingredients:

- 1 (15 ounce) can kidney beans, drained
- 1 (15.5 ounce) can garbanzo beans, drained
- 1 lemon, zested and juiced
- 1 medium tomato, chopped
- 1 teaspoon capers, rinsed and drained
- 1/2 cup chopped fresh parsley
- 1/2 teaspoon salt, or to taste
- 1/4 cup chopped red onion
- 3 tablespoons extra virgin olive oil

Directions for Cooking:

1) In a salad bowl, whisk well lemon juice, olive oil and salt until dissolved.

2) Stir in garbanzo, kidney beans, tomato, red onion, parsley, and capers. Toss well to coat.

3) Allow flavors to mix for 30 minutes by setting in the fridge.

4) Mix again before serving.

Nutrition Information:

Calories per serving: 329; Protein: 12.1g; Carbs: 46.6g; Fat: 12.0g

Garbanzo and Lentil Soup

Serves: 8, Cooking Time: 90 minutes

Ingredients:

- 1 14.5-oz can petite diced tomatoes, undrained
- 2 15-oz cans Garbanzo beans, rinsed and drained
- 1 cup lentils
- 6 cups vegetable broth
- ¼ tsp ground cayenne pepper
- ½ tsp ground cumin
- 1 tsp turmeric
- 1 tsp garam masala
- 1 tsp minced garlic
- 2 tsp grated fresh ginger
- 1 cup diced carrots
- 1 cup chopped celery
- 2 onions, chopped

Directions for Cooking:

1) On medium-high fire, place a heavy bottomed large pot and grease with cooking spray.
2) Add onions and sauté until tender, around three to four minutes.
3) Add celery and carrots. Cook for another five minutes.
4) Add cayenne pepper, cumin, turmeric, ginger, garam masala and garlic, cook for half a minute.
5) Add diced tomatoes, garbanzo beans, lentils and vegetable broth. Bring to a boil.
6) Once boiling, slow fire to a simmer and cook while covered for 90 minutes. Occasionally stir soup.
7) If you want a thicker and creamier soup, you can puree ½ of the pot's content and mix in.
8) Once lentils are soft, turn off fire and serve.

Nutrition Information:

Calories per serving: 196; Protein: 10.1g; Carbs: 33.3g; Fat: 3.6g

Greek Farro Salad

Serves: 4, Cooking Time: 15 minutes

Farro Ingredients:

- ½ teaspoon fine-grain sea salt
- 1 cup farro, rinsed
- 1 tablespoon olive oil
- 2 garlic cloves, pressed or minced

Salad Ingredients:

- ½ small red onion, chopped and then rinsed under water to mellow the flavor
- 1 avocado, sliced into strips
- 1 cucumber, sliced into thin rounds
- 15 pitted Kalamata olives, sliced into rounds
- 1-pint cherry tomatoes, sliced into rounds
- 2 cups cooked chickpeas (or one 14-ounce can, rinsed and drained)
- 5 ounces mixed greens
- Lemon wedges

Herbed Yogurt Ingredients:

- ⅛ teaspoon salt
- 1 ¼ cups plain Greek yogurt
- 1 ½ tablespoon lightly packed fresh dill, roughly chopped
- 1 ½ tablespoon lightly packed fresh mint, torn into pieces
- 1 tablespoon lemon juice (about ½ lemon)
- 1 tablespoon olive oil

Directions for Cooking:

1) In a blender, blend and puree all herbed yogurt ingredients and set aside.
2) Then cook the farro by placing in a pot filled halfway with water. Bring to a boil, reduce fire to a simmer and cook for 15 minutes or until farro is tender. Drain well. Mix in salt, garlic, and olive oil and fluff to coat.
3) Evenly divide the cooled farro into 4 bowls. Evenly divide the salad ingredients on the 4 farro bowl. Top with ¼ of the yogurt dressing.
4) Serve and enjoy.

Nutrition Information:

Calories per serving: 428; Protein: 17.7g; Carbs: 47.6g; Fat: 24.5g

Garlicky Lemon-Parsley Hummus

Serves: 8, Cooking Time: 0 minutes

Ingredients:

- ¼ cup tahini
- ¼ teaspoon fine grain sea salt
- ⅓ cup fresh lemon juice
- ¾ cup chopped parsley
- 1 tablespoon olive oil, plus more for drizzling
- 1 ½ cans (15 ounces each) chickpeas, rinsed and drained
- 5 cloves garlic, peeled and roughly chopped
- Dash freshly ground black pepper

Directions for Cooking:

1) Place all ingredients in a blender and puree until smooth and creamy.
2) Transfer to a bowl and adjust seasoning if needed.
3) If dip dries up, just add more olive oil and mix well.
4) Serve and enjoy with carrot sticks.

Nutrition Information:

Calories per serving: 131; Protein: 4.9g; Carbs: 13.8g; Fat: 7.0g

Goat Cheese 'n Red Beans Salad

Serves: 6, Cooking Time: 0 minutes

Ingredients:

- 2 cans of Red Kidney Beans, drained and rinsed well
- Water or vegetable broth to cover beans
- 1 bunch parsley, chopped
- 1 1/2 cups red grape tomatoes, halved
- 3 cloves garlic, minced
- 3 tablespoons olive oil
- 3 tablespoons lemon juice
- 1/2 teaspoon salt
- 1/2 teaspoon white pepper
- 6 ounces goat cheese, crumbled

Directions for Cooking:

1) In a large bowl, combine beans, parsley, tomatoes and garlic.
2) Add olive oil, lemon juice, salt and pepper.
3) Mix well and refrigerate until ready to serve.
4) Spoon into individual dishes topped with crumbled goat cheese.

Nutrition Information:

Calories per serving: 385; Protein: 22.5g; Carbs: 44.0g; Fat: 15.0g

Hummus – A Bean Dip Recipe

Serves: 12, Cooking Time: 0 minutes

Ingredients:

- ¼ tsp cumin
- 1 bunch parsley
- 1 tsp paprika
- 1 tsp sea salt
- 2 ½ cups chickpeas
- 2 garlic cloves, peeled and crushed
- 2 lemons, juiced
- 3 tbsp extra virgin olive oil
- 3 tbsp tahini

Directions for Cooking:

1) Add olive oil, lemon juice, tahini, salt, ang garlic cloves in a blender. Puree until smooth and creamy.
2) Add chickpeas. Puree until smooth and creamy.
3) Transfer to a bowl.
4) Drizzle with more olive oil. Sprinkle paprika and parsley.
5) Serve and enjoy as a dip.

Nutrition Information:

Calories per serving: 215; Protein: 9.4g; Carbs: 28.2g; Fat: 8.0g

Italian White Bean Soup

Serves: 4, Cooking Time: 50 minutes

Ingredients:

- 1 (14 ounce) can chicken broth
- 1 bunch fresh spinach, rinsed and thinly sliced
- 1 clove garlic, minced
- 1 stalk celery, chopped
- 1 tablespoon lemon juice
- 1 tablespoon vegetable oil
- 1 onion, chopped
- 1/4 teaspoon ground black pepper
- 1/8 teaspoon dried thyme
- 2 (16 ounce) cans white kidney beans, rinsed and drained
- 2 cups water

Directions for Cooking:

1) Place a pot on medium-high fire and heat pot for a minute. Add oil and heat for another minute.
2) Stir in celery and onion. Sauté for 7 minutes.
3) Stir in garlic and cook for another minute.
4) Add water, thyme, pepper, chicken broth, and beans. Cover and simmer for 15 minutes.
5) Remove 2 cups of the bean and celery mixture with a slotted spoon and set aside.
6) With an immersion blender, puree remaining soup in pot until smooth and creamy.
7) Return the 2 cups of bean mixture. Stir in spinach and lemon juice. Cook for 2 minutes until heated through and spinach is wilted.
8) Serve and enjoy.

Nutrition Information:
Calories per serving: 245; Protein: 12.0g; Carbs: 38.1g; Fat: 4.9g

Kidney and Black Bean Chicken Soup

Serves: 10, Cooking Time: 7 hours

Ingredients:

- 2 chicken breasts fillets, skinless, cut into 1-inch cubes
- ½ cup freshly chopped cilantro
- Salt to taste
- ½ tsp black pepper
- ½ tsp cayenne pepper
- 1 tsp cumin
- 1 tbsp chili powder
- Juice from 1 lime
- 1 cup fresh or frozen corn kernels
- 2 ½ cups chicken broth, low sodium, fat-free
- 1 14.5-oz can diced tomatoes
- 1 4.5-oz can diced green chili peppers
- 1 15-oz can kidney beans, rinsed and drained
- 1 15-oz can black beans, rinsed and drained
- 1 clove garlic, minced
- ½ cup diced onion

Directions for Cooking:

1) In slow cooker, add all ingredients.
2) Cover and cook on low settings for six to eight hours.
3) When done, transfer to serving bowls and enjoy.

Nutrition Information:
Calories per serving: 192; Protein: 20.0g; Carbs: 21.0g; Fat: 12.8g

Kidney Beans and Beet Salad

Serves: 4, Cooking Time: 15 minutes

Ingredients:

- 1 14.5-ounce can kidney beans, drained and rinsed
- 1 tablespoon pomegranate syrup or juice
- 2 tablespoons olive oil
- 4 beets, scrubbed and stems removed
- 4 green onions, chopped
- Juice of 1 lemon
- Salt and pepper to taste

Directions for Cooking:

1) Bring a pot of water to boil and add beets. Simmer for 10 minutes or until tender. Drain beets and place in ice bath for 5 minutes.
2) Peel bets and slice in halves.

3) Toss to mix the pomegranate syrup, olive oil, lemon juice, green onions, and kidney beans in a salad bowl.
4) Stir in beets. Season with pepper and salt to taste.

5) Serve and enjoy.
Nutrition Information:
Calories per serving: 175; Protein: 6.0g; Carbs: 22.0g; Fat: 7.0g

Kidney Bean and Chickpea Salad

Serves: 10, Cooking Time: 0 minutes
Ingredients:

- ¼ cup lemon juice
- ¼ teaspoon ground cinnamon
- ½ cup chopped fresh mint
- ½ cup extra-virgin olive oil
- 1 15-ounce can chickpeas, rinsed
- 1 cup finely diced carrot
- 1 small clove garlic, peeled and minced
- 1 teaspoon kosher salt, divided
- 1½ cups chopped fresh parsley
- 2 15-ounce cans dark red kidney beans, rinsed

- 2 tablespoons ground cumin

Directions for Cooking:
1) In a salad bowl, whisk well lemon juice, cinnamon, olive oil, garlic, salt, parsley, and cumin.
2) Stir in remaining ingredients and toss well to coat in the dressing.
3) Serve and enjoy.

Nutrition Information:
Calories per serving: 221; Protein: 6.0g; Carbs: 22.0g; Fat: 12.0g

Kidney Bean and Parsley-Lemon Salad

Serves: 6, Cooking Time: 0 minutes
Ingredients:

- ¼ cup lemon juice (about 1 ½ lemons)
- ¼ cup olive oil
- ¾ cup chopped fresh parsley
- ¾ teaspoon salt
- 1 can (15 ounces) chickpeas, rinsed and drained, or 1 ½ cups cooked chickpeas
- 1 medium cucumber, peeled, seeded and diced
- 1 small red onion, diced
- 2 cans (15 ounces each) red kidney beans, rinsed and drained, or 3 cups cooked kidney beans
- 2 stalks celery, sliced in half or thirds lengthwise and chopped
- 2 tablespoons chopped fresh dill or mint

- 3 cloves garlic, pressed or minced
- Small pinch red pepper flakes

Directions for Cooking:
1) Whisk well in a small bowl the pepper flakes, salt, garlic, and lemon juice until emulsified.
2) In a serving bowl, combine the prepared kidney beans, chickpeas, onion, celery, cucumber, parsley and dill (or mint).
3) Drizzle salad with the dressing and toss well to coat.
4) Serve and enjoy.

Nutrition Information:
Calories per serving: 228; Protein: 8.5g; Carbs: 26.2g; Fat: 11.0g

Mushroom Chickpea Marsala

Serves: 4, Cooking Time: 20 minutes
Ingredients:

- 2 tbsp olive oil
- 8 oz. baby portobello mushrooms, sliced
- 2 garlic cloves, minced
- 1 cup dry Marsala wine
- 2 tbsp lemon juice, or to taste
- 1 tsp rubbed sage

- 1/2 tsp black pepper
- 1/4 tsp salt
- 2 tbsp chopped fresh parsley
- 1-14 oz. can or 1 3/4 cups cooked chickpeas, rinsed and drained

Directions for Cooking:

1) On medium fire, place a large saucepan and heat oil.
2) Add mushrooms, cover and cook for 5 minutes.
3) Stir in garlic and cook for 2 minutes.
4) Add wine, lemon juice, sage, salt and pepper. Deglaze pot.
5) Simmer for 10 minutes while covered.
6) Add chickpeas and mix well. Cook for 3 minutes.
7) Remove pot from fire and stir in parsley.
8) Serve and enjoy.

Nutrition Information:
Calories per serving: 159; Protein: 6.1g; Carbs: 16.8g; Fat: 8.5g

Rice and Chickpea Stew

Serves: 6, Cooking Time: 60 minutes
Ingredients:
- ½ cup chopped fresh cilantro
- ¼ tsp freshly ground pepper
- ¼ tsp salt
- 2/3 cup brown basmati rice
- 3 cups peeled and diced sweet potato
- 2 15-oz cans chickpeas, rinsed
- 4 cups reduced-sodium chicken broth
- 1 cup orange juice
- 2 tsp ground coriander
- 2 tsp ground cumin
- 3 medium onions, halved and thinly sliced
- 1 tbsp extra virgin olive oil

Directions for Cooking:
1) On medium fire, place a large nonstick fry pan and heat oil.
2) Sauté onions for 8 minutes or until soft and translucent.
3) Add coriander and cumin, sauté for half a minute.
4) Add broth and orange juice.
5) Add salt, rice, sweet potato, and chickpeas.
6) Bring to a boil, once boiling lower fire to a simmer, cover and cook.
7) Stir occasionally, cook for 45 minutes or until potatoes and rice are tender.
8) Season with pepper.
9) Stew will be thick, if you want a less thick soup, just add water and adjust salt and pepper to taste.
10) To serve, garnish with cilantro.

Nutrition Information:
Calories per serving: 332; Protein: 13.01g; Carbs: 55.5g; Fat: 7.5g

Roasted Chickpea-Cauliflower Stew

Serves: 6, Cooking Time: 50 minutes
Ingredients:
- 1 tsp ground coriander
- 1 tsp Sweet paprika
- 1 tsp cayenne pepper (optional)
- 1 whole head cauliflower, divided into small florets
- Salt and pepper
- Private Reserve extra virgin olive oil
- 1 large sweet onion, chopped
- 6 garlic cloves, chopped
- 1 1/2 tsp ground turmeric
- 1 1/2 tsp ground cumin
- 1 1/2 tsp ground cinnamon
- 1/2 tsp ground green cardamom
- 5 medium-sized bulk carrots, peeled, cut into 1 1/2" pieces
- 1/2 cup parsley leaves, stems removed, roughly chopped
- 1 28-oz can diced tomatoes with its juice
- 2 14-oz cans chickpeas, drained and rinsed

Directions for Cooking:
1) Preheat the oven to 475 degrees F.
2) Mix well all the spices in a small bowl.
3) Lightly oil a baking sheet and spread carrots and cauliflower. Season with salt and pepper. Add a little more than 1/2 of the spice mixture. Drizzle generously with olive oil, then toss well to mix.
4) Pop in the oven and bake until soft, around 20 minutes.
5) Heat 2 tbsp olive oil in a large cast iron pan on medium-high fire.

6) Sauté onion for 3 minutes. Stir in garlic and the remaining spices. Sauté for 2-3 more minutes.
7) Stir in canned tomatoes and chickpeas. Season with salt and pepper. Bring to a boil, then reduce heat to medium- low. Cover and simmer for 5 minutes.

8) Stir in the roasted cauliflower and carrots. Cover and cook for another 15-20 minutes. Stir occasionally and add a little water if needed.
9) Garnish with fresh parsley, serve and enjoy.

Nutrition Information:
Calories per serving: 407; Protein: 12.1g; Carbs: 38.9g; Fat: 25.3g

Saffron Green Bean-Quinoa Soup

Serves: 6, Cooking Time: 20 minutes
Ingredients:
- 2 tablespoons extra virgin olive oil
- 1 large leek, white and light green parts only, halved, washed, and sliced
- 2 cloves garlic, minced
- 8 ounces fresh green beans, trimmed and chopped into 1" pieces
- 2 large pinches saffron, or one capsule
- 15 ounces chickpeas and liquid (do not rinse!)
- 1 large tomato, seeded and chopped into 1" pieces
- salt and freshly ground pepper, to taste
- freshly chopped basil, for serving
- 1 large carrot, chopped into 1/2" pieces
- 1 large celery stalk, chopped into 1/2" pieces
- 1 large zucchini, chopped into 1/2" pieces
- 1/2 cup quinoa, rinsed
- 4-5 cups vegetable stock

Directions for Cooking:
1) Place a large pot on medium fire and heat olive oil for 2 minutes.
2) Stir in celery and carrots. Cook for 6 minutes or until soft.
3) Mix in garlic and leek. Sauté for 3 minutes.
4) Add the zucchini and green beans, and sauté 1 minute more.
5) Pour in broth and saffron. Bring to a boil. Stir in chickpeas and quinoa. Cook until quinoa is soft, around 11 minutes while covered.
6) Stir in the diced tomato and salt and pepper, to taste, and remove from heat.
7) Serve the soup with the freshly chopped basil and enjoy!

Nutrition Information:
Calories per serving: 196; Protein: 7.9g; Carbs: 26.6g; Fat: 7.5g

Simply Good Chickpeas Recipe

Serves: 8, Cooking Time: 95 minutes
Ingredients:
- 1 14.5-oz can of petite diced tomatoes, undrained
- 2 15-oz cans garbanzo beans, rinsed and drained
- 1 cup lentils
- 6 cups vegetable broth or stock
- ¼ tsp ground cayenne pepper
- ½ tsp ground cumin
- 1 tsp turmeric
- 1 tsp garam masala
- 1 tsp minced garlic
- 2 tsp grated fresh ginger
- 1 cup diced carrots
- 1 cup chopped celery
- 2 onions, chopped

- 1 tbsp olive oil

Directions for Cooking:
1) On medium-high fire, set a large soup pot and heat oil.
2) Add onions and cook until tender around 3-4 minutes.
3) Add celery and carrots, continue sautéing for 5 minutes.
4) Add garlic, cayenne pepper, cumin, turmeric and garam masala and cook until heated through.
5) Add tomatoes, garbanzo beans, lentils and broth. Cook while covered for 90 minutes or until lentils are tender.

6) If desired, you can puree half of the soup to make a thick broth.
7) Serve while hot.

Nutrition Information:
Calories per serving: 211; Protein: 10.1g; Carbs: 33.3g; Fat: 5.3g

Spicy Sweet Red Hummus

Serves: 8, Cooking Time: 0 minutes
Ingredients:
- 1 (15 ounce) can garbanzo beans, drained
- 1 (4 ounce) jar roasted red peppers
- 1 1/2 tablespoons tahini
- 1 clove garlic, minced
- 1 tablespoon chopped fresh parsley
- 1/2 teaspoon cayenne pepper
- 1/2 teaspoon ground cumin
- 1/4 teaspoon salt
- 3 tablespoons lemon juice

Directions for Cooking:
1) In a blender, add all ingredients and process until smooth and creamy.
2) Adjust seasoning to taste if needed.
3) Can be stored in an airtight container for up to 5 days.

Nutrition Information:
Calories per serving: 64; Protein: 2.5g; Carbs: 9.6g; Fat: 2.2g

Sun-Dried Tomatoes and Chickpeas

Serves: 6, Cooking Time: 22 minutes
Ingredients:
- 1 red bell pepper
- 1/2 cup parsley, chopped
- 1/4 cup red wine vinegar
- 2 14.5-ounce cans chickpeas, drained and rinsed
- 2 cloves garlic, chopped
- 2 cups water
- 2 tablespoons extra-virgin olive oil
- 4 sun-dried tomatoes
- Salt to taste

Directions for Cooking:
1) Lengthwise, slice bell pepper in half. Place on baking sheet with skin side up. Broil on top rack for 5 minutes until skin is blistered.
2) In a brown paper bag, place the charred bell pepper halves. Fold bag and leave in there for 10 minutes. Remove pepper and peel off skin. Slice into thin strips.
3) Meanwhile, microwave 2 cups of water to boiling. Add the sun-dried tomatoes and leave in to reconstitute for 10 minutes. Drain and slice into thin strips.
4) Whisk well olive oil, garlic, and red wine vinegar.
5) Mix in parsley, sun-dried tomato, bell pepper, and chickpeas.
6) Season with salt to taste and serve.

Nutrition Information:
Calories per serving: 195; Protein: 8.0g; Carbs: 26.0g; Fat: 7.0g

Sweet Potato-Chickpea Cajun Patties

Serves: 5, Cooking Time: 8 minutes
Ingredients:
- 1 1/2 cups old-fashioned rolled oats
- 1 1/2 tbsp Cajun seasoning
- 1 cup cooked and pureed sweet potato
- 1 large egg
- 1/2 cup diced onion
- 1/2 cup red bell pepper
- 1/4 cup diced celery
- 1/4 tsp cayenne
- 1/4 tsp garlic powder
- 1-2 cloves garlic, smashed and minced
- 2 cups chickpeas, rinsed and drained
- 2 tsp extra virgin olive oil
- salt and pepper to taste

Directions for Cooking:
1) Boil sweet potato until tender. Discard skin and puree in a blender.

2) Place pureed sweet potato in a large bowl.
3) Add chickpeas in blender and pulse to desired texture and not too creamy.
4) Next pulse one and a half cups of oats until flour-like. Add to the sweet potato mixture.
5) On medium-high fire, place a saucepan and heat oil for 2 minutes. Sauté celery, bell pepper and onion for 5 minutes. Stir in garlic and cook for another 2 minutes. Transfer to bowl.
6) In a small bowl, whisk egg, salt, cayenne pepper, garlic powder, and Cajun seasoning.
7) With hands, mix well chickpea mixture. Pour eggs and continue mixing well.
8) Evenly divide into 5. Form each into a burger pattie.
9) Cook for 4 minutes per side or until lightly browned.
10) Serve and enjoy with burger buns and desired condiment.

Nutrition Information:
Calories per serving: 269; Protein: 11.0g; Carbs: 43.0g; Fat: 6.0g

Three Bean Salad

Serves: 6, Cooking Time: 0 minutes
Ingredients:
- 1 can, 15.5 can Garbanzo Beans, rinsed
- 1 can, 15.5 can Kidney Beans, rinsed
- 1 clove garlic, minced
- 1 large Shallot, minced
- 1 tsp Salt
- 1/3 cup Apple Cider Vinegar
- 1/4 tsp Pepper
- 2 cups Green Beans, freshly blanched if possible or 1 can cut green beans
- 2 Tbsp Sugar
- 2 Tbsp olive Oil

Directions for Cooking:

1) In a small bowl, whisk together shallots, garlic, pepper, salt, oil, and sugar.
2) In a large bowl stir together kidney, garbanzo, and green beans.
3) Drizzle olive oil dressing and toss well to coat.
4) Cover and place in the fridge to chill to allow the flavors to meld.
5) Mix well before serving.

Nutrition Information:
Calories per serving: 210; Protein: 9.1g; Carbs: 30.2g; Fat: 6.2g

White Bean and Tuna Salad

Serves: 4, Cooking Time: 8 minutes
Ingredients:
- 1 (12 ounce) can solid white albacore tuna, drained
- 1 (16 ounce) can Great Northern beans, drained and rinsed
- 1 (2.25 ounce) can sliced black olives, drained
- 1 teaspoon dried oregano
- 1/2 teaspoon finely grated lemon zest
- 1/4 medium red onion, thinly sliced
- 3 tablespoons lemon juice
- 3/4-pound green beans, trimmed and snapped in half
- 4 large hard-cooked eggs, peeled and quartered
- 6 tablespoons extra-virgin olive oil
- Salt and ground black pepper, to taste

Directions for Cooking:

1) Place a saucepan on medium-high fire. Add a cup of water and the green beans. Cover and cook for 8 minutes. Drain immediately once tender.
2) In a salad bowl, whisk well oregano, olive oil, lemon juice, and lemon zest. Season generously with pepper and salt and mix until salt is dissolved.
3) Stir in drained green beans, tuna, beans, olives, and red onion. Mix thoroughly to coat.
4) Adjust seasoning to taste.
5) Spread eggs on top.
6) Serve and enjoy.

Nutrition Information:
Calories per serving: 551; Protein: 36.3g; Carbs: 33.4g; Fat: 30.3g

Chapter 9 Seafood Recipes

Avocado Peach Salsa on Grilled Swordfish

Serves: 2 , Cook Time: 10 minutes

Swordfish Marinade Ingredients:
- 1 garlic clove, minced
- 1 lemon juice
- 1 tbsp apple cider vinegar
- 1 tbsp olive oil
- 1 tsp honey
- 2 swordfish fillets (around 4oz each)
- pinch cayenne pepper
- pinch of pepper and salt

Salsa Ingredients:
- ¼ red onion, finely chopped
- ½ cup cilantro, finely chopped
- 1 avocado, halved and diced
- 1 garlic clove, minced
- 2 peaches, seeded and diced
- juice of 1 lime
- Salt to taste

Directions for Cooking:
1) In a shallow dish, mix all swordfish marinade ingredients except fillet. Mix well then add fillets to marinate. Place in refrigerator for at least an hour.
2) Meanwhile create salsa by mixing all salsa ingredients in a medium bowl. Put in the refrigerator to cool.
3) Preheat grill and grill fish on medium fire after marinating until cooked around 4 minutes per side.
4) Place each cooked fillet on one serving plate, top with half of salsa, serve and enjoy.

Nutrition Information:
Calories per serving: 416; Carbohydrates: 21g; Protein: 30g; Fat: 23.5g

Baked Cod Crusted with Herbs

Serves: 4 , Cook Time: 10 minutes

Ingredients:
- ¼ cup honey
- ¼ tsp salt
- ½ cup panko
- ½ tsp pepper
- 1 tbsp extra virgin olive oil
- 1 tbsp lemon juice
- 1 tsp dried basil
- 1 tsp dried parsley
- 1 tsp rosemary
- 4 pieces of 4-oz cod fillets

Directions for Cooking:
1) With olive oil, grease a 9 x 13-inch baking pan and preheat oven to 375 degrees F.
2) In a zip top bag mix panko, rosemary, salt, pepper, parsley and basil.
3) Evenly spread cod fillets in prepped dish and drizzle with lemon juice.
4) Then brush the fillets with honey on all sides. Discard remaining honey if any.
5) Then evenly divide the panko mixture on top of cod fillets.
6) Pop in the oven and bake for ten minutes or until fish is cooked.
7) Serve and enjoy.

Nutrition Information:
Calories per serving: 137; Protein: 5g; Fat: 2g; Carbs: 21g

Baked Cod Fillets with Sauce

Serves: 4 , Cook Time: 15 minutes

Ingredients:
- Pepper and salt to taste
- 2 tablespoons minced parsley
- 1 lemon, sliced into ¼-inch thick circles
- 1 lemon, juiced and zested
- 4 garlic cloves, crushed, peeled, and minced
- ¼ cup olive oil

- 4 Cod fillets

Directions for Cooking:

1) Bring oven to 425 degrees F.
2) Mix parsley, lemon juice, lemon zest, garlic, and olive oil in a small bowl. Mix well and then season with pepper and salt to taste.
3) Prepare a large baking dish by greasing it with cooking spray.
4) Evenly lay the cod fillets on the greased dish. Season generously with pepper and salt.
5) Pour the bowl of garlic sauce from step 2 on top of cod fillets.
6) Top the cod fillets with the thinly sliced lemon.
7) Pop in the preheated oven and bake until flaky, around 13 to 15 minutes.
8) Remove from oven, transfer to dishes, serve, and enjoy.

Nutrition Information:
Calories per Serving: 200; Fat: 12g; Protein: 21g; Carbs: 2g

Berries and Grilled Calamari

Serves: 4, Cook Time: 5 minutes

Ingredients:

- ¼ cup dried cranberries
- ¼ cup extra virgin olive oil
- ¼ cup olive oil
- ¼ cup sliced almonds
- ½ lemon, juiced
- ¾ cup blueberries
- 1 ½ pounds calamari tube, cleaned
- 1 granny smith apple, sliced thinly
- 1 tablespoon fresh lemon juice
- 2 tablespoons apple cider vinegar
- 6 cups fresh spinach
- Freshly grated pepper to taste
- Sea salt to taste

Directions for Cooking:

1) In a small bowl, make the vinaigrette by mixing well the tablespoon of lemon juice, apple cider vinegar, and extra virgin olive oil. Season with pepper and salt to taste. Set aside.
2) Turn on the grill to medium fire and let the grates heat up for a minute or two.
3) In a large bowl, add olive oil and the calamari tube. Season calamari generously with pepper and salt.
4) Place seasoned and oiled calamari onto heated grate and grill until cooked or opaque. This is around two minutes per side.
5) As you wait for the calamari to cook, you can combine almonds, cranberries, blueberries, spinach, and the thinly sliced apple in a large salad bowl. Toss to mix.
6) Remove cooked calamari from grill and transfer on a chopping board. Cut into ¼-inch thick rings and throw into the salad bowl.
7) Drizzle with vinaigrette and toss well to coat salad.
8) Serve and enjoy!

Nutrition Information:
Calories per Serving: 567; Fat: 24.5g; Protein: 54.8g; Carbs: 30.6g

Breaded and Spiced Halibut

Serves: 4, Cook Time: 15 minutes

Ingredients:

- ¼ cup chopped fresh chives
- ¼ cup chopped fresh dill
- ¼ tsp ground black pepper
- ¾ cup panko breadcrumbs
- 1 tbsp extra-virgin olive oil
- 1 tsp finely grated lemon zest
- 1 tsp sea salt
- 1/3 cup chopped fresh parsley
- 4 pieces of 6-oz halibut fillets

Directions for Cooking:

1) Line a baking sheet with foil, grease with cooking spray and preheat oven to 400 degrees F.
2) In a small bowl, mix black pepper, sea salt, lemon zest, olive oil, chives, dill, parsley and breadcrumbs. If needed add more salt to taste. Set aside.

3) Meanwhile, wash halibut fillets on cold tap water. Dry with paper towels and place on prepared baking sheet.
4) Generously spoon crumb mixture onto halibut fillets. Ensure that fillets are covered with crumb mixture. Press down on crumb mixture onto each fillet.

5) Pop into the oven and bake for 10-15 minutes or until fish is flaky and crumb topping are already lightly browned.

Nutrition Information:
Calories per serving: 336.4; Protein: 25.3g; Fat: 25.3g; Carbs: 4.1g

Coconut Salsa on Chipotle Fish Tacos

Serves: 4, Cook Time: 10 minutes
Ingredients:
- ¼ cup chopped fresh cilantro
- ½ cup seeded and finely chopped plum tomato
- 1 cup peeled and finely chopped mango
- 1 lime cut into wedges
- 1 tbsp chipotle Chile powder
- 1 tbsp safflower oil
- 1/3 cup finely chopped red onion
- 10 tbsp fresh lime juice, divided
- 4 6-oz boneless, skinless cod fillets
- 5 tbsp dried unsweetened shredded coconut
- 8 pcs of 6-inch tortillas, heated

Directions for Cooking:
1) Whisk well Chile powder, oil, and 4 tbsp lime juice in a glass baking dish. Add cod and

marinate for 12 – 15 minutes. Turning once halfway through the marinating time.
2) Make the salsa by mixing coconut, 6 tbsp lime juice, cilantro, onions, tomatoes and mangoes in a medium bowl. Set aside.
3) On high, heat a grill pan. Place cod and grill for four minutes per side turning only once.
4) Once cooked, slice cod into large flakes and evenly divide onto tortilla.
5) Evenly divide salsa on top of cod and serve with a side of lime wedges.

Nutrition Information:
Calories per serving: 477; Protein: 35.0g; Fat: 12.4g; Carbs: 57.4g

Crazy Saganaki Shrimp

Serves: 4, Cook Time: 10 minutes
Ingredients:
- ¼ tsp salt
- ½ cup Chardonnay
- ½ cup crumbled Greek feta cheese
- 1 medium bulb. fennel, cored and finely chopped
- 1 small Chile pepper, seeded and minced
- 1 tbsp extra virgin olive oil
- 12 jumbo shrimps, peeled and deveined with tails left on
- 2 tbsp lemon juice, divided
- 5 scallions sliced thinly
- Pepper to taste

Directions for Cooking:
1) In medium bowl, mix salt, lemon juice and shrimp.
2) On medium fire, place a saganaki pan (or large nonstick saucepan) and heat oil.

3) Sauté Chile pepper, scallions, and fennel for 4 minutes or until starting to brown and is already soft.
4) Add wine and sauté for another minute.
5) Place shrimps on top of fennel, cover and cook for 4 minutes or until shrimps are pink.
6) Remove just the shrimp and transfer to a plate.
7) Add pepper, feta and 1 tbsp lemon juice to pan and cook for a minute or until cheese begins to melt.
8) To serve, place cheese and fennel mixture on a serving plate and top with shrimps.

Nutrition Information:
Calories per serving: 310; Protein: 49.7g; Fat: 6.8g; Carbs: 8.4g

Crisped Coco-Shrimp with Mango Dip

Serves: 4, Cook Time: 20 minutes

Ingredients:

- 1 cup shredded coconut
- 1 lb. raw shrimp, peeled and deveined
- 2 egg whites
- 4 tbsp tapioca starch
- Pepper and salt to taste

Mango Dip Ingredients:

- 1 cup mango, chopped
- 1 jalapeño, thinly minced
- 1 tsp lime juice
- 1/3 cup coconut milk
- 3 tsp raw honey

Directions for Cooking:

1) Preheat oven to 400 degrees F.
2) Ready a pan with wire rack on top.
3) In a medium bowl, add tapioca starch and season with pepper and salt.
4) In a second medium bowl, add egg whites and whisk.
5) In a third medium bowl, add coconut.
6) To ready shrimps, dip first in tapioca starch, then egg whites, and then coconut. Place dredged shrimp on wire rack. Repeat until all shrimps are covered.
7) Pop shrimps in the oven and roast for 10 minutes per side.
8) Meanwhile make the dip by adding all ingredients in a blender. Puree until smooth and creamy. Transfer to a dipping bowl.
9) Once shrimps are golden brown, serve with mango dip.

Nutrition Information:

Calories per Serving: 294.2; Protein: 26.6g; Fat: 7g; Carbs: 31.2g

Cucumber-Basil Salsa on Halibut Pouches

Serves: 4, Cook Time: 17 minutes

Ingredients:

- 1 lime, thinly sliced into 8 pieces
- 2 cups mustard greens, stems removed
- 2 tsp olive oil
- 4 – 5 radishes trimmed and quartered
- 4 4-oz skinless halibut filets
- 4 large fresh basil leaves
- Cayenne pepper to taste – optional
- Pepper and salt to taste

Salsa Ingredients:

- 1 ½ cups diced cucumber
- 1 ½ finely chopped fresh basil leaves
- 2 tsp fresh lime juice
- Pepper and salt to taste

Directions for Cooking:

1) Preheat oven to 400 degrees F.
2) Prepare parchment papers by making 4 pieces of 15 x 12-inch rectangles. Lengthwise, fold in half and unfold pieces on the table.
3) Season halibut fillets with pepper, salt and cayenne—if using cayenne.
4) Just to the right of the fold going lengthwise, place ½ cup of mustard greens. Add a basil leaf on center of mustard greens and topped with 1 lime slice. Around the greens, layer ¼ of the radishes. Drizzle with ½ tsp of oil, season with pepper and salt. Top it with a slice of halibut fillet.
5) Just as you would make a calzone, fold parchment paper over your filling and crimp the edges of the parchment paper beginning from one end to the other end. To seal the end of the crimped parchment paper, pinch it.
6) Repeat process to remaining ingredients until you have 4 pieces of parchment papers filled with halibut and greens.
7) Place pouches in a baking pan and bake in the oven until halibut is flaky, around 15 to 17 minutes.
8) While waiting for halibut pouches to cook, make your salsa by mixing all salsa ingredients in a medium bowl.
9) Once halibut is cooked, remove from oven and make a tear on top. Be careful of the steam as it is very hot. Equally divide salsa and spoon ¼ of salsa on top of halibut through the slit you have created.
10) Serve and enjoy.

Nutrition Information:

Calories per serving: 335.4; Protein: 20.2g; Fat: 16.3g; Carbs: 22.1g

Curry Salmon with Mustard

Serves: 4, Cook Time: 8 minutes

Ingredients:

- ¼ tsp ground red pepper or chili powder
- ¼ tsp ground turmeric
- ¼ tsp salt
- 1 tsp honey
- 1/8 tsp garlic powder or 1 clove garlic minced
- 2 tsp. whole grain mustard
- 4 pcs 6-oz salmon fillets

Directions for Cooking:

1) In a small bowl mix well salt, garlic powder, red pepper, turmeric, honey and mustard.
2) Preheat oven to broil and grease a baking dish with cooking spray.
3) Place salmon on baking dish with skin side down and spread evenly mustard mixture on top of salmon.
4) Pop in the oven and broil until flaky around 8 minutes.

Nutrition Information:

Calories per Serving: 324; Fat: 18.9 g; Protein: 34 g; Carbs: 2.9 g

Dijon Mustard and Lime Marinated Shrimp

Serves: 8 , Cook Time: 10 minutes

Ingredients:

- ½ cup fresh lime juice, plus lime zest as garnish
- ½ cup rice vinegar
- ½ tsp hot sauce
- 1 bay leaf
- 1 cup water
- 1 lb. uncooked shrimp, peeled and deveined
- 1 medium red onion, chopped
- 2 tbsp capers
- 2 tbsp Dijon mustard
- 3 whole cloves

Directions for Cooking:

1) Mix hot sauce, mustard, capers, lime juice and onion in a shallow baking dish and set aside.
2) Bring to a boil in a large saucepan bay leaf, cloves, vinegar and water.
3) Once boiling, add shrimps and cook for a minute while stirring continuously.
4) Drain shrimps and pour shrimps into onion mixture.
5) For an hour, refrigerate while covered the shrimps.
6) Then serve shrimps cold and garnished with lime zest.

Nutrition Information:

Calories per serving: 232.2; Protein: 17.8g; Fat: 3g; Carbs: 15g

Dill Relish on White Sea Bass

Serves: 4 , Cook Time: 12 minutes

Ingredients:

- 1 ½ tbsp chopped white onion
- 1 ½ tsp chopped fresh dill
- 1 lemon, quartered
- 1 tsp Dijon mustard
- 1 tsp lemon juice
- 1 tsp pickled baby capers, drained
- 4 pieces of 4-oz white sea bass fillets

Directions for Cooking:

1) Preheat oven to 375 degrees F.
2) Mix lemon juice, mustard, dill, capers and onions in a small bowl.
3) Prepare four aluminum foil squares and place 1 fillet per foil.
4) Squeeze a lemon wedge per fish.
5) Evenly divide into 4 the dill spread and drizzle over fillet.
6) Close the foil over the fish securely and pop in the oven.
7) Bake for 10 to 12 minutes or until fish is cooked through.
8) Remove from foil and transfer to a serving platter, serve and enjoy.

Nutrition Information:

Calories per serving: 115; Protein: 7g; Fat: 1g; Carbs: 12g

Easy Broiled Lobster Tails

Serves: 2, Cook Time: 10 minutes
Ingredients:

- 1 6-oz frozen lobster tails
- 1 tbsp olive oil
- 1 tsp lemon pepper seasoning

Directions for Cooking:

1) Preheat oven broiler.
2) With kitchen scissors, cut thawed lobster tails in half lengthwise.
3) Brush with oil the exposed lobster meat. Season with lemon pepper.
4) Place lobster tails in baking sheet with exposed meat facing up.
5) Place on top broiler rack and broil for 10 minutes until lobster meat is lightly browned on the sides and center meat is opaque.
6) Serve and enjoy.

Nutrition Information:
Calories per Serving: 175.6; Protein: 3g; Fat: 10g; Carbs: 18.4g

Easy Fish Curry

Serves: 4, Cook Time: 20 minutes
Ingredients:

- Juice of half a lime
- A handful of coriander leaves
- ½ pound white fish cut into large strips
- Salt and pepper to taste
- 2 tomatoes, chopped
- ½ cup coconut milk
- 15 curry leaves
- 1 teaspoon turmeric, ground
- 2 teaspoon curry powder
- 2 tablespoon ginger, grated
- 3 cloves garlic, sliced
- 1 onion, chopped
- 2 tablespoon olive oil

Directions for Cooking:

1) Heat oil in a medium saucepan. Sauté the onion over medium heat until translucent.
2) Add the ginger and garlic and cook for a minute before adding the curry powder, curry leaves and turmeric. Continue cooking for a minute before adding the coconut milk.
3) Add the chopped tomatoes and simmer for 5 minutes or until the tomatoes are soft.
4) Add the fish and season with salt and pepper to taste. Cook for 8 minutes before adding the lime juice and coriander leaves.
5) Serve warm.

Nutrition Information:
Calories per Serving: 213; Fat: 14.7g; Protein: 12.3g; Carbs: 10.5g

Easy Seafood French Stew

Serves: 12, Cooking Time: 45 minutes
Bouillabaisse Ingredients:

- Pepper and Salt
- 1/2 lb. littleneck clams
- 1/2 lb. mussels
- 1 lb. shrimp, peeled and deveined
- 1 large lobster
- 2 lbs. assorted small whole fresh fish, scaled and cleaned
- 2 tbsp parsley, finely chopped
- 2 tbsp garlic, chopped
- 1 cup fennel, julienned
- Juice and zest of one orange
- 3 cups tomatoes, peeled, seeded, and chopped
- 1 cup leeks, julienned
- Pinch of Saffron

Stew Ingredients:

- 1 cup white wine
- Water
- 1 lb. fish bones
- 2 sprigs thyme
- 8 peppercorns
- 1 bay leaf
- 3 cloves garlic
- Salt and pepper
- 1/2 cup chopped celery
- 1/2 cup chopped onion
- 2 tbsp olive oil

Directions for Cooking:

1) Do the stew: Heat oil in a large saucepan. Sauté the celery and onions for 3 minutes. Season with pepper and salt. Stir in the garlic and cook for about a minute. Add the thyme, peppercorns, and bay leaves. Stir in the wine, water and fish bones. Let it boil then before reducing to a simmer. Take the pan off the fire and strain broth into another container.

2) For the Bouillabaisse: Bring the strained broth to a simmer and stir in the parsley, leeks, orange juice, orange zest, garlic, fennel, tomatoes and saffron. Sprinkle with pepper and salt. Stir in the lobsters and fish. Let it simmer for eight minutes before stirring in the clams, mussels and shrimps. For six minutes, allow to cook while covered before seasoning again with pepper and salt.

3) Assemble in a shallow dish all the seafood and pour the broth over it.

Nutrition Information:

Calories per serving: 348; Carbs: 20.0g; Protein: 31.8g; Fat: 15.2g

Fresh and No-Cook Oysters

Serves: 4, Cook Time: 5 minutes

Ingredients:

- 2 lemons
- 24 medium oysters
- tabasco sauce

Directions for Cooking:

1) If you are a newbie when it comes to eating oysters, then I suggest that you blanch the oysters before eating.

2) For some, eating oysters raw is a great way to enjoy this dish because of the consistency and juiciness of raw oysters. Plus, adding lemon juice prior to eating the raw oysters cooks it a bit.

3) So, to blanch oysters, bring a big pot of water to a rolling boil. Add oysters in batches of 6-10 pieces. Leave on boiling pot of water between 3-5 minutes and remove oysters right away.

4) To eat oysters, squeeze lemon juice on oyster on shell, add tabasco as desired and eat.

Nutrition Information:

Calories per Serving: 247; Protein: 29g; Fat: 7g; Carbs: 17g

Orange Herbed Sauced White Bass

Serves: 6, Cook Time: 33 minutes

Ingredients:

- ¼ cup thinly sliced green onions
- ½ cup orange juice
- 1 ½ tbsp fresh lemon juice
- 1 ½ tbsp olive oil
- 1 large onion, halved, thinly sliced
- 1 large orange, unpeeled, sliced
- 3 tbsp chopped fresh dill
- 6 3-oz skinless white bass fillets
- Additional unpeeled orange slices

Directions for Cooking:

1) Grease a 13 x 9-inch glass baking dish and preheat oven to 400 degrees F.

2) Arrange orange slices in single layer on baking dish, top with onion slices, seasoned with pepper and salt plus drizzled with oil.

3) Pop in the oven and roast for 25 minutes or until onions are tender and browned.

4) Remove from oven and increased oven temperature to 450 degrees F.

5) Push onion and orange slices on sides of dish and place bass fillets in middle of dish. Season with 1 ½ tbsp dill, pepper and salt. Arrange onions and orange slices on top of fish and pop into the oven.

6) Roast for 8 minutes or until salmon is opaque and flaky.

7) In a small bowl, mix 1 ½ tbsp dill, lemon juice, green onions and orange juice.

8) Transfer salmon to a serving plate, discard roasted onions, drizzle with the newly made orange sauce and garnish with fresh orange slices.

9) Serve and enjoy.

Nutrition Information:

Calories per serving: 312.42; Protein: 84.22; Fat: 23.14; Carbs: 33.91g

Garlic Roasted Shrimp with Zucchini Pasta

Serves: 2, Cook Time: 10 minutes

Ingredients:

- 2 medium-sized zucchinis, cut into thin strips or spaghetti noodles
- Salt and pepper to taste
- 1 lemon, zested and juiced
- 2 garlic cloves, minced
- 2 tablespoon olive oil
- 8 ounces shrimps, cleaned and deveined

Directions for Cooking:

1) Preheat the oven to 400 degrees F.
2) In a mixing bowl, mix all ingredients except the zucchini noodles. Toss to coat the shrimp.
3) Bake for 10 minutes until the shrimps turn pink.
4) Add the zucchini pasta then toss.

Nutrition Information:

Calories per Serving: 299; Fat: 23.2g; Protein: 14.3g; Carbs: 10.9g

Ginger Scallion Sauce over Seared Ahi

Serves: 4, Cook Time: 6 minutes

Ingredients:

- 1 bunch scallions, bottoms removed, finely chopped
- 1 tbsp rice wine vinegar
- 1 tbsp. Bragg's liquid amino
- 16-oz ahi tuna steaks
- 2 tbsp. fresh ginger, peeled and grated
- 3 tbsp. olive oil, melted
- Pepper and salt to taste

Directions for Cooking:

1) In a small bowl mix together vinegar, 2 tbsp. oil, soy sauce, ginger and scallions. Put aside.
2) On medium fire, place a large saucepan and heat remaining oil. Once oil is hot and starts to smoke, sear tuna until deeply browned or for two minutes per side.
3) Place seared tuna on a serving platter and let it stand for 5 minutes before slicing into 1-inch thick strips.
4) Drizzle ginger-scallion mixture over seared tuna, serve and enjoy.

Nutrition Information:

Calories per Serving: 247; Protein: 29g; Fat: 1g; Carbs: 8g

Healthy Poached Trout

Serves: 2, Cooking Time: 10 minutes

Ingredients:

- 1 8-oz boneless, skin on trout fillet
- 2 cups chicken broth or water
- 2 leeks, halved
- 6-8 slices lemon
- salt and pepper to taste

Directions for Cooking:

1) On medium fire, place a large nonstick skillet and arrange leeks and lemons on pan in a layer. Cover with soup stock or water and bring to a simmer.
2) Meanwhile, season trout on both sides with pepper and salt. Place trout on simmering pan of water. Cover and cook until trout is flaky, around 8 minutes.
3) In a serving platter, spoon leek and lemons on bottom of plate, top with trout and spoon sauce into plate. Serve and enjoy.

Nutritional Information:

Calories per serving: 360.2; Protein: 13.8g; Fat: 7.5g; Carbs: 51.5g

Leftover Salmon Salad Power Bowls

Serves: 1, Cook Time: 10 minutes
Ingredients:

- ½ cup raspberries
- ½ cup zucchini, sliced
- 1 lemon, juice squeezed
- 1 tablespoon balsamic glaze
- 2 sprigs of thyme, chopped
- 2 tablespoon olive oil
- 4 cups seasonal greens
- 4 ounces leftover grilled salmon
- Salt and pepper to taste

Directions for Cooking:
1) Heat oil in a skillet over medium flame and sauté the zucchini. Season with salt and pepper to taste.
2) In a mixing bowl, mix all ingredients together.
3) Toss to combine everything.
4) Sprinkle with nut cheese.

Nutrition Information:
Calories per Serving: 450.3; Fat: 35.5 g; Protein: 23.4g; Carbs: 9.3 g

Lemon-Garlic Baked Halibut

Serves: 2, Cook Time: 15 minutes
Ingredients:

- 1 large garlic clove, minced
- 1 tbsp chopped flat leaf parsley
- 1 tsp olive oil
- 2 5-oz boneless, skin-on halibut fillets
- 2 tsp lemon zest
- Juice of ½ lemon, divided
- Salt and pepper to taste

Directions for Cooking:
1) Grease a baking dish with cooking spray and preheat oven to 400 degrees F.
2) Place halibut with skin touching the dish and drizzle with olive oil.
3) Season with pepper and salt.
4) Pop into the oven and bake until flaky around 12-15 minutes.
5) Remove from oven and drizzle with remaining lemon juice, serve and enjoy with a side of salad greens.

Nutrition Information:
Calories per serving: 315.3; Protein: 14.1g; Fat: 10.5g; Carbs: 36.6g

Minty-Cucumber Yogurt Topped Grilled Fish

Serves: 4, Cook Time: 8 minutes
Ingredients:

- ¼ cup 2% plain Greek yogurt
- ¼ tsp + 1/8 tsp salt
- ¼ tsp black pepper
- ½ green onion, finely chopped
- ½ tsp dried oregano
- 1 tbsp finely chopped fresh mint leaves
- 3 tbsp finely chopped English cucumber
- 4 5-oz cod fillets
- Cooking oil as needed

Directions for Cooking:
1) Brush grill grate with oil and preheat grill to high.
2) Season cod fillets on both sides with pepper, ¼ tsp salt and oregano.
3) Grill cod for 3 minutes per side or until cooked to desired doneness.
4) Mix thoroughly 1/8 tsp salt, onion, mint, cucumber and yogurt in a small bowl.
5) Serve cod with a dollop of the dressing. This dish can be paired with salad greens or brown rice.

Nutrition Information:
Calories per serving: 253.5; Protein: 25.5g; Fat: 1g; Carbs: 5g

One-Pot Seafood Chowder

Serves: 3, Cooking Time: 10 minutes

Ingredients:

- 3 cans coconut milk
- 1 tablespoon garlic, minced
- salt and pepper to taste
- 3 cans clams, chopped
- 2 cans shrimps, canned
- 1 package fresh shrimps, shelled and deveined
- 1 can corn, drained
- 4 large potatoes, diced
- 2 carrots, peeled and chopped
- 2 celery stalks, chopped

Directions for Cooking:

1) Place all ingredients in a pot and give a good stir to mix everything.
2) Close the lid and turn on the heat to medium.
3) Bring to a boil and allow to simmer for 10 minutes.
4) Place in individual containers.
5) Put a label and store in the fridge.
6) Allow to warm at room temperature before heating in the microwave oven.

Nutrition Information:
Calories per serving: 532; Carbs: 92.5g; Protein: 25.3g; Fat: 6.7g

Orange Rosemary Seared Salmon

Serves: 4, Cook Time: 10 minutes

Ingredients:

- ½ cup chicken stock
- 1 cup fresh orange juice
- 1 tablespoon olive oil
- 1 tablespoon tapioca starch
- 2 garlic cloves, minced
- 2 tablespoon fresh lemon juice
- 2 teaspoon fresh rosemary, minced
- 2 teaspoon orange zest
- 4 salmon fillets, skins removed
- Salt and pepper to taste

Directions for Cooking:

1) Season the salmon fillet on both sides.
2) In a skillet, heat olive oil over medium-high heat. Cook the salmon fillets for 5 minutes on each side. Set aside.
3) In a mixing bowl, combine the orange juice, chicken stock, lemon juice and orange zest.
4) In the skillet, sauté the garlic and rosemary for 2 minutes and pour the orange juice mixture. Bring to a boil. Lower the heat to medium low and simmer. Season with salt and pepper to taste.
5) Pour the sauce all over the salmon fillet then serve.

Nutrition Information:
Calories per Serving: 493; Fat: 17.9g; Protein: 66.7g; Carbs: 12.8g

Red Peppers & Pineapple Topped Mahi-Mahi

Serves: 4, Cook Time: 30 minutes

Ingredients:

- ¼ tsp black pepper
- ¼ tsp salt
- 1 cup whole wheat couscous
- 1 red bell pepper, diced
- 2 1/3 cups low sodium chicken broth
- 2 cups chopped fresh pineapple
- 2 tbsp. chopped fresh chives
- 2 tsp. olive oil
- 4 pieces of skinless, boneless mahi mahi (dolphin fish) fillets (around 4-oz each)

Directions for Cooking:

1) On high fire, add 1 1/3 cups broth to a small saucepan and heat until boiling. Once boiling, add couscous. Turn off fire, cover and set aside to allow liquid to be fully absorbed around 5 minutes.
2) On medium-high fire, place a large nonstick saucepan and heat oil.
3) Season fish on both sides with pepper and salt. Add mahi mahi to hot pan and pan fry until

golden around one minute each side. Once cooked, transfer to plate.

4) On same pan, sauté bell pepper and pineapples until soft, around 2 minutes on medium-high fire.
5) Add couscous to pan along with chives, and remaining broth.

6) On top of the mixture in pan, place fish. With foil, cover pan and continue cooking until fish is steaming and tender underneath the foil, around 3-5 minutes.

Nutrition Information:
Calories per serving: 302; Protein: 43.1g; Fat: 4.8g; Carbs: 22.0g

Pan Fried Tuna with Herbs and Nut

Serves: 4, Cook Time: 5 minutes
Ingredients:
- ¼ cup almonds, chopped finely
- ¼ cup fresh tangerine juice
- ½ tsp fennel seeds, chopped finely
- ½ tsp ground pepper, divided
- ½ tsp sea salt, divided
- 1 tbsp olive oil
- 2 tbsp. fresh mint, chopped finely
- 2 tbsp. red onion, chopped finely
- 4 pieces of 6-oz Tuna steak cut in half

Directions for Cooking:
1) Mix fennel seeds, olive oil, mint, onion, tangerine juice and almonds in small bowl. Season with ¼ each of pepper and salt.

2) Season fish with the remaining pepper and salt.
3) On medium-high fire, place a large nonstick fry pan and grease with cooking spray.
4) Pan fry tuna until desired doneness is reached or for one minute per side.
5) Transfer cooked tuna in serving plate, drizzle with dressing and serve.

Nutrition Information:
Calories per Serving: 272; Fat: 9.7 g; Protein: 42 g; Carbohydrates: 4.2 g

Scallops in Wine 'n Olive Oil

Serves: 4, Cook Time: 8 minutes
Ingredients:
- ¼ tsp salt
- ½ cup dry white wine
- 1 ½ lbs. large sea scallops
- 1 ½ tsp chopped fresh tarragon
- 2 tbsp olive oil
- Black pepper – optional

Directions for Cooking:
1) On medium-high fire, place a large nonstick fry pan and heat oil.

2) Add scallops and fry for 3 minutes per side or until edges are lightly browned. Transfer to a serving plate.
3) On same pan, add salt, tarragon and wine while scraping pan to loosen browned bits.
4) Turn off fire.
5) Pour sauce over scallops and serve.

Nutrition Information:
Calories per Serving: 205.2; Fat: 8 g; Protein: 28.6 g; Carbohydrates: 4.7 g

Paprika Salmon and Green Beans

Serves: 3, Cook Time: 20 minutes
Ingredients:
- ¼ cup olive oil
- ½ tablespoon onion powder
- ½ teaspoon bouillon powder
- ½ teaspoon cayenne pepper
- 1 tablespoon smoked paprika

- 1-pound green beans
- 2 teaspoon minced garlic
- 3 tablespoon fresh herbs
- 6 ounces of salmon steak
- Salt and pepper to taste

Directions for Cooking:
1) Preheat the oven to 400 degrees F.
2) Grease a baking sheet and set aside.
3) Heat a skillet over medium low heat and add the olive oil. Sauté the garlic, smoked paprika, fresh herbs, cayenne pepper and onion powder. Stir for a minute then let the mixture sit for 5 minutes. Set aside.
4) Put the salmon steaks in a bowl and add salt and the paprika spice mixture. Rub to coat the salmon well.
5) Place the salmon on the baking sheet and cook for 18 minutes.
6) Meanwhile, blanch the green beans in boiling water with salt.
7) Serve the beans with the salmon.

Nutrition Information:
Calories per Serving: 945.8; Fat: 66.6 g; Protein: 43.5 g; Carbs: 43.1 g

Pecan Crusted Trout

Serves: 4, Cook Time: 12 minutes
Ingredients:
- ½ cup crushed pecans
- ½ tsp grated fresh ginger
- 1 egg, beaten
- 1 tsp crush dried rosemary
- 1 tsp salt
- 4 4-oz trout fillets
- Black pepper to taste
- cooking spray
- Whole wheat flour, as needed

Directions for Cooking:
1) Grease baking sheet lightly with cooking spray and preheat oven to 400 degrees F.
2) In a shallow bowl, combine black pepper, salt, rosemary and pecans. In another shallow bowl, add whole wheat flour. In a third bowl, add beaten egg.
3) To prepare fish, dip in flour until covered well. Shake off excess flour. Then dip into beaten egg until coated well. Let excess egg drip off before dipping trout fillet into pecan crumbs. Press the trout lightly onto pecan crumbs to make it stick to the fish.
4) Place breaded fish onto prepared pan. Repeat process for remaining fillets.
5) Pop into the oven and bake for 10 to 12 minutes or until fish is flaky.

Nutrition Information:
Calories per Serving: 329; Fat: 19g; Protein: 26.95g; Carbs: 3g

Pesto and Lemon Halibut

Serves: 4, Cook Time: 10 minutes
Ingredients:
- 1 tbsp fresh lemon juice
- 1 tbsp lemon rind, grated
- 2 garlic cloves, peeled
- 2 tbsp olive oil
- ¼ cup Parmesan Cheese, freshly grated
- 2/3 cups firmly packed basil leaves
- 1/8 tsp freshly ground black pepper
- ¼ tsp salt, divided
- 4 pcs 6-oz halibut fillets

Directions for Cooking:
1) Preheat grill to medium fire and grease grate with cooking spray.
2) Season fillets with pepper and 1/8 tsp salt. Place on grill and cook until halibut is flaky around 4 minutes per side.
3) Meanwhile, make your lemon pesto by combining lemon juice, lemon rind, garlic, olive oil, Parmesan cheese, basil leaves and remaining salt in a blender. Pulse mixture until finely minced but not pureed.
4) Once fish is done cooking, transfer to a serving platter, pour over the lemon pesto sauce, serve and enjoy.

Nutrition Information:
Calories per Serving: 277.4; Fat: 13g; Protein: 38.7g; Carbs: 1.4g

Roasted Halibut with Banana Relish

Serves: 4, Cook Time: 12 minutes

Ingredients:

- ¼ cup cilantro
- ½ tsp freshly grated orange zest
- ½ tsp kosher salt, divided
- 1 lb. halibut or any deep-water fish
- 1 tsp ground coriander, divided into half
- 2 oranges (peeled, segmented and chopped)
- 2 ripe bananas, diced
- 2 tbsp lime juice

Directions for Cooking:

1) In a pan, prepare the fish by rubbing ½ tsp coriander and ¼ tsp kosher salt.
2) Place in a baking sheet with cooking spray and bake for 8 to 12 minutes inside a 450-degree Fahrenheit preheated oven.
3) Prepare the relish by stirring the orange zest, bananas, chopped oranges, lime juice, cilantro and the rest of the salt and coriander in a medium bowl.
4) Spoon the relish over the roasted fish.
5) Serve and enjoy.

Nutrition Information:

Calories per serving: 245.7; Protein: 15.3g; Fat: 6g; Carbs: 21g

Seafood Stew Cioppino

Serves: 6,.Cook Time: 40 minutes

Ingredients:

- ¼ cup Italian parsley, chopped
- ¼ tsp dried basil
- ¼ tsp dried thyme
- ½ cup dry white wine like pinot grigio
- ½ lb. King crab legs, cut at each joint
- ½ onion, chopped
- ½ tsp red pepper flakes (adjust to desired spiciness)
- 1 28-oz can crushed tomatoes
- 1 lb. mahi mahi, cut into ½-inch cubes
- 1 lb. raw shrimp
- 1 tbsp olive oil
- 2 bay leaves
- 2 cups clam juice
- 50 live clams, washed
- 6 cloves garlic, minced
- Pepper and salt to taste

Directions for Cooking:

1) On medium fire, place a stockpot and heat oil.
2) Add onion and for 4 minutes sauté until soft.
3) Add bay leaves, thyme, basil, red pepper flakes and garlic. Cook for a minute while stirring a bit.
4) Add clam juice and tomatoes. Once simmering, place fire to medium low and cook for 20 minutes uncovered.
5) Add white wine and clams. Cover and cook for 5 minutes or until clams have slightly opened.
6) Stir pot then add fish pieces, crab legs and shrimps. Do not stir soup to maintain the fish's shape. Cook while covered for 4 minutes or until clams are fully opened; fish and shrimps are opaque and cooked.
7) Season with pepper and salt to taste.
8) Transfer Cioppino to serving bowls and garnish with parsley before serving.

Nutrition Information:

Calories per Serving: 371; Carbs: 15.5 g; Protein: 62 g; Fat: 6.8 g

Simple Cod Piccata

Serves: 3 , Cook Time: 15 minutes

Ingredients:

- ¼ cup capers, drained
- ½ teaspoon salt
- ¾ cup chicken stock
- 1/3 cup almond flour
- 1-pound cod fillets, patted dry
- 2 tablespoon fresh parsley, chopped
- 2 tablespoon grapeseed oil
- 3 tablespoon extra-virgin oil
- 3 tablespoon lemon juice

Directions for Cooking:

1) In a bowl, combine the almond flour and salt.
2) Dredge the fish in the almond flour to coat. Set aside.
3) Heat a little bit of olive oil to coat a large skillet. Heat the skillet over medium-high heat. Add grapeseed oil. Cook the cod for 3 minutes on each side to brown. Remove from the plate and place on a paper towel-lined plate.
4) In a saucepan, mix together the chicken stock, capers and lemon juice. Simmer to reduce the sauce to half. Add the remaining grapeseed oil.
5) Drizzle the fried cod with the sauce and sprinkle with parsley.

Nutrition Information:

Calories per Serving: 277.1; Fat: 28.3 g; Protein: 1.9 g; Carbs: 3.7 g

Smoked Trout Tartine

Serves: 4, Cook Time: 0 minutes

Ingredients:

- ½ 15-oz can cannellini beans
- ½ cup diced roasted red peppers
- ¾ lb. smoked trout, flaked into bite-sized pieces
- 1 stalk celery, finely chopped
- 1 tbsp extra virgin olive oil
- 1 tsp chopped fresh dill
- 1 tsp Dijon mustard
- 2 tbsp capers, rinsed and drained
- 2 tbsp freshly squeezed lemon juice
- 2 tsp minced onion
- 4 large whole grain bread, toasted
- Dill sprigs – for garnish
- Pinch of sugar

Directions for Cooking:

1) Mix sugar, mustard, olive oil and lemon juice in a big bowl.
2) Add the rest of the ingredients except for toasted bread.
3) Toss to mix well.
4) Evenly divide fish mixture on top of bread slices and garnish with dill sprigs.
5) Serve and enjoy.

Nutrition Information:

Calories per serving: 348.1; Protein: 28.2 g; Fat: 10.1g; Carbs: 36.1g

Steamed Mussels Thai Style

Serves: 4, Cook Time: 15 minutes

Ingredients:

- ¼ cup minced shallots
- ½ tsp Madras curry
- 1 cup dry white wine
- 1 small bay leaf
- 1 tbsp chopped fresh basil
- 1 tbsp chopped fresh cilantro
- 1 tbsp chopped fresh mint
- 2 lbs. mussel, cleaned and debearded
- 2 tbsp olive oil
- 4 medium garlic cloves, minced

Directions for Cooking:

1) In a large heavy bottomed pot, on medium-high fire add to pot the curry powder, bay leaf, wine plus the minced garlic and shallots. Bring to a boil and simmer for 3 minutes.

2) Add the cleaned mussels, stir, cover, and cook for 3 minutes.
3) Stir mussels again, cover, and cook for another 2 or 3 minutes. Cooking is done when majority of shells have opened.
4) With a slotted spoon, transfer cooked mussels in a large bowl. Discard any unopened mussels.

5) Continue heating pot with sauce. Add oil and the chopped herbs.
6) Season with pepper and salt to taste.
7) Once good, pour over mussels, serve and enjoy.

Nutrition Information:
Calories per Serving: 407.2; Protein: 43.4g; Fat: 21.2g; Carbs: 10.8g

Tasty Tuna Scaloppine

Serves: 4, Cook Time: 10 minutes
Ingredients:
- ¼ cup chopped almonds
- ¼ cup fresh tangerine juice
- ½ tsp fennel seeds
- ½ tsp ground black pepper, divided
- ½ tsp salt
- 1 tbsp extra virgin olive oil
- 2 tbsp chopped fresh mint
- 2 tbsp chopped red onion
- 4 6-oz sushi-grade Yellowfin tuna steaks, each split in half horizontally
- Cooking spray

Directions for Cooking:

1) In a small bowl mix fennel seeds, olive oil, mint, onion, tangerine juice, almonds, ¼ tsp pepper and ¼ tsp salt. Combine thoroughly.
2) Season fish with remaining salt and pepper.
3) On medium-high fire, place a large nonstick pan and grease with cooking spray. Pan fry fish in two batches cooking each side for a minute.
4) Fish is best served with a side of salad greens or a half cup of cooked brown rice.

Nutrition Information:
Calories per serving: 405; Protein: 27.5g; Fat: 11.9g; Carbs: 27.5

Thyme and Lemon on Baked Salmon

Serves: 2, Cook Time: 25 minutes
Ingredients:
- 1 32-oz salmon fillet
- 1 lemon, sliced thinly
- 1 tbsp capers
- 1 tbsp fresh thyme
- Olive oil for drizzling
- Pepper and salt to taste

Directions for Cooking:
1) In a foil line baking sheet, place a parchment paper on top.
2) Place salmon with skin side down on parchment paper.

3) Season generously with pepper and salt.
4) Place capers on top of fillet. Cover with thinly sliced lemon.
5) Garnish with thyme.
6) Pop in cold oven and bake for 25 minutes at 400 degrees F settings.
7) Serve right away and enjoy.

Nutrition Information:
Calories per Serving: 684.4; Protein: 94.3g; Fat: 32.7g; Carbs: 4.3g

Warm Caper Tapenade on Cod

Serves: 4, Cook Time: 30 minutes

Ingredients:

- ¼ cup chopped cured olives
- ¼ tsp freshly ground pepper
- 1 ½ tsp chopped fresh oregano
- 1 cup halved cherry tomatoes
- 1 lb. cod fillet
- 1 tbsp capers, rinsed and chopped
- 1 tbsp minced shallot
- 1 tsp balsamic vinegar
- 3 tsp extra virgin olive oil, divided

Directions for Cooking:

1) Grease baking sheet with cooking spray and preheat oven to 450 degrees F.
2) Place cod on prepared baking sheet. Rub with 2 tsp oil and season with pepper.
3) Roast in oven for 15 to 20 minutes or until cod is flaky.
4) While waiting for cod to cook, on medium fire, place a small fry pan and heat 1 tsp oil.
5) Sauté shallots for a minute.
6) Add tomatoes and cook for two minutes or until soft.
7) Add capers and olives. Sauté for another minute.
8) Add vinegar and oregano. Turn off fire and stir to mix well.
9) Evenly divide cod into 4 servings and place on a plate.
10) To serve, top cod with Caper-Olive-Tomato Tapenade and enjoy.

Nutrition Information:

Calories per Serving: 107; Fat: 2.9g; Protein: 17.6g; Carbs: 2.0g

Yummy Salmon Panzanella

Serves: 4, Cook Time: 10 minutes

Ingredients:

- ¼ cup thinly sliced fresh basil
- ¼ cup thinly sliced red onion
- ¼ tsp freshly ground pepper, divided
- ½ tsp salt
- 1 lb. center cut salmon, skinned and cut into 4 equal portions
- 1 medium cucumber, peeled, seeded, and cut into 1-inch slices
- 1 tbsp capers, rinsed and chopped
- 2 large tomatoes, cut into 1-inch pieces
- 2 thick slices day old whole grain bread, sliced into 1-inch cubes
- 3 tbsp extra virgin olive oil
- 3 tbsp red wine vinegar
- 8 Kalamata olives, pitted and chopped

Directions for Cooking:

1) Grease grill grate and preheat grill to high.
2) In a large bowl, whisk 1/8 tsp pepper, capers, vinegar, and olives. Add oil and whisk well.
3) Stir in basil, onion, cucumber, tomatoes, and bread.
4) Season both sides of salmon with remaining pepper and salt.
5) Grill on high for 4 minutes per side.
6) Into 4 plates, evenly divide salad, top with grilled salmon, and serve.

Nutrition Information:

Calories per Serving: 383; Fat: 20.6g; Protein: 34.8g; Carbs: 13.6g

Chapter 10 Poultry and Meat Recipes

Avocado-Orange Grilled Chicken

Serves: 4 , Cooking Time: 12 minutes

Ingredients:
- ¼ cup fresh lime juice
- ¼ cup minced red onion
- 1 avocado
- 1 cup low fat yogurt
- 1 small red onion, sliced thinly
- 1 tbsp honey
- 2 oranges, peeled and sectioned
- 2 tbsp chopped cilantro
- 4 pieces of 4-6oz boneless, skinless chicken breasts
- Pepper and salt to taste

Directions for Cooking:
1) In a large bowl mix honey, cilantro, minced red onion and yogurt.
2) Submerge chicken into mixture and marinate for at least 30 minutes.
3) Grease grate and preheat grill to medium-high fire.
4) Remove chicken from marinade and season with pepper and salt.
5) Grill for 6 minutes per side or until chicken is cooked and juices run clear.
6) Meanwhile, peel avocado and discard seed. Chop avocados and place in bowl. Quickly add lime juice and toss avocado to coat well with juice.
7) Add cilantro, thinly sliced onions and oranges into bowl of avocado, mix well.
8) Serve grilled chicken and avocado dressing on the side.

Nutrition Information:
Calories per Serving: 422.2; Carbs: 26.4g; Protein: 48.1g; Fat: 13.8g

Braised Beef in Oregano-Tomato sauce

Serves: 12, Cooking Time: 1 hour and 30 minutes

Ingredients:
- 2 onions, chopped
- 3 celery stalks, diced
- 4 cloves garlic, minced
- 2 (28-ounce) cans Italian-style stewed tomatoes
- 1 cup dry red wine
- 1 teaspoon dried oregano
- 1 teaspoon salt
- 3 pounds boneless beef chuck roast, cut into 1-1/2-inch cubes
- 1/2 cup chopped fresh parsley
- 1/4 cup vegetable oil
- 3/4 teaspoon black pepper

Directions for Cooking:
1) Place a pot on medium-high fire and heat for 2 minutes.
2) Add oil and heat for another 2 minutes.
3) Add beef and brown on all sides. Around 12 minutes.
4) Add onions, celery, and garlic, and sauté 5 minutes or until vegetables are tender. Add remaining ingredients and bring to a boil.
5) Reduce heat to low, cover, and simmer for 60 minutes or until beef is fork tender.

Nutrition Information:
Calories per Serving: 285; Carbs: 7.4g; Protein: 31.7g; Fats: 14.6g

Balsamic Chicken with Roasted Tomatoes

Serves: 2, Cooking Time: 20 minutes

Ingredients:
- ½ medium onion, chopped
- 1 cup mushrooms, chopped
- 1 tablespoon honey
- 1-pint cherry tomatoes, halved
- 2 chicken thighs, skins removed
- 2 tablespoon extra-virgin olive oil

- 3 tablespoon balsamic vinegar
- Fresh parsley, chopped
- Salt and pepper to taste

Directions for Cooking:
1) Preheat the oven to 400 degrees F.
2) In a greased baking sheet, place the tomatoes and drizzle with honey and oil. Season with salt and pepper and cook in the oven for 20 minutes.
3) Meanwhile, heat 1 tablespoon of olive oil in a skillet. Sauté the mushrooms and onions for 12 minutes until softened. Add the chicken then season with salt and pepper. Add the balsamic glaze and reduce the heat to low. Let it simmer for 15 minutes or until the chicken is cooked through.
4) Assemble by placing tomatoes in the plate, add a chicken thigh and spoon the mushroom and pan drippings.
5) Garnish with parsley.

Nutrition Information:
Calories per Serving: 217.7; Carbs: 39.2g; Protein: 6.0g; Fat: 4.1g

Beef Rice Bowl Mediterranean Style

Serves: 4, Cooking Time: 15 minutes
Ingredients:
- 1 lb. ground beef
- 1 tbsp dried dill
- 2 tsp salt
- 1 1/2 tsp dried oregano
- 1 tsp ground black pepper
- 2/3 cup water
- 2 cups cooked brown rice
- 4 tbsp Hummus
- 4 tbsp Crumbled feta
- Cucumber slices
- 4 Pita wedges

Yogurt Sauce Ingredients:
- 1 5.3-oz container full-fat plain Greek yogurt
- 1 tbsp extra-virgin olive oil
- 1/4 tsp dried dill
- 2 cloves garlic, minced
- Half of a cucumber, peeled, seeded, and roughly chopped
- Salt and pepper to taste

Directions for Cooking:
1) In a blender, puree all yogurt sauce ingredients until smooth and creamy. Transfer to a bowl and refrigerate. If needed adjust seasoning to taste.
2) Add beef to a skillet set over medium-high heat. Brown the beef, breaking it up into smaller pieces and crumble as it cooks, for 10 minutes. Drain the fat.
3) Evenly scatter dried dill, salt, dried oregano, and black pepper over top of the beef.
4) Raise heat to high and pour water over top. Once the water begins to bubble, reduce heat to low and let the beef simmer until the water has reduced, around 15 minutes.
5) To make the bowls, evenly divide brown rice, cucumber slices, hummus, pita and feta into 4 bowls. Evenly divide beef into bowls. Top with the dressing.
6) Serve and enjoy.

Nutrition Information:
Calories per Serving: 472; Carbs: 35.7g; Protein: 34.4g; Fats: 20.3g

Beef Skewers with Smoked Paprika-Bean Dip

Serves: 4, Cooking Time: 30 minutes
Beef Ingredients:
- 1 teaspoon garlic-pepper seasoning
- 1/4 teaspoon smoked paprika
- 1-pound beef Top Sirloin Steak Boneless, cut 1 inch thick

Smoked Paprika-Bean Dip Ingredients:
- 1 can 15.5-ounces cannellini beans, rinsed, drained
- 1 clove garlic, chopped
- 1 tablespoon plus 2 teaspoons extra virgin olive oil, divided
- 1 tablespoon sherry or balsamic vinegar
- 1/2 teaspoon salt
- 1/2 teaspoon smoked paprika
- 2 tablespoons water

Directions for Cooking:

1) Soak sixteen 6-inch bamboo skewers in water 10 minutes; drain.
2) Meanwhile cut beef steak crosswise into 1/4-inch thick strips, season with ¼ tsp paprika and garlic-pepper seasoning. Let it marinate for at least 10 minutes.
3) Thread beef, weaving back and forth, onto each skewer.
4) Place skewers on a rack on a pan and broil for 4 minutes per side.
5) Meanwhile, make the dip by adding all ingredients in a blender. Puree until smooth and creamy. Adjust seasoning to taste if needed.
6) Serve beef skewers with bean dip.

Nutrition Information:
Calories per Serving: 272; Carbs: 16.0g; Protein: 32.0g; Fats: 12.0g

Bell Peppers on Chicken Breasts

Serves: 6, Cooking Time: 30 minutes

Ingredients:

- ¼ tsp freshly ground black pepper
- ½ tsp salt
- 1 large red bell pepper, cut into ¼-inch strips
- 1 large yellow bell pepper, cut into ¼-inch strips
- 1 tbsp olive oil
- 1 tsp chopped fresh oregano
- 2 1/3 cups coarsely chopped tomato
- 2 tbsp finely chopped fresh flat-leaf parsley
- 20 Kalamata olives
- 3 cups onion sliced crosswise
- 6 4-oz skinless, boneless chicken breast halves, cut in half horizontally
- Cooking spray

Directions for Cooking:

1) On medium-high fire, place a large nonstick fry pan and heat oil. Once oil is hot, sauté onions until soft and translucent, around 6 to 8 minutes.
2) Add bell peppers and sauté for another 10 minutes or until tender.
3) Add black pepper, salt and tomato. Cook until tomato juice has evaporated, around 7 minutes.
4) Add olives, oregano and parsley, cook until heated through around 1 to 2 minutes. Transfer to a bowl and keep warm.
5) Wipe pan with paper towel and grease with cooking spray. Return to fire and place chicken breasts. Cook for three minutes per side or until desired doneness is reached. If needed, cook chicken in batches.
6) When cooking the last batch of chicken is done, add back the previous batch of chicken and the onion-bell pepper mixture and cook for a minute or two while tossing chicken to coat well in the onion-bell pepper mixture.
7) Serve and enjoy.

Nutrition Information:
Calories per Serving: 261.8; Carbs: 11.0g; Protein: 36.0g; Fat: 8.2g

Brussels Sprouts and Paprika Chicken Thighs

Serves: 4, Cooking Time: 25 minutes

Ingredients:

- ½ tsp ground pepper, divided
- ¾ tsp salt, divided
- 1 lb. Brussels sprouts, trimmed and halved
- 1 lemon, sliced
- 1 tbsp smoked paprika
- 1 tsp dried thyme
- 2 cloves garlic, minced
- 3 tbsp extra virgin olive oil, divided
- 4 large bone-in chicken thighs, skin removed
- 4 small shallots, quartered

Directions for Cooking:

1) Preheat oven to 450 degrees F and position rack to lower third in oven.
2) On a large and rimmed baking sheet, mix ¼ tsp pepper, ¼ tsp salt, 2 tbsp oil, lemon, shallots, and Brussels sprouts.
3) With a chef's knife, mash ½ tsp salt and garlic to form a paste.

4) In small bowl, mix ¼ tsp pepper, 1 tbsp oil, thyme, paprika, and garlic paste. Rub all over chicken and place around Brussels sprouts in pan.
5) Pop in the oven and roast for 20 to 25 minutes or until chicken is cooked and juices run clear.

6) Serve and enjoy.

Nutrition Information:
Calories per Serving: 416.4; Carbs: 14.7g; Protein: 29.1g; Fat: 26.8g

Bulgur and Chicken Skillet

Serves: 4, Cooking Time: 40 minutes

Ingredients:
- 4 (6-oz.) skinless, boneless chicken breasts
- 1 tablespoon olive oil, divided
- 1 cup thinly sliced red onion
- 1 tablespoon thinly sliced garlic
- 1 cup unsalted chicken stock
- 1 tablespoon coarsely chopped fresh dill
- 1/2 teaspoon freshly ground black pepper, divided
- 1/2 cup uncooked bulgur
- 2 teaspoons chopped fresh or 1/2 tsp. dried oregano
- 4 cups chopped fresh kale (about 2 1/2 oz.)
- 1/2 cup thinly sliced bottled roasted red bell peppers
- 2 ounces feta cheese, crumbled (about 1/2 cup)
- 3/4 teaspoon kosher salt, divided

Directions for Cooking:

1) Place a cast iron skillet on medium-high fire and heat for 5 minutes. Add oil and heat for 2 minutes.
2) Season chicken with pepper and salt to taste.
3) Brown chicken for 4 minutes per side and transfer to a plate.
4) In same skillet, sauté garlic and onion for 3 minutes. Stir in oregano and bulgur and toast for 2 minutes.
5) Stir in kale and bell pepper, cook for 2 minutes. Pour in stock and season well with pepper and salt.
6) Return chicken to skillet and turn off fire. Pop in a preheated 400 degrees F oven and bake for 15 minutes.
7) Remove form oven, fluff bulgur and turn over chicken. Let it stand for 5 minutes.
8) Serve and enjoy with a sprinkle of feta cheese.

Nutrition Information:
Calories per Serving: 369; Carbs: 21.0g; Protein: 45.0g; Fats: 11.3g

Cashew Beef Stir Fry

Serves: 8, Cooking Time: 15 minutes

Ingredients:
- ¼ cup coconut aminos
- 1 ½ pound ground beef
- 1 cup raw cashews
- 1 green bell pepper, julienned
- 1 red bell pepper, julienned
- 1 small can water chestnut, sliced
- 1 small onion, sliced
- 1 tablespoon garlic, minced
- 2 tablespoon ginger, grated
- 2 teaspoon olive oil
- Salt and pepper to taste

Directions for Cooking:

1) Heat a skillet over medium heat then add raw cashews. Toast for a couple of minutes or until slightly brown. Set aside.
2) In the same skillet, add the olive oil and sauté the ground beef for 5 minutes or until brown.
3) Add the garlic, ginger and season with coconut aminos. Stir for one minute before adding the onions, bell peppers and water chestnuts. Cook until the vegetables are almost soft.
4) Season with salt and pepper to taste.
5) Add the toasted cashews last.

Nutrition Information:
Calories per Serving: 324.8; Carbs: 12.4g; Protein: 19.3g; Fat: 22.0g

Chicken and Avocado Lettuce Wraps

Serves: 3, Cooking Time: 5 minutes
Ingredients:
- 2 tablespoons cilantro chopped
- 2 tablespoons lime juice
- 1 tablespoon lemon juice
- ½ cups avocado, pitted and mashed
- 1 cup cooked chicken, shredded
- 6 leaves of Romaine lettuce
- 1 cup grape tomatoes, halved
- 1/8 teaspoon black pepper
- 1/8 teaspoon salt

Directions for Cooking:
1) In a mixing bowl, mix together the avocado, lime juice, lemon juice and stir to combine.
2) Add the chicken and cilantro. Season with salt and pepper to taste.
3) Spoon into the lettuce leaves and add chopped tomatoes.

Nutrition Information:
Calories per Serving: 134.7; Carbs: 4.9g; Protein: 14.6g; Fat: 6.3g

Chicken and Hazelnut Mash

Serves: 2, Cooking Time: 45 minutes
Ingredients:
- ¼ cup thick coconut milk
- ½ cup hazelnut, crushed
- 1 medium-sized boneless chicken breast, sliced in half
- 1 medium-sized butternut squash, halved and deseeded
- 1 orange, juiced
- 6 cups baby spinach leaves, chopped
- Salt and pepper to taste

Directions for Cooking:
1) Preheat the oven to 350 degrees F.
2) Sprinkle the butternut squash with salt and paper and place them face down in a baking pan. Put the chicken breasts in the same baking pan. Squeeze orange juice over the chicken. Bake for 35 minutes until both squash and chicken are cooked through.
3) Meanwhile, sauté spinach in a skillet and cook for 3 minutes or until wilted.
4) In another pan, toast the crushed hazelnuts over medium heat.
5) Once the chicken and squash are cooked, it is time to assemble everything.
6) Scoop the squash and shred the chicken and put them in a mixing bowl. Add the hazelnut, spinach and coconut cream. Mix until well combined.
7) Place in a baking dish and cook in the broiler for 1o minutes or until the top takes on a golden brown.

Nutrition Information:
Calories per Serving: 584.8; Carbs: 40.7g; Protein: 40.7g; Fat: 28.8g

Chicken Breasts with Stuffing

Serves: 8, Cooking Time: 37 minutes
Ingredients:
- ¼ cup crumbled feta cheese
- 1 large bell pepper, halved and seeded
- 1 tbsp minced fresh basil
- 2 tbsp finely chopped, pitted Kalamata olives
- 8 pcs of 6-oz boneless and skinless chicken breasts

Directions for Cooking:
1) In a greased baking sheet place bell pepper with skin facing up and pop into a preheated broiler on high. Broil until blackened around 15 minutes. Remove from broiler and place right away into a re-sealable bag, seal and leave for 15 minutes.
2) After, peel bell pepper and mince. Preheat grill to medium-high fire.
3) In a medium bowl, mix well basil, olives, cheese and bell pepper.
4) Form a pocket on each chicken breast by creating a slit through the thickest portion; add 2 tbsp bell pepper mixture and seal with a

wooden pick. (At this point, you can stop and freeze chicken and just thaw when needed for grilling already)

5) Season chicken breasts with pepper and salt.

6) Grill for six minutes per side, remove from grill and cover loosely with foil and let stand for 10 minutes before serving.

Nutrition Information:
Calories per Serving: 201.1; Carbs: 1.8g; Protein: 35.2g; Fat: 5.9g

Chicken Dish from West Africa

Serves: 6, Cooking Time: 85 minutes
Ingredients:
- ¼ cup apple cider vinegar
- ¼ cup lemon juice
- ¼ cup olive oil
- ¼ tsp ground allspice
- ½ tsp pepper
- ½ tsp salt
- 1 jalapeno pepper, seeds removed, diced
- 1 lime cut into wedges
- 1 tbsp zest of lemon
- 2 bay leaves
- 2 lbs. bone in, skin on drumsticks and chicken thighs
- 4 onions, sliced
- 6 cloves garlic, minced

Directions for Cooking:
1) In wide and shallow bowl with lid, combine allspice, salt, pepper, bay leaves, jalapeno, garlic, lemon zest, lemon juice, vinegar and oil. Mix well.
2) Add chicken, cover and marinate in the ref. Ensuring to turn chicken in two hours.

Chicken is best left overnight or for at least 4 hours.

3) Once you are done marinating, grease a roasting pan and preheat oven to 400 degrees F.
4) Remove chicken from marinade and arrange on prepared pan. Pop in the oven and bake until juices run clear around 35-40 minutes.
5) Meanwhile, discard 3/4s of the marinade while reserving onions. Then place a nonstick pan on low fire and add remaining marinade with bay leaves and onions. Sauté for 45 minutes until caramelized while stirring every once in a while.
6) To serve, place baked chicken on a serving plate drizzled with caramelized onion sauce and lime wedges on the side.
7) Also best eaten with plain white rice.

Nutrition Information:
Calories per Serving: 489.2; Carbs: 13.5g; Protein: 32.3g; Fat: 34.0g

Chicken in A Bowl

Serves: 2, Cooking Time: 10 minutes
Ingredients:
- ½ cup cooked chicken, cut into strips
- 1 head of cabbage, chopped
- 1 tablespoon olive oil
- 1 tablespoon sesame oil
- 1/3 cup coconut aminos
- 2 garlic cloves, minced
- 2 large carrots, cut into strips
- 4 green onions, diced

Directions for Cooking:
1) Heat olive oil in a skillet over medium-high heat.

2) Sauté the cabbage then add the carrots. Continue sautéing until soft. If it gets too dry, add a little bit of water.
3) Season with sesame oil and coconut aminos.
4) Add the garlic and cook for five minutes.
5) Throw in the chicken strips and toss the green onions.

Nutrition Information:
Calories per Serving: 373.7; Carbs: 25.1g; Protein: 10.5g; Fat: 25.7g

Chicken Soup Filipino Style

Serves: 4, Cooking Time: 45 minutes

Ingredients:
- 1 whole chicken, around 2 lbs, cut into 10-pieces
- Hot pepper leaves
- 2 tbsp fish sauce
- 1 thumb ginger, cut into strips
- 1 medium sized onion, chopped
- 1 tbsp garlic, minced
- ½ small green papaya, peeled and cut into wedges
- 5 cups chicken broth
- 1 tbsp corn oil
- Pepper and salt to taste

Directions for Cooking:
1) In a heavy bottomed medium pot, heat oil on medium-high fire.
2) Once oil is hot, sauté garlic and ginger for a minute or until garlic begins to brown lightly.
3) Add onions, sauté for 3 to 5 minutes or until soft and translucent.
4) Add chicken and sauté for ten minutes.
5) Season with pepper and salt.
6) Add 2 cups of Chicken broth or water to pot, cover and cook chicken for another ten minutes.
7) Add papaya wedges and remaining liquid. Cover and cook until papaya is soft.
8) Once papaya is soft, add fish sauce and hot pepper leaves, and cook while covered for another minute.
9) Adjust seasoning to taste, serve and enjoy.

Nutrition Information:
Calories per serving: 334; Carbs: 10.8g; Protein: 47.9g; Fat: 10.4g

Chicken Thighs with Butternut Squash

Serves: 6, Cooking Time: 30 minutes

Ingredients:
- ½ pound bacon
- 3 cups butternut squash, cubed
- 6 boneless chicken thighs
- A sprig of fresh sage, chopped
- Extra olive oil for frying
- Salt and pepper to taste

Directions for Cooking:
1) Preheat the oven to 425 degrees F.
2) In a skillet, fry the bacon over medium heat until crisp. Set aside then crumble.
3) In the same skillet, sauté the butternut squash and season with salt and pepper to taste. Once the squash is cooked, remove from the skillet and set aside.
4) Using the same skillet, add olive oil and cook the chicken thighs for 10 minutes on each side.
5) Season with salt and pepper and add the squash back.
6) Remove the skillet from the stove and bake in the oven for 15 minutes.
7) Garnish with bacon.

Nutrition Information:
Calories per Serving: 315.3; Carbs: 11.3g; Protein: 25.0g; Fat: 18.9g

Creamy Chicken-Spinach Skillet

Serves: 4, Cooking Time: 17 minutes

Ingredients:
- 1 lb. boneless skinless chicken breast sliced into cutlets
- 1 medium onion diced
- 12 oz roasted red peppers finely diced
- 2 1/2 cups chicken stock divided
- 2 cups fresh baby spinach leaves
- 2 cups freshly cooked pasta
- 2 tbsp olive oil
- 4 garlic cloves minced
- 7 oz cream cheese try to find an herb/garlic flavored one!
- Salt and pepper

Directions for Cooking:
1) Place a saucepan on medium-high fire and heat for 2 minutes. Add oil and heat for a minute, swirling to coat pan.
2) Add chicken to pan, season with pepper and salt to taste. Cook chicken on high fire for 3 minutes per side.
3) Lower fire to medium and stir in onions, red peppers, and garlic. Sauté for 5 minutes and deglaze pot with a little bit of stock.
4) Whisk in chicken stock and cream cheese. Cook and mix until thoroughly combined.
5) Stir in spinach and adjust seasoning to taste. Cook for 2 minutes or until spinach is wilted.
6) Serve and enjoy.

Nutrition Information:
Calories per Serving: 484; Carbs: 33.0g; Protein: 36.0g; Fats: 22.0g

Easy Chicken with Capers Skillet

Serves: 4, Cooking Time: 35 minutes
Ingredients:
- 4 boneless skinless chicken breast halves (6 ounces each)
- 1/4 teaspoon salt
- 1/4 teaspoon pepper
- 3 tablespoons olive oil
- 1-pint grape tomatoes
- 16 pitted Greek or ripe olives, sliced
- 3 tablespoons capers, drained

Directions for Cooking:
1) Place a cast iron skillet on medium-high fire and heat for 5 minutes.
2) Meanwhile, season chicken with pepper and salt.
3) Add oil to pan and heat for another minute. Add chicken and increase fire to high. Brown sides for 4 minutes per side.
4) Lower fire to medium and add capers and tomatoes.
5) Bake uncovered in a 475 degrees F preheated oven for 12 minutes.
6) Remove from oven and let it sit for 5 minutes before serving.

Nutrition Information:
Calories per Serving: 336; Carbs: 6.0g; Protein: 36.0g; Fats: 18.0g

Easy Stir-Fried Chicken

Serves: 3, Cooking Time: 12 minutes
Ingredients:
- ¼ lb. brown mushrooms
- ¼ medium onion, sliced thinly
- 1 large orange bell pepper
- 1 tbsp soy sauce
- 1 tbsp virgin olive oil
- 2 7-oz skinless and boneless chicken breast

Directions for Cooking:
1) On medium-high fire, place a nonstick saucepan and heat olive oil.
2) Add soy sauce, onion powder, mushrooms, bell pepper and chicken.
3) Stir fry for 8 to 10 minutes.
4) Remove from pan and serve.

Nutrition Information:
Calories per Serving: 184; Carbs: 7.0g; Protein: 32.0g; Fat: 10.0g

Fruit Slaw Topped Grilled Chops

Serves: 4, Cooking Time: 20 minutes
Ingredients:
- 1 tsp ground coriander
- 1 tsp ground cumin
- 1 tsp ground paprika
- 1 tsp sea salt
- 4 bone-in pork chops, around 1 – 1 ½ inches thick

Slaw Ingredients:
- ¼ tsp ground chipotle powder

- 1 lb. assorted firm stone fruit (apricots, plums, and peaches preferably)
- 1 tsp lime juice
- 1 tsp lime zest
- A pinch of salt

Directions for Cooking:
1) Grease grate and preheat grill to medium-high fire.
2) In a small bowl, mix well paprika, coriander, cumin and salt. Rub spice evenly on all sides of pork chops.
3) Grill pork chops per side for five minutes. Remove from grill, transfer to a plate and loosely tent with foil and let it stand for at least 10 minutes.
4) Meanwhile, slice the firm stone fruits thin strips and place in a bowl.
5) Add salt, lime juice, lime zest, and chipotle powder into bowl, and toss well to coat.
6) To serve, place one pork chop per plate and top with ¼ of the fruit slaw mixture.

Nutrition Information:
Calories per Serving: 388.4; Carbs: 14.5g; Protein: 42.1g; Fat: 18.0g

Greek Chicken Stew

Serves: 8, Cooking Time: 1 hour and 15minutes
Ingredients:
- 10 smalls shallots, peeled
- 1 cup olive oil
- 1 (4 pound) whole chicken, cut into pieces
- 2 cloves garlic, finely chopped
- ½ cup red wine
- 1 cup tomato sauce
- 2 tablespoons chopped fresh parsley
- salt and ground black pepper to taste
- 1 pinch dried oregano, or to taste
- 2 bay leaves
- 1 ½ cups chicken stock, or more if needed

Directions for Cooking:
1) In a large pot, fill half full of water and bring to a boil. Lightly salt the water and once boiling add shallots and boil uncovered for 3 minutes. Drain and quickly place on an ice bath for 5 minutes. Drain well.
2) In same pot, heat for 3 minutes and add oil. Heat for 3 minutes.
3) Add chicken and shallots. Cook 15 minutes.
4) Add chopped garlic and cook for another 3 minutes or until garlic starts to turn golden.
5) Add red wine and tomato sauce. Deglaze pot.
6) Stir in bay leaves, oregano, pepper, salt, and parsley. Cook for 3 minutes.
7) Stir in chicken stock.
8) Cover and simmer for 40 minutes while occasionally stirring pot.
9) Serve and enjoy while hot with a side of rice if desired.

Nutrition Information:
Calories per Serving: 574; Carbs: 6.8g; Protein: 31.8g; Fats: 45.3g

Greek Styled Lamb Chops

Serves: 4, Cook Time: 4 minutes
Ingredients:
- ¼ tsp black pepper
- ½ tsp salt
- 1 tbsp bottled minced garlic
- 1 tbsp dried oregano
- 2 tbsp lemon juice
- 8 pcs of lamb loin chops, around 4 oz
- Cooking spray

Direction:
1) Preheat broiler.
2) In a big bowl or dish, combine the black pepper, salt, minced garlic, lemon juice and oregano. Then rub it equally on all sides of the lamb chops.
3) Then coat a broiler pan with the cooking spray before placing the lamb chops on the pan and broiling until desired doneness is reached or for four minutes.

Nutrition Information:
Calories per Serving: 131.9; Carbs: 2.6g; Protein: 17.1g; Fat: 5.9g

Grilled Chicken Breasts

Serves: 4, Cooking Time: 15 minutes

Ingredients:

- 4 boneless skinless chicken breast halves
- 3 tablespoons lemon juice
- 3 tablespoons olive oil
- 3 tablespoons chopped fresh parsley
- 3 garlic cloves, crushed and minced
- 1 teaspoon paprika
- 1 /2 teaspoon dried oregano
- 1/2 teaspoon salt
- 1/2 teaspoon pepper

Directions for Cooking:

1) In a large Ziplock bag, mix well oregano, paprika, garlic, parsley, olive oil, and lemon juice.

2) Pierce chicken with knife several times and sprinkle with salt and pepper.

3) Add chicken to bag and marinate 20 minutes or up to two days in the fridge.

4) Remove chicken from bag and grill for 5 minutes per side in a 350 degrees F preheated grill.

5) Remove chicken from grill and let it stand on a plate for 5 minutes before slicing.

6) Serve and enjoy with a side of rice or salad.

Nutrition Information:
Calories per Serving: 485; Carbs: 2.7g; Protein: 72.8g; Fats: 19.3g

Huntsman's Beef Stew

Serves: 4, Cooking Time: 50 minutes

Ingredients:

- 1 large onion, sliced in semi circles
- Pepper and salt to taste
- 1 tsp garlic powder
- 1 tsp oregano
- 1 tbsp olive oil
- 2 cups baby carrots, julienned
- 1 cup fresh blueberries
- 2 lbs. beef meat, cubed
- A splash of Worcestershire sauce
- ½ cup red wine
- Enough water

Directions for Cooking:

1) In a large heavy bottomed pot, heat olive oil. Brown beef for ten minutes.

2) Add onions, Worcestershire sauce, red wine, garlic, oregano, pepper, salt, and water to cover meat.

3) Cook on medium fire while covered for 30 minutes. Fifteen minutes into cooking time, add carrots.

4) Once 30 minutes is up, add berries. Cook for another 10 minutes.

5) Serve and enjoy.

Nutrition Information:
Calories per Serving: 561; Carbs: 16.9g; Protein: 61.6g; Fat: 27.8g

Grilled Veggies and Chicken

Serves: 3, Cooking Time: 20 minutes

Ingredients:

- ¼ teaspoon cayenne pepper
- ½ teaspoon garlic granules
- ½ teaspoon onion powder
- 1 cup organic tomatoes, blended
- 1 red onion
- 1 red pepper, chopped
- 1 tablespoon vinegar
- 1 teaspoon Italian seasoning
- 1 teaspoon rosemary
- 1 yellow squash, chopped
- 1 zucchini, chopped
- 1-pound organic chicken breast
- 2 cups fresh cherry tomatoes, halved
- 4 tablespoon extra-virgin olive oil
- Pepper to taste
- Salt to taste

Directions for Cooking:

1) Marinade the chicken by mixing together 1 tablespoon of extra virgin olive oil, Italian seasoning, and rosemary. Season with salt the set aside for at least 2 hours.
2) In another bowl, make the salad by combining the red onion, fresh cherry tomatoes, red pepper, squash and zucchini. Add 1 tablespoon of extra virgin olive oil and season with salt and pepper to taste. Place inside a greased tinfoil then set aside.
3) Prepare the grill and heat it to 350 degrees F. Cook the chicken breast and let it cook for 7 minutes on each side. Place the tinfoil with the veggies on the grill and cook it for five to 7 minutes.
4) Meanwhile, make the vinaigrette my combining the cayenne pepper, onion powder, garlic granules, vinegar and blended organic tomatoes in a food processor. Add 2 tablespoon of extra virgin olive oil and season with salt and pepper to taste.

Nutrition Information:
Calories per Serving: 363.6; Carbs: 14.2g; Protein: 45.2g; Fat: 14.0g

Kefta Styled Beef Patties

Serves: 2, Cook Time: 8 minutes
Ingredients:
- ¼ cup cilantro, fresh
- ¼ cup plus 2 tbsp fresh parsley, chopped and divided
- ½ cup plain Greek yogurt, fat-free
- ½ tsp freshly ground black pepper
- ½ tsp ground cinnamon
- ½ tsp salt
- 1 lb ground sirloin
- 1 tbsp fresh lemon juice
- 1 tbsp peeled and chopped ginger
- 1 tsp ground cumin
- 2 cups thinly sliced English cucumber
- 2 pcs of 6-inch pita, quartered
- 2 tsps ground coriander

Directions for Cooking:
1) On medium-high fire, preheat a grill pan coated with cooking spray.
2) In a medium bowl, mix together cinnamon, salt, cumin, coriander, ginger, cilantro, parsley and beef. Then divide the mixture equally into four parts and shaping each portion into a patty ½ inch thick.
3) Then place patties on pan cooking each side for three minutes or until desired doneness is achieved.
4) In a separate bowl, toss together vinegar and cucumber.
5) In a small bowl, whisk together pepper, juice, 2 tbsp parsley and yogurt.
6) Serve each patty on a plate with ½ cup cucumber mixture and 2 tbsp of the yogurt sauce.

Nutrition Information:
Calories per Serving: 480.5; Carbs: 23.1g; Protein: 54.5g; Fat: 18.9g

Kumquat and Chicken Tagine

Serves: 6, Cooking Time: 1 hour and 20 minutes
Ingredients:
- ½ tsp ground pepper
- ½ tsp salt
- ¾ tsp ground cinnamon
- 1 ½ tbsp honey
- 1 14-oz can vegetable broth
- 1 15-oz can chickpeas, rinsed
- 1 tbsp extra virgin olive oil
- 1 tbsp minced fresh ginger
- 1 tsp ground coriander
- 1 tsp ground cumin
- 1/8 tsp ground cloves
- 12-oz kumquats, seeded and roughly chopped
- 2 lbs. boneless, skinless chicken thighs, trimmed of fat and cut into 2-inch pieces
- 2 onions, thinly sliced
- 4 cloves garlic, slivered

Directions for Cooking:
1) Preheat oven to 375 degrees F.
2) On medium fire, place a heatproof casserole and heat oil.

3) Add onions and sauté for 4 minutes or until soft.
4) Add ginger and garlic, sauté for another minute.
5) Add chicken and sauté for 8 minutes.
6) Season with cloves, pepper, salt, cinnamon, cumin, and coriander. Sauté for a minute or until aromatic.
7) Add honey, chickpeas, kumquats, and broth. Bring to a boil and turn off fire.
8) Cover casserole and pop in the oven. Bake for an hour while stirring every after 15-minute intervals.

Nutrition Information:
Calories per Serving: 412.6; Carbs: 32.1g; Protein: 43.0g; Fat: 18.7g

Lamb Burger on Arugula

Serves: 6, Cooking Time: 6 minutes
Ingredients:
- ½ oz fresh mint, divided
- 1 tbsp salt
- 2 lbs. ground lamb
- 2 tbsp shelled and salted Pistachio nuts
- 3 oz dried apricots, diced
- 3 oz Feta crumbled – you can omit if you do not eat dairy
- 4 cups arugula

Directions for Cooking:
1) In a bowl, with your hands blend feta, salt, ½ of fresh mint (diced), apricots and ground lamb.
2) Then form into balls or patties with an ice cream scooper. Press ball in between palm of hands to flatten to half an inch. Do the same for remaining patties.
3) In a nonstick thick pan on medium fire, place patties without oil and cook for 3 minutes per side or until lightly browned. Flip over once and cook the other side.
4) Meanwhile, arrange 1 cup of arugula per plate. Total of 4 plates.
5) Divide evenly and place cooked patties on top of arugula.
6) In a food processor, process until finely chopped the remaining mint leaves and nuts.
7) Sprinkle on top of patties, serve and enjoy.

Nutrition Information:
Calories per Serving: 458.2; Carbs: 12.0g; Protein: 23.8g; Fat: 35.0g

Lamb with Spinach Sauce

Serves: 8, Cooking Time: 3 hours
Ingredients:
- ¼ cup full fat coconut milk
- ½ cup diced tomatoes
- 1 ½ tbsp garam masala
- 1 tbsp ground cumin
- 1 tsp ground turmeric
- 2 lbs. boneless lamb meat
- 2 medium onions, thinly sliced
- 2 tbsp ground coriander
- 2 tbsp olive oil
- 3 tbsp minced ginger
- 3 tsp kosher salt, divided
- 30-oz frozen spinach, defrosted and squeezed dry
- 4 cloves of garlic, minced
- Freshly ground black pepper
- Juice from ½ of a lemon

Directions for Cooking:
1) Preheat oven to 300 degrees F.
2) On medium-high fire, place a large Dutch oven and heat olive oil.
3) With paper towels, dry lamb meat. Season with 1 tsp salt.
4) Once olive oil is hot, sear lamb meat on all sides in batches. Transfer seared lamb into a plate with a slotted spoon.
5) Once all meat is done searing, lower fire to medium and sauté onions until soft and translucent.
6) Add turmeric, coriander, cumin, ginger, and garlic. Sauté until fragrant around a minute.
7) Add tomatoes, cook for 3 minutes.
8) Add coconut milk and simmer until sauce is thickened.

9) Puree sauce with a stick blender. Return lamb meat.
10) Add 2 cups water and 2 tsp salt. Bring to a boil.
11) Once boiling, mix and scrape bottom of pot, cover, and pop in the oven.
12) Bake until meat is tender, around 2 ½ hours.
13) Serve and enjoy while still hot.

Nutrition Information:
Calories per Serving: 174.5; Carbs: 7.3g; Protein: 27.7g; Fat: 9.0g

La Paz Batchoy (Beef Noodle Soup La Paz Style)

Serves: 4, Cooking Time: 25 minutes

Ingredients:
- 4 cups zucchini, spiral
- 1 cup carrots, spiral
- 1 cup jicama, spiral
- 2 pcs Beef Knorr Cubes
- 8 cups water
- 2 tbsp fish sauce
- freshly ground pepper to taste
- 3 stalks green onions, chopped
- ¼ lb beef, thinly sliced
- 4 tbsp ground pork rinds (chicharon), divided
- 2 hardboiled eggs, halved

Directions for Cooking:
1) In a pot, bring water to a boil. Add Knorr cubes and fish sauce.
2) With a strainer, dip into the boiling water the zucchini noodles and cook for 3 minutes. Remove from water, drain and arrange into 4 bowls. If needed, you can cook zucchini noodles in batches.
3) Next, cook the carrots in the boiling pot of water using a strainer still. Around 2-3 minutes, drain and arrange on top of the zucchini noodles.
4) Do the same with jicama, cook in the pot, drain and arrange equally into the bowls.
5) Do the same for the thinly sliced beef. Cook for 5-10 minutes in the boiling pot of soup, swirling the strainer occasionally to ensure uniform cooking for the beef. Arrange equally on the 4 bowls.
6) Sprinkle 1 tbsp of ground pork rinds on each bowl, topped by chopped green onions, ½ hardboiled egg and freshly ground pepper.
7) Taste the boiling pot of soup and adjust to your taste. It should be slightly saltier than the usual so that the noodles will absorb the excess salt once you pour it into the bowls. Add more fish sauce to make it salty or add water to make the pot less salty. Keep soup on a rolling boil before pouring 1-2 cups of soup on each bowl. Serve right away.

Nutrition Information:
Calories per serving: 106; Carbs: 7.8g; Protein: 10.4g; Fat: 4.0g

Lettuce Tacos with Chipotle Chicken

Serves: 4, Cooking Time: 20 minutes

Ingredients:
- ½ avocado, sliced
- ½ teaspoon cumin
- 1 can tomatoes
- 1 cup skinless chicken, cut into strips
- 1 head lettuce, leaves separated and washed
- 1 red onion, sliced
- 1 tablespoon chopped chipotle in adobo sauce
- 1 tablespoon olive oil
- 2 pickled jalapenos, chopped
- A handful coriander leaves
- A pinch of brown sugar
- Fresh tomatoes, sliced for garnish
- Lime wedges for garnish
- Salt and pepper to taste

Directions for Cooking:
1) Heat the olive oil in a skillet and fry the chicken until they are golden brown. Set aside.
2) In the same pan, fry the onions until they become soft. Add the canned tomatoes, chipotle, cumin and sugar. Let it simmer for 15 minutes until the tomatoes become soft and thickened.

3) Add the chicken to the sauce and cook for 5 minutes.
4) Assemble the tacos by putting the chicken inside the lettuce wraps. Garnish with lime wedges, fresh tomatoes, avocado, jalapeno and coriander leaves.

Nutrition Information:
Calories per Serving: 218.2; Carbs: 13.0g; Protein: 20.4g; Fat: 9.4g

Light Beef Soup

Serves: 8, Cooking Time: 1 hour and 10 minutes
Ingredients:
- 1 tablespoon olive oil
- 1 large onion, chopped
- 2 cloves of garlic, minced
- 2 stalks celery, sliced
- 1-pound beef chuck, bones removed and cut into cubes
- salt and pepper to taste
- 2 carrots, peeled and diced
- 8 ounces mushrooms, sliced
- ½ teaspoon dried thyme
- 2 cups beef broth
- 2 cups chicken broth
- 2 cups water
- 1 bay leaf

Directions for Cooking:

1) Heat the oil in a pot and sauté the onion, garlic, and celery until fragrant.
2) Stir in the beef chuck and season with salt and pepper.
3) Add the rest of the ingredients.
4) Close the lid and bring to a boil.
5) Allow to simmer for 60 minutes until the beef is soft.
6) Place in individual containers.
7) Put a label and store in the fridge.
8) Allow to thaw at room temperature before heating in the microwave oven.

Nutrition Information:
Calories per serving: 252; Carbs: 10.5g; Protein: 17.2g; Fat: 15.7g

Meatball Gyro Pita Sandwich

Serves: 4, Cooking Time: 30 minutes
Ingredients:
- 1 cup Greek yogurt
- 1/4 cup cucumber, grated
- 4 teaspoons minced garlic, divided
- 1 teaspoon extra-virgin olive oil
- 1 tablespoon fresh dill
- 1 teaspoon sea salt, divided and more to taste
- 1/2 teaspoon cracked black pepper, divided and more to taste
- 1 tablespoon fresh lemon juice
- 1-pound ground chuck
- 1/4 cup Italian breadcrumbs
- 1 large egg
- 3 tablespoons chopped flat leaf Italian parsley, divided
- 1/2 teaspoon ground cumin
- 1 cup cucumbers, diced finely
- 1 cup finely diced tomatoes
- 1/2 cup finely diced red onion
- 4 flatbreads

Directions for Cooking:
1) First make the tzatziki sauce by combining ¼ tsp pepper, ½ tsp salt, 1 tbsp fresh dill, 1 tsp olive oil, 1 tsp minced garlic, ¼ cup grated cucumber, 1 tbsp fresh lemon juice, and 1 cup Greek yogurt. Mix well in a Ball jar, adjust seasoning to taste if needed, cover, and refrigerate until ready to use. Best when made at least a day ahead.
2) Preheat the oven to 425°F.
3) In a large mixing bowl, combine 1-pound ground chuck, 1/4 cup dry Italian breadcrumbs, 1 large egg, 2 tablespoons chopped fresh flat-leaf Italian parsley, 1 tablespoon freshly minced garlic, 1/2 teaspoon ground cumin, 1/2 teaspoon sea salt, and 1/4 teaspoon freshly cracked black pepper.
4) Mix well to combine and then form into 16 equal sized meatballs.

5) Place meatballs on a lightly greased baking sheet and bake in the pre-heated oven for 16 minutes or until cooked through and no longer pink inside. When done, remove from oven and let it rest for 5 minutes.
6) While the meatballs are cooking, mix well a tbsp of parsley, red onions, tomatoes, and cucumbers in a bowl. Season with pepper and salt.
7) Toast flatbread in toaster oven for 5 minutes.

8) To assemble, place about 4 meatballs down the center of each flatbread. Spoon a generous amount of Tzatziki sauce on the center next to the meatballs and top with a heaping spoonful of the tomato-cucumber salad. Wrap up and enjoy!

Nutrition Information:
Calories per Serving: 540; Carbs: 51.0g; Protein: 33.0g; Fats: 22.0g

Mediterranean Beef Skewers

Serves: 8, Cooking Time: 8 minutes
Ingredients:
- 2 lbs. beef sirloin, cut into cubes
- 3 garlic cloves, minced
- 1 tbsp fresh lemon zest
- 1 tbsp fresh parsley, minced
- 2 tsp fresh thyme, minced
- 2 tsp fresh rosemary, minced
- 2 tsp dried oregano
- 4 tbsp olive oil
- 2 tbsp fresh lemon juice
- Sea salt and freshly ground black

Directions for Cooking:
1) In a bowl, mix all the ingredients except for beef. Mix well and season to taste.

2) Add the beef to the herb mixture and let marinate for at least half an hour.
3) Preheat your grill to medium-high.
4) Remove the meat from the marinade, and slide onto wood or metal skewers.
5) Cook on the grill for 6 to 8 minutes, turning every 2 minutes.
6) Remove from the heat and let rest for 5 minutes before serving.

Nutrition Information:
Calories per Serving: 331; Carbs: 0.5g; Protein: 30.5g; Fats: 23.0g

Mouth-Watering Lamb Stew

Serves: 4, Cooking Time: 180 minutes
Ingredients:
- ½ cup golden raisins
- 1 cup dates, cut in half
- 1 cup dried figs, cut in half
- 1 lb. lamb shoulder, trimmed of fat and cut into 2-inch cubes
- 1 onion, minced
- 1 tbsp fresh coriander, roughly chopped
- 1 tbsp honey, optional
- 1 tbsp olive oil
- 1 tbsp Ras el Hanout
- 2 cloves garlic, minced
- 2 cups beef stock or lamb stock
- Pepper and salt to taste

Ras el Hanout Ingredients:
- ¼ tsp ground cloves
- ½ tsp ground black pepper
- 1 tsp ground turmeric

- 1 tsp ground nutmeg
- 1 tsp ground allspice
- 1 tsp ground cinnamon
- 2 tsp ground mace
- 2 tsp ground cardamom
- 2 tsp ground ginger
- ½ tsp anise seeds' 1/2 tsp ground cayenne pepper

Directions for Cooking:
1) Preheat oven to 300°F.
2) In small bowl, add all Ras el Hanout ingredients and mix thoroughly. Just get what the ingredients need and store remaining in a tightly lidded spice jar.
3) On high fire, place a heavy bottomed medium pot and heat olive oil. Once hot, brown lamb pieces on each side for around 3 to 4 minutes.

4) Lower fire to medium high and add remaining ingredients, except for the coriander.
5) Mix well. Season with pepper and salt to taste. Cover pot and bring to a boil.
6) Once boiling, turn off fire, and pop pot into oven.
7) Bake uncovered for 2 to 2.5 hours or until meat is fork tender.
8) Once meat is tender, remove from oven.
9) To serve, sprinkle fresh coriander, and enjoy.

Nutrition Information:
Calories per Serving: 633.4; Carbs: 78.1g; Protein: 33.0g; Fat: 21.0g

Mini Bell Pepper Mediterranean Chicken Bake

Serves: 4, Cooking Time: 40 minutes
Ingredients:
- 1 tbsp dried oregano
- 1 tsp freshly ground black pepper
- 1 tsp Himalayan salt
- 1 tsp smoked paprika
- 2 green onions, sliced
- 2 jalapeño peppers, seeded and sliced
- 2 large boneless, skinless chicken breasts
- 2 medium tomatoes, diced
- 6 mini bell peppers of assorted colors, seeded and chopped
- The juice of 1 lime

Directions for Cooking:
1) Preheat your oven to 450 degrees F.
2) In baking dish, mix all spices. Add chicken and cover well with spices.
3) Arrange the vegetables around the chicken.
4) Cover dish with foil and bake for 35 minutes.
5) Set the oven to broil, remove the foil and broil for 2 minutes.
6) Slice the chicken breasts on a diagonal and serve, topped with vegetables.

Nutrition Information:
Calories per Serving: 293; Carbs: 14.1g; Protein: 45.1g; Fats: 5.5g

Mustard Chops with Apricot-Basil Relish

Serves: 4, Cooking Time: 12 minutes
Ingredients:
- ¼ cup basil, finely shredded
- ¼ cup olive oil
- ½ cup mustard
- ¾ lb. fresh apricots, stone removed, and fruit diced
- 1 shallot, diced small
- 1 tsp ground cardamom
- 3 tbsp raspberry vinegar
- 4 pork chops
- Pepper and salt

Directions for Cooking:
1) Make sure that pork chops are defrosted well. Season with pepper and salt. Slather both sides of each pork chop with mustard. Preheat grill to medium-high fire.
2) In a medium bowl, mix cardamom, olive oil, vinegar, basil, shallot, and apricots. Toss to combine and season with pepper and salt, mixing once again.
3) Grill chops for 5 to 6 minutes per side. As you flip, baste with mustard.
4) Serve pork chops with the Apricot-Basil relish and enjoy.

Nutrition Information:
Calories per Serving: 486.5; Carbs: 7.3g; Protein: 42.1g; Fat: 32.1g

Olive Oil Drenched Lemon Chicken

Serves: 4, Cooking Time: 60 minutes
Ingredients:
- 1 lemon, thinly sliced
- 1 red bell pepper, cut into 1-inch wide strips
- 1 red onion, cut into 1-inch wedges
- 1 tablespoon dried oregano
- 1/2 teaspoon coarsely ground black pepper
- 1/4 cup olive oil

- 2 tablespoons fresh lemon juice
- 2 tablespoons fresh lemon zest
- 3/4 teaspoon salt
- 4 large cloves garlic, pressed
- 4 skinless, boneless chicken breast halves
- 8 baby red potatoes, halved

Directions for Cooking:
1) Preheat oven to 400 degrees F.
2) In a bowl, mix well pepper, salt, oregano, garlic, lemon zest, lemon juice, and olive oil.
3) In a 9 x 13-inch casserole dish, evenly spread chicken in a single layer. Brush lemon juice mixture over chicken.
4) In a bowl mix well lemon slices, red onion, bell pepper, and potatoes. Drizzle remaining olive oil sauce and toss well to coat. Arrange vegetables and lemon slices around chicken breasts in baking dish.
5) Bake for 50 minutes; brush chicken and vegetables with pan drippings halfway through cooking time.
6) Let chicken rest for ten minutes before serving.

Nutrition Information:
Calories per Serving: 517; Carbs: 65.1g; Protein: 30.8g; Fats: 16.7g

Oregano-Smoked Paprika Baked Chicken

Serves: 2, Cooking Time: 40 minutes
Ingredients:
- 1 tbsp dried oregano
- 1 tsp freshly ground black pepper
- 1 tsp Himalayan salt
- 1 tsp smoked paprika
- 2 green onions, sliced
- 2 jalapeño peppers, seeded and sliced
- 2 large boneless, skinless chicken breasts (about 400g/14oz each)
- 2 medium tomatoes, diced
- 6 mini bell peppers of assorted colors, seeded and chopped
- The juice of 1 lime

Directions for Cooking:
1) Preheat oven to 450 degrees F.
2) Mix all the spices in a small bowl. Rub all over chicken breasts.
3) Lightly grease an oven-proof dish with olive oil.
4) Place the chicken breasts in the dish and arrange the vegetables around it.
5) Cover with aluminum foil and bake for 35 minutes.
6) Set the oven to broil, remove the foil and cook under the broiler about 5 minutes, or until the chicken becomes golden brown.
7) Let the chicken rest for 5 minutes before slicing and serving.

Nutrition Information:
Calories per Serving: 286; Carbs: 14.1g; Protein: 45.1g; Fats: 5.5g

Paprika and Feta Cheese on Chicken Skillet

Serves: 6, Cooking Time: 35 minutes
Ingredients:
- ¼ cup black olives, sliced in circles
- ½ teaspoon coriander
- ½ teaspoon paprika
- 1 ½ cups diced tomatoes with the juice
- 1 cup yellow onion, chopped
- 1 teaspoon onion powder
- 2 garlic cloves, peeled and minced
- 2 lb. free range organic boneless skinless chicken breasts
- 2 tablespoons feta cheese
- 2 tablespoons olive oil
- Crushed red pepper to taste
- Salt and black pepper to taste

Directions for Cooking:
1) Preheat oven to 400 degrees F.
2) Place a cast-iron pan on medium-high fire and heat for 5 minutes. Add oil and heat for 2 minutes more.
3) Meanwhile in a large dish, mix well pepper, salt, crushed red pepper, paprika, coriander, and onion powder. Add chicken and coat well in seasoning.
4) Add chicken to pan and brown sides for 4 minutes per side. Increase fire to high.

5) Stir in garlic and onions. Lower fire to medium and mix well.
6) Pop pan in oven and bake for 15 minutes.
7) Remove from oven, turnover chicken and let it stand for 5 minutes before serving.

Nutrition Information:
Calories per Serving: 232; Carbs: 5.0g; Protein: 33.0g; Fats: 8.0g

Pepper Steak Taco

Serves: 4, Cooking Time: 20 minutes
Ingredients:
- ¼ cup grated low fat Monterey Jack
- ½ avocado, sliced
- ½ cup fresh frozen corn kernels
- ½ red onion, sliced
- ½ tsp mild chili powder
- 1 lb. flank or hanger steak
- 1 tsp salt
- 2 garlic cloves, crushed
- 2 tbsp chopped fresh cilantro
- 2 tbsp sliced pickled jalapenos
- 3 bell pepper, 1 each red, yellow and orange, sliced thinly
- 3 tsp vegetable oil
- 8 small corn tortillas, warmed
- Juice of 1 lime, plus lime wedges for serving

Directions for Cooking:
1) In a re-sealable plastic bag, mix chili powder, garlic, salt and lime juice until salt is dissolved. Add steak and marinate for at least 30 minutes while making sure to flip over or toss around steak halfway through the marinating time.
2) On high fire, place a large saucepan and heat 2 tsp oil. Once hot, sauté bell peppers and red onion for 5 minutes. Add corn and continue sautéing for another 3 to 5 minutes. Transfer veggies to a bowl and keep warm.
3) With paper towel, wipe skillet and return to medium-high fire. Heat remaining teaspoon of oil. Once hot add steak in pan in a single layer and cook 4 minutes per side for medium rare. Remove from fire and let it rest for 5minutes on a chopping board before cutting into thin slices.
4) To make tortilla, layer jalapenos, cilantro, Monterey Jack, avocado, steak and veggies. Best serve with a dollop of sour cream.

Nutrition Information:
Calories per Serving: 419.7; Carbs: 36.2g; Protein: 31.6g; Fat: 16.5g

Pita Chicken Burger with Spicy Yogurt

Serves: 4, Cook Time: 15 minutes
Ingredients:
- ½ cup chopped green onions
- ½ cup diced tomato
- ½ cup plain low-fat yogurt
- ½ tsp coarsely ground black pepper
- 1 ½ tsp chopped fresh oregano
- 1 lb ground chicken
- 1 tbsp olive oil
- 1 tbsp Greek or Moroccan seasoning blend
- 1/3 cup Italian seasoned breadcrumbs
- 2 cups shredded lettuce
- 2 large egg whites, lightly beaten
- 2 tsps grated lemon rind, divided
- 4 pcs of 6-inch pitas, cut in half

Directions for Cooking:
1) Mix thoroughly the ground chicken, 1 tsp lemon rind, egg whites, black pepper, Greek or Moroccan seasoning and green onions. Equally separate into eight parts and shaping each part into ¼ inch thick patty.
2) Put fire on medium high and place a large skillet. Fry the patties until browned or for two mins each side. Then slow the fire to medium, cover the skillet and continue cooking for another four minutes.
3) In a small bowl, mix thoroughly the oregano, yogurt and 1 tsp lemon rind.
4) To serve, spread the mixture on the pita, add cooked patty, 1 tbsp tomato and ¼ cup lettuce.

Nutrition Information:
Calories per Serving: 434.3; Carbs: 44g; Protein: 30.6g; Fat: 15.1g

Roasted Leg of Lamb

Serves: 8, Cooking Time: 120 minutes

Ingredients:

- ¼ cup + 1 tbsp olive oil, divided
- ½ tbsp garlic powder
- 1 cup almond flour
- 1 large red onion, roughly chopped
- 1 tbsp fresh parsley, chopped
- 1 tbsp fresh rosemary, chopped
- 2 apples, cored and sliced
- 2 heads of garlic, ¼ inch of top end removed to show individual cloves
- 2 sweet potatoes, diced
- 2 tbsp fresh tarragon, chopped
- 2 tbsp fresh thyme, chopped
- 4 lbs. leg of lamb, bone in
- 5 tbsp Dijon mustard
- Pepper and salt to taste

Directions for Cooking:

1) Let leg of lamb sit in room temperature for an hour. Then pat dry with a paper towel.
2) Grease a roasting pan and preheat oven to 400 degrees F.
3) Mix well the pepper, salt, ¼ cup olive oil, garlic powder, all the chopped herbs and almond flour in a medium bowl.
4) With mustard, coat leg of lamb. Then with a basting brush, coat leg of lamb with the herb mixture all around.
5) Pop in the oven and roast for 30 minutes. Then reduce oven temperature to 350 degrees F and remove lamb.
6) Add veggies and apple. Season with pepper, salt and remaining olive oil and return to oven.
7) Bake for 1 ½ hours for a medium rare meat around 130oF when thermometer is inserted into lamb.
8) Remove from oven and let lamb rest for 20 minutes before carving.

Nutrition Information:
Calories per Serving: 568.2; Carbs: 17.6g; Protein: 61.0g; Fat: 28.2g

Sirloin Rolls with Brussels Sprouts

Serves: 2, Cooking Time: 50 minutes

Ingredients:

- ½ fennel bulb cut into thick slices
- 1 tsp olive oil
- 2 cups Brussels sprouts, bottoms trimmed off and quartered
- 2 pieces of ½ lb. each sirloin steak
- 3 fennel fronds
- Pepper and salt to taste

Filling Ingredients:

- ½ cup Brussels sprouts, bottoms trimmed off and halved
- ½ fennel bulb, roughly chopped
- 1 tsp oregano
- 1 tsp rosemary
- 1 tsp sage
- 2 garlic cloves

Directions for Cooking:

1) Preheat oven to 375 degrees F.
2) In a blender, puree all filling ingredients.
3) With a mallet, pound steaks until ½-inch thick. Divide into two the pureed filling ingredients and spread on each steak. Roll steak and secure ends with a toothpick.
4) In a large roasting pan, place fennel and Brussels sprouts slices. Season with pepper, salt, and olive oil. Toss well to coat. Arrange sprouts and fennel on the side of pan.
5) Place steaks in middle of roasting pan and season with pepper and salt.
6) Roast for 35 to 40 minutes. Remove steak if desired doneness is reached and let it rest as you continue to roast veggies for another 5 to 10 minutes.

Nutrition Information:
Calories per Serving: 635.6; Carbs: 48.0g; Protein: 82.2g; Fat: 28.7g

Spicy Chicken Vegetable Soup

Serves: 4, Cooking Time: 25 minutes
Ingredients:

- 1-pound skinless chicken breast
- 3 bay leaves
- ½ teaspoon red chili pepper flakes
- ½ teaspoon sea salt
- 1 teaspoon dried basil
- 1 garlic clove, minced
- 1 can diced tomatoes
- 1 small onion, diced
- 1 ½ cups sweet potatoes, cubed
- 2 cups frozen vegetable mix
- 2 cups chicken broth
- 1 jar spicy tomato sauce

Directions for Cooking:

1) In a Dutch oven, put all ingredients and mix until well combined.
2) Season with salt and pepper to taste.
3) Let it simmer for 15 minutes. Cook for 10 minutes more.
4) Serve warm.

Nutrition Information:
Calories per Serving: 250; Carbs: 23.5g; Protein: 30.9g; Fat: 3.8g

Stewed Chicken Greek Style

Servers: 10, Cook Time: 1 hour and 15 minutes
Ingredients:

- ½ cup red wine
- 1 ½ cups chicken stock or more if needed
- 1 cup olive oil
- 1 cup tomato sauce
- 1 pc, 4lbs whole chicken cut into pieces
- 1 pinch dried oregano or to taste
- 10 small shallots, peeled
- 2 bay leaves
- 2 cloves garlic, finely chopped
- 2 tbsp chopped fresh parsley
- 2 tsps almond oil
- Salt and ground black pepper to taste

Directions for Cooking:

1) Bring to a boil a large pot of lightly salted water. Mix in the shallots and let boil uncovered until tender for around three minutes. Then drain the shallots and dip in cold water until no longer warm.
2) In another large pot over medium fire, heat almond oil and olive oil until bubbling and melted. Then sauté in the chicken and shallots for 15 minutes or until chicken is cooked and shallots are soft and translucent. Then add the chopped garlic and cook for three mins more.
3) Then add bay leaves, oregano, salt and pepper, parsley, tomato sauce and the red wine and let simmer for a minute before adding the chicken stock. Stir before covering and let cook for 50 minutes on medium-low fire or until chicken is tender.

Nutrition Information:
Calories per Serving: 644.8; Carbs: 8.2g; Protein: 62.1g; Fat: 40.4g

Sun-Dried Tomatoes 'n Artichoke Chicken

Serves: 4, Cooking Time: 20 minutes
Ingredients:

- 4 (6-oz.) skinless, boneless chicken breasts
- 1 tablespoon olive oil, divided
- 1 cup thinly sliced red onion
- 1 tablespoon thinly sliced garlic
- 1 cup unsalted chicken stock
- 1 tablespoon coarsely chopped fresh dill
- 1/2 teaspoon freshly ground black pepper, divided
- 1/2 cup uncooked bulgur
- 2 teaspoons chopped fresh or 1/2 tsp. dried oregano
- 4 cups chopped fresh kale (about 2 1/2 oz.)
- 1/2 cup thinly sliced bottled roasted red bell peppers
- 2 ounces feta cheese, crumbled (about 1/2 cup)

- 3/4 teaspoon kosher salt, divided

Directions for Cooking:
1) Season chicken with salt and pepper and then on a large plate, dredge chicken in flour.
2) On medium-high fire, heat 2 tablespoons of olive oil in a large skillet.
3) Brown chicken for 4 minutes per side. Transfer chicken to a plate.
4) In same skillet, stir in artichokes, sun-dried tomatoes, capers, 3 tbsp olive oil and lemon juice. Sauté for 3 minutes.
5) Push the vegetables to the sides of the skillet and add the chicken back.
6) Cook the chicken and the vegetables for 10 minutes, covered and on medium low fire.

Nutrition Information:
Calories per Serving: 552; Carbs: 33.0g; Protein: 43.0g; Fats: 28.0g

Sweet Potato and Chicken Patties

Serves: 7, Cooking Time: 4 hours and 10 minutes

Ingredients:
- ½ medium sweet potato, chopped
- ½ teaspoon sea salt
- 1 clove of garlic, minced
- 1 egg
- 1 pound skinless and boneless chicken, chopped finely
- 1 tablespoon fresh rosemary, chopped
- 1 teaspoon Dijon mustard
- 1 teaspoon paprika powder
- 2 ½ cups kale, chopped
- 2 green onions, chopped
- 2 tablespoon coconut flour

Directions for Cooking:
1) Heat oil in a large skillet and sauté the green onions for five minutes.
2) Add the sweet potatoes and cook for 5 minutes until almost tender.
3) Mix in the kale and cook until the kale has wilted. Set aside.
4) In a mixing bowl, mix together the chicken and season with salt, paprika, mustard, garlic and rosemary. Add the egg, coconut flour and sweet potato mix.
5) Cover with plastic wrap and refrigerate for 4 hours.
6) Make patties out of the chicken mixture.
7) Cook the patties in a hot skillet for 5 minutes each side.

Nutrition Information:
Calories per Serving: 238.8; Carbs: 35.2g; Protein: 12.8g; Fat: 5.2g

Tender Beef in Tomato Sauce

Serves: 4, Cooking Time: 35 minutes

Ingredients:
- 1 lb. beef, cut into 1-inch cubes
- 1/4 cup extra virgin olive oil
- 1 onion, chopped
- 2 red bell peppers, chopped
- 1 orange bell pepper, chopped
- salt and pepper to taste
- 1 cup tomato sauce
- 2 cloves garlic, smashed
- 2 tomatoes, sliced
- 3 carrots, peeled and cut into 2-inch lengths
- 2 small potatoes, peeled and quartered

Directions for Cooking:
1) In a heavy bottomed pot, heat pot for 2 minutes. Add oil and heat on medium fire for 5 minutes.
2) Meanwhile, season beef generously with salt and pepper.
3) Add to pot and brown for 10 minutes.
4) Stir in garlic and cook for a minute. Add tomatoes and onion. Cook for 3 minutes.
5) Stir in tomato sauce and simmer for 20 minutes while stirring occasionally.
6) Add bell peppers and adjust seasoning to taste. Continue simmering for 8 more minutes until peppers are crisp tender.
7) Serve and enjoy.

Nutrition Information:
Calories per Serving: 388; Carbs: 26.6g; Protein: 26.6g; Fats: 20.5g

Tender Beef in Tomato-Artichoke Stew

Serves: 6, Cooking Time: 2 hours

Ingredients:

- 1 (14 ounce) can artichoke hearts, drained and halved
- 1 (14.5 ounce) can diced tomatoes
- 1 (15 ounce) can tomato sauce
- 1 (32 fluid ounce) container beef broth
- 1 bay leaf
- 1 onion, diced
- 1 tablespoon grapeseed oil
- 1 teaspoon dried basil
- 1 teaspoon dried oregano
- 1 teaspoon dried parsley
- 1/2 cup pitted and roughly chopped
- 1/2 teaspoon ground cumin
- 2 pounds stewing beef
- 4 cloves garlic, chopped or more to taste
- Kalamata olives (optional)

Directions for Cooking:

1) Place a pot on medium-high fire and heat for 3 minutes. Add oil and heat for 2 minutes.
2) Brown beef and cook for 15 minutes.
3) Add all ingredients, deglaze pot, and mix well.
4) Once boiling, lower fire to a simmer, cover, and cook for 60 minutes. Occasionally stirring pot.
5) If needed cook for 30 minutes more to desired beef tenderness.
6) Adjust seasoning if needed.
7) Serve and enjoy.

Nutrition Information:

Calories per Serving: 416; Carbs: 14.1g; Protein: 29.9g; Fats: 26.2g

Tenderloin Steaks with Onions

Serves: 4, Cooking Time: 20 minutes

Ingredients:

- ¼ tsp ground black pepper
- ½ tsp salt, divided
- 1 large red onion, sliced into rings and separated
- 1 tsp dried thyme
- 2 tbsp honey
- 2 tbsp red wine vinegar
- 4 pcs of 4-oz beef tenderloin steaks, trimmed

Directions for Cooking:

1) On medium-high fire, place a large nonstick fry pan and grease with cooking spray.
2) Add onion, cover and cook for three minutes.
3) Add ¼ tsp salt, honey and vinegar. Stir to mix and reduce fire to medium low.
4) Simmer until sauce has thickened around 8 minutes. Stir constantly. Turn off fire.
5) In an oven safe pan, grease with cooking spray add beef. Season with pepper, thyme and remaining salt.
6) Pop into a preheated broiler on high and broil for 4 minutes. Remove from oven and turnover tenderloin pieces. Return to oven and broil for another 4 minutes or until desired doneness is achieved.
7) Transfer to a serving plate and pour onion sauce over.
8) Serve and enjoy.

Nutrition Information:

Calories per Serving: 283; Carbs: 12.6g; Protein: 32.5g; Fat: 11.4g

Vegetable Lover's Chicken Soup

Serves: 4, Cooking Time: 20 minutes

Ingredients:

- 1 ½ cups baby spinach
- 2 tbsp orzo (tiny pasta)
- ¼ cup dry white wine
- 1 14oz low sodium chicken broth
- 2 plum tomatoes, chopped
- 1/8 tsp salt
- ½ tsp Italian seasoning
- 1 large shallot, chopped
- 1 small zucchini, diced
- 8-oz chicken tenders
- 1 tbsp extra virgin olive oil

Directions for Cooking:

1) In a large saucepan, heat oil over medium heat and add the chicken. Stir occasionally for 8 minutes until browned. Transfer in a plate. Set aside.
2) In the same saucepan, add the zucchini, Italian seasoning, shallot and salt and stir often until the vegetables are softened, around 4 minutes.
3) Add the tomatoes, wine, broth and orzo and increase the heat to high to bring the mixture to boil. Reduce the heat and simmer.
4) Add the cooked chicken and stir in the spinach last.
5) Serve hot.

Nutrition Information:

Calories per Serving: 207; Carbs: 14.8g; Protein: 12.2g; Fat: 11.4g

Yummy Turkey Meatballs

Serves: 4, Cooking Time: 25 minutes

Ingredients:

- ¼ yellow onion, finely diced
- 1 14-oz can of artichoke hearts, diced
- 1 lb. ground turkey
- 1 tsp dried parsley
- 1 tsp oil
- 4 tbsp fresh basil, finely chopped
- Pepper and salt to taste

Directions for Cooking:

1) Grease a cookie sheet and preheat oven to 350 degrees F.
2) On medium fire, place a nonstick medium saucepan and sauté artichoke hearts and diced onions for 5 minutes or until onions are soft.
3) Remove from fire and let cool.
4) Meanwhile, in a big bowl, mix with hands parsley, basil and ground turkey. Season to taste.
5) Once onion mixture has cooled add into the bowl and mix thoroughly.
6) With an ice cream scooper, scoop ground turkey and form into balls, makes around 6 balls.
7) Place on prepped cookie sheet, pop in the oven and bake until cooked through around 15-20 minutes.
8) Remove from pan, serve and enjoy.

Nutrition Information:

Calories per Serving: 328; Carbs: 11.8g; Protein: 33.5g; Fat: 16.3g

Chapter 11 Fruits and Sweets Recipes

Amazing Avocado Smoothie

Serves: 2, Cooking Time: 5 minutes

Ingredients:

- ½ avocado, pitted and sliced
- 3 celery stalks
- 1 lime
- 3 tablespoons maple syrup
- Fresh mint leaves, for garnish
- 1 tablespoon linseed

Directions for Cooking:

1) Place the avocado, celery stalks, and lime in a blender.
2) Add in maple syrup.
3) Blend until smooth.
4) Pour in glass containers.
5) Place in the fridge to chill for at least 30 minutes.
6) Serve chilled.

Nutrition Information:

Calories per serving: 180.2; Carbs: 27.1g; Protein: 1.3g; Fat: 7.4g

Apple and Walnut Salad

Serves: 6, Cooking Time: 5 minutes

Ingredients:

- Juice from ½ orange
- Zest from ½ orange, grated
- 2 tablespoons honey
- 1 tablespoon olive oil
- 4 medium Gala apples, cubed
- 8 dried apricots, chopped
- ¼ cup walnuts, toasted and chopped

Directions for Cooking:

1) In a small bowl, whisk together the orange juice, zest, honey, and olive oil. Set aside.
2) In a larger bowl, toss the apples, apricots, and walnuts.
3) Drizzle with the vinaigrette and toss to coat all Ingredients.
4) Serve chilled.

Nutrition Information:

Calories per serving: 178; Carbs: 30g; Protein: 1g; Fat: 6g

Banana Kale Smoothie

Serves: 3, Cooking Time: 5 minutes

Ingredients:

- 2 cups kale leaves
- 1 cup almond milk
- ½ cup crushed ice
- 1 banana, peeled
- 1 apple, peeled and cored
- A dash of cinnamon

Directions for Cooking:

1) Place all Ingredients in a blender.
2) Blend until smooth.
3) Pour in a glass container and allow to chill in the fridge for at least 30 minutes.

Nutrition Information:

Calories per serving: 175.4; Carbs: 32.1g; Protein: 2.3g; Fat: 4.2g

Delectable Strawberry Popsicle

Serves: 5, Cooking Time: 10 minutes

Ingredients:

- 2 ½ cups fresh strawberry
- ½ cup almond milk

Directions for Cooking:

1) Blend all ingredients until smooth.
2) Pour into the popsicle molds with sticks and freeze for at least 4 hours.
3) Serve chilled.

Nutrition Information:

Calories per serving: 37.7; Carbs: 7.7g; Protein: 0.6g; Fat:0.5 g

Banana-Peanut Butter Oatmeal Smoothie

Serves: 4, Cooking Time: 5 minutes

Ingredients:
- 2 bananas
- 1 cup skim milk
- 1 cup non-fat Greek yogurt
- 1 cup rolled oats
- ¼ cup natural peanut butter
- 1 teaspoon cinnamon
- 2 scoops of crushed ice

Directions for Cooking:
1) Place all Ingredients in a blender.
2) Pulse until smooth.
3) Serve immediately.

Nutrition Information:
Calories per serving: 335.06; Carbs: 49.44g; Protein: 15.2g; Fat: 8.5g

Beetroot Apple Smoothie

Serves: 3, Cooking Time: 5 minutes

Ingredients:
- 1 boiled beetroot, peeled
- 2 teaspoons minced ginger
- 1 tablespoon lemon juice
- 1 apple, peeled and cored
- 1 carrot, peeled and sliced
- 1 pear, peeled and cored
- 1 cup ice

Directions for Cooking:
1) Place all Ingredients in a blender.
2) Blend until smooth.
3) Pour in a glass container.
4) Serve immediately.

Nutrition Information:
Calories per serving: 192.1; Carbs: 29.9g; Protein: 2.6g; Fat: 6.9g

Blueberry Frozen Yogurt

Serves: 6, Cooking Time: 30 minutes

Ingredients:
- 1-pint blueberries, fresh
- 2/3 cup honey
- 1 small lemon, juiced and zested
- 2 cups yogurt, chilled

Directions for Cooking:
1) In a saucepan, combine the blueberries, honey, lemon juice, and zest.
2) Heat over medium heat and allow to simmer for 15 minutes while stirring constantly.
3) Once the liquid has reduced, transfer the fruits in a bowl and allow to cool in the fridge for another 15 minutes.
4) Once chilled, mix together with the chilled yogurt.

Nutrition Information:
Calories per serving: 248.9; Carbs:52.2 g; Protein:3.5 g; Fat: 2.9g

Delectable Mango Smoothie

Serves: 2 , Cooking Time: 5 minutes

Ingredients:
- 2 cups diced mango
- 1 carrot, peeled and sliced roughly
- 1 orange, peeled and segmented
- Fresh mint leaves

Directions for Cooking:
1) Place the mango, carrot, and oranges in a blender.
2) Pulse until smooth.
3) Pour in a glass container and allow to chill before serving.
4) Garnish with mint leaves on top.

Nutrition Information:
Calories per serving: 148.7; Carbs: 33.6g; Protein: 2g; Fat: 0.7.

Deliciously Cold Lychee Sorbet

Serves: 4, Cooking Time: 5 minutes
Ingredients:
- 2 cups fresh lychees, pitted and sliced
- 2 tablespoons honey
- Mint leaves for garnish

Directions for Cooking:
1) Place the lychee slices and honey in a food processor.
2) Pulse until smooth.
3) Pour in a container and place inside the fridge for at least two hours.
4) Scoop the sorbet and serve with mint leaves.

Nutrition Information:
Calories per serving: 162; Carbs: 38.9g; Protein: 0.7g; Fat: 0.4

Dragon Fruit, Pear, and Spinach Salad

Serves: 4, Cooking Time: 3 minutes
Ingredients:
- 5 ounces spinach leaves, torn
- 1 dragon fruit, peeled then cubed
- 2 pears, peeled then cubed
- 10 ounces organic goat cheese
- 1 cup pecan, halves
- 6 ounces blackberries
- 6 ounces raspberries
- 8 tablespoons olive oil
- 8 tablespoons red wine vinegar
- 1 tablespoon poppy seeds

Directions for Cooking:
1) In a mixing bowl, combine all Ingredients except for the poppy seeds.
2) Place inside the fridge and allow to chill before serving.
3) Sprinkle with poppy seeds on top before serving.

Nutrition Information:
Calories per serving:149.9; Carbs: 27.2g; Protein: 3.3g; Fat: 3.1g

Greek Yogurt Muesli Parfaits

Serves: 4, Cooking Time: 10 minutes
Ingredients:
- 4 cups Greek yogurt
- 1 cup whole wheat muesli
- 2 cups fresh berries of your choice

Directions for Cooking:
1) Layer the four glasses with Greek yogurt at the bottom, muesli on top, and berries.
2) Repeat the layers until the glass is full.
3) Place in the fridge for at least 2 hours to chill.

Nutrition Information:
Calories per serving: 272; Carbs: 36g; Protein:23 g; Fat: 4g

Easy Fruit Compote

Serves: 2, Cooking Time: 15 minutes
Ingredients:
- 1-pound fresh fruits of your choice
- 2 tablespoons maple syrup
- A dash of salt

Directions for Cooking:
1) Slice the fruits thinly and place them in a saucepan.
2) Add the honey and salt.
3) Heat the saucepan over medium low heat and allow the fruits to simmer for 15 minutes or until the liquid has reduced.
4) Make sure that you stir constantly to prevent the fruits from sticking at the bottom of your pan and eventually burning.
5) Transfer in a lidded jar.
6) Allow to cool.
7) Serve with slices of whole wheat bread or vegan ice cream.

Nutrition Information:
Calories per serving:232.6; Carbs: 56.8g; Protein: 0.9g; Fat: 0.2g

Five Berry Mint Orange Infusion

Serves: 12, Cooking Time: 10 minutes
Ingredients:
- ½ cup water
- 3 orange pekoe tea bags
- 3 sprigs of mint
- 1 cup fresh strawberries
- 1 cup fresh golden raspberries
- 1 cup fresh raspberries
- 1 cup blackberries
- 1 cup fresh blueberries
- 1 cup pitted fresh cherries
- 1 bottle Sauvignon Blanc
- ½ cup pomegranate juice, natural
- 1 teaspoon vanilla

Directions for Cooking:
1) In a saucepan, bring water to a boil over medium heat. Add the tea bags, mint and stir. Let it stand for 10 minutes.
2) In a large bowl, combine the rest of the ingredients.
3) Put in the fridge to chill for at least 3 hours.

Nutrition Information:
Calories per serving: 146.7; Carbs: 32.1g; Protein: 1.2g; Fat: 1.5g

Fruit Salad with Orange Blossom Water

Serves: 8, Cooking Time: 3 minutes
Ingredients:
- 4 oranges, peeled and cut into bite-sized pieces
- 8 dried figs, quartered
- 2 Medjool dates, pitted then chopped
- ½ cup pomegranate seeds
- 2 tablespoons honey
- 2 tablespoons orange blossom water
- 2 bananas, peeled and sliced
- ¼ cup pistachio nuts, shelled and chopped

Directions for Cooking:
1) In a large mixing bowl, toss in all the ingredients except for the pistachio nuts.
2) Let the fruits rest in the fridge for at least 8 hours before serving.
3) Garnish with chopped pistachios before serving.

Nutrition Information:
Calories per serving: 202; Carbs: 43g; Protein: 3g; Fat: 2g

Mediterranean Baked Apples

Serves: 4, Cooking Time: 25 minutes
Ingredients:
- 1.5 pounds apples, peeled and sliced
- Juice from ½ lemon
- A dash of cinnamon

Directions for Cooking:
1) Preheat the oven to 250 degrees F.
2) Line a baking sheet with parchment paper then set aside.
3) In a medium bowl, apples with lemon juice and cinnamon.
4) Place the apples on the parchment paper-lined baking sheet.
5) Bake for 25 minutes until crisp.

Nutrition Information:
Calories per serving: 100; Carbs: 23.9g; Protein: 0.5g; Fat: 0.3g

Mediterranean Diet Cookie Recipe

Serves: 12, Cooking Time: 40 minutes
Ingredients:
- 1 tsp vanilla extract
- ½ tsp salt
- 4 large egg whites
- 1 ¼ cups sugar
- 2 cups toasted and skinned hazelnuts

Directions for Cooking:

1) Preheat oven to 325 degrees F and position oven rack in the center. Then line with baking paper your baking pan.
2) In a food processor, finely grind the hazelnuts and then transfer into a medium sized bowl.
3) In a large mixing bowl, on high speed beat salt and egg whites until stiff and there is formation of peaks. Then gently fold in the ground nut and vanilla until thoroughly mixed.
4) Drop a spoonful of the mixture onto prepared pan and bake the cookies for twenty minutes or until lightly browned per batch. Bake 6 cookies per cookie sheet.
5) Let it cool on pan for five minutes before removing.

Nutrition Information:
Calorie per Servings: 173; Carbs: 23.0g; Protein: 3.1g; Fats: 7.6g

Mediterranean Style Fruit Medley

Serves: 7, Cooking Time: 5 minutes
Ingredients:
- 4 fuyu persimmons, sliced into wedges
- 1 ½ cups grapes, halved
- 8 mint leaves, chopped
- 1 tablespoon lemon juice
- 1 tablespoon honey
- ½ cups almond, toasted and chopped

Directions for Cooking:
1) Combine all Ingredients in a bowl.
2) Toss then chill before serving.

Nutrition Information:
Calories per serving:176; Carbs: 32g; Protein: 3g; Fat: 4g

Mediterranean Watermelon Salad

Serves: 6, Cooking Time: 2 minutes
Ingredients:
- 6 cups mixed salad greens, torn
- 3 cups watermelon, seeded and cubed
- ½ cup onion, sliced
- 1 tablespoon extra-virgin olive oil
- 1/3 cup feta cheese, crumbled
- Cracked black pepper

Directions for Cooking:
1) In a large bowl, mix all ingredients.
2) Toss to combine everything.
3) Allow to chill before serving.

Nutrition Information:
Calories per serving: 93.6; Carbs: 15.2g; Protein: 1.9g; Fat: 2.8g

Melon Cucumber Smoothie

Serves: 2, Cooking Time: 5 minutes
Ingredients:
- ½ cucumber
- 2 slices of melon
- 2 tablespoons lemon juice
- 1 pear, peeled and sliced
- 3 fresh mint leaves
- ½ cup almond milk

Directions for Cooking:
1) Place all Ingredients in a blender.
2) Blend until smooth.
3) Pour in a glass container and allow to chill in the fridge for at least 30 minutes.

Nutrition Information:
Calories per serving: 278.9; Carbs: 59.3g; Protein: 5.7g; Fat: 2.1g

Peanut Banana Yogurt Bowl

Serves: 4, Cooking Time: 15 minutes

Ingredients:

- 4 cups Greek yogurt
- 2 medium bananas, sliced
- ¼ cup creamy natural peanut butter
- ¼ cup flax seed meal
- 1 teaspoon nutmeg

Directions for Cooking:

1) Divide the yogurt between four bowls and top with banana, peanut butter, and flax seed meal.
2) Garnish with nutmeg.
3) Chill before serving.

Nutrition Information:

Calories per serving: 377; Carbs: 47.7g; Protein: 22.7g; Fat: 10.6g

Pomegranate and Lychee Sorbet

Serves: 6, Cooking Time: 5 minutes

Ingredients:

- ¾ cup dragon fruit cubes
- 8 lychees, peeled and pitted
- Juice from 1 lemon
- 3 tablespoons stevia sugar
- 2 tablespoons pomegranate seeds

Directions for Cooking:

1) In a blender, combine, the dragon fruit, lychees, lemon, and stevia sugar.
2) Pulse until smooth.
3) Pour the mixture in a container with lid and place inside the fridge.
4) Allow sorbet to harden for at least 8 hours.
5) Sprinkle with pomegranate seeds before serving.

Nutrition Information:

Calories per serving:140; Carbs: 30.4g; Protein: 1.9g; Fat: 1.2g

Pomegranate Granita with Lychee

Serves: 7, Cooking Time: 5 minutes

Ingredients:

- 2 cups pomegranate juice, organic and sugar-free
- 1 cup water
- ½ cup lychee syrup
- 2 tablespoons lemon juice
- 4 mint leaves
- 1 cup fresh lychees, pitted and sliced

Directions for Cooking:

1) Place all ingredients in a large pitcher.
2) Place inside the fridge to cool before serving.

Nutrition Information:

Calories per serving: 100; Carbs: 23.8g; Protein: 0.4g; Fat: 0.4g

Roasted Berry and Honey Yogurt Pops

Serves: 8, Cooking Time: 15 minutes

Ingredients:

- 12 ounces mixed berries
- A dash of sea salt
- 2 tablespoons honey
- 2 cups whole Greek yogurt
- ½ small lemon, juice

Directions for Cooking:

1) Preheat the oven to 350 degrees F.
2) Line a baking sheet with parchment paper then set aside.
3) In a medium bowl, toss the berries with sea salt and honey.
4) Pour the berries on the prepared baking sheet.
5) Roast for 30 minutes while stirring halfway.

6) While the fruit is roasting, blend the Greek yogurt and lemon juice. Add honey to taste if desired.
7) Once the berries are done, cool for at least ten minutes.
8) Fold the berries into the yogurt mixture.
9) Pour into popsicle molds and allow to freeze for at least 8 hours.
10) Serve chilled.

Nutrition Information:
Calories per serving: 183; Carbs: 24.8g; Protein: 3.2g; Fat: 7.9g

Scrumptious Cake with Cinnamon

Serves: 8, Cooking Time: 40 minutes
Ingredients:
- 1 lemon
- 4 eggs
- 1 tsp cinnamon
- ¼ lb. sugar
- ½ lb. ground almonds

Directions for Cooking:
1) Preheat oven to 350 degrees F. Then grease a cake pan and set aside.
2) On high speed, beat for three minutes the sugar and eggs or until the volume is doubled.
3) Then with a spatula, gently fold in the lemon zest, cinnamon and almond flour until well mixed.
4) Then pour batter on prepared pan and bake for forty minutes or until golden brown.
5) Let cool before serving.

Nutrition Information:
Calorie per Servings: 266; Carbs: 21.1g; Protein: 8.8g; Fats: 16.3g

Smoothie Bowl with Dragon Fruit

Serves: 4, Cooking Time: 5 minutes
Ingredients:
- ¼ of dragon fruit, peeled and sliced
- 1 cup frozen berries
- 2 cups baby greens (mixed)
- ½ cup coconut meat

Directions for Cooking:
1) Place all Ingredients in a blender and pulse until smooth.
2) Place on a bowl and allow to cool in the fridge for at least 20 minutes.
3) Garnish with whatever fruits or nuts available in your fridge.

Nutrition Information:
Calories per serving: 201; Carbs: 19g; Protein: 5g; Fat: 13g

Soothing Red Smoothie

Serves: 2, Cooking Time: 3 minutes
Ingredients:
- 4 plums, pitted
- ¼ cup raspberry
- ¼ cup blueberry
- 1 tablespoon lemon juice
- 1 tablespoon linseed oil

Directions for Cooking:
1) Place all Ingredients in a blender.
2) Blend until smooth.
3) Pour in a glass container and allow to chill in the fridge for at least 30 minutes.

Nutrition Information:
Calories per serving: 212.7; Carbs: 36.4g; Protein: 0.8g; Fat: 7.1g

Strawberry and Avocado Medley

Serves: 4, Cooking Time: 5 minutes

Ingredients:
- 2 cups strawberry, halved
- 1 avocado, pitted and sliced
- 2 tablespoons slivered almonds

Directions for Cooking:
1) Place all Ingredients in a mixing bowl.
2) Toss to combine.
3) Allow to chill in the fridge before serving.

Nutrition Information:
Calories per serving: 116.2; Carbs: 9.9g; Protein: 1.6g; Fat: 7.8g

Strawberry Banana Greek Yogurt Parfaits

Serves: 4, Cooking Time: 5 minutes

Ingredients:
- 1 cup plain Greek yogurt, chilled
- 1 cup pepitas
- ½ cup chopped strawberries
- ½ banana, sliced

Directions for Cooking:
1) In a parfait glass, add the yogurt at the bottom of the glass.
2) Add a layer of pepitas, strawberries, and bananas.
3) Continue to layer the Ingredients: until the entire glass is filled.

Nutrition Information:
Calories per serving:359.8; Carbs: 69.6g; Protein: 18.1g; Fat: 1g

Summertime Fruit Salad

Serves: 6, Cooking Time: 5 minutes

Ingredients:
- 1-pound strawberries, hulled and sliced thinly
- 3 medium peaches, sliced thinly
- 6 ounces blueberries
- 1 tablespoon fresh mint, chopped
- 2 tablespoons lemon juice
- 1 tablespoon honey
- 2 teaspoons balsamic vinegar

Directions for Cooking:
1) In a salad bowl, combine all ingredients.
2) Gently toss to coat all ingredients.
3) Chill for at least 30 minutes before serving.

Nutrition Information:
Calories per serving: 154.2; Carbs: 22.8g; Protein: 8.1g; Fat: 3.4g

Sweet Tropical Medley Smoothie

Serves: 4, Preparation Time: 10 minutes, Cooking Time: 5 minutes

Ingredients:
- 1 banana, peeled
- 1 sliced mango
- 1 cup fresh pineapple
- ½ cup coconut water

Directions for Cooking:
1) Place all Ingredients in a blender.
2) Blend until smooth.
3) Pour in a glass container and allow to chill in the fridge for at least 30 minutes.

Nutrition Information:
Calories per serving:82.1 ; Carbs: 18.6g; Protein: 0.8g; Fat: 0.5g

CPSIA information can be obtained
at www.ICGtesting.com
Printed in the USA
LVHW020509121220
674004LV00009B/133